PCEP

Perinatal Continuing Education Program

Maternal and Fetal Care

4th Edition

BOOK 2

American Academy of Pediatrics

DEDICATED TO THE HEALTH OF ALL CHILDREN®

American Academy of Pediatrics Publishing Staff

Mary Lou White, *Chief Product and Services Officer/SVP, Membership, Marketing, and Publishing*

Mark Grimes, *Vice President, Publishing*

Heather Babiar, MS, *Senior Editor, Professional/Clinical Publishing*

Jason Crase, *Senior Manager, Production and Editorial Services*

Theresa Wiener, *Production Manager, Clinical and Professional Publications*

Peg Mulcahy, *Manager, Art Direction and Production*

Linda Smessaert, *Director, Marketing*

Published by the American Academy of Pediatrics
345 Park Blvd
Itasca, IL 60143
Telephone: 630/626-6000
Facsimile: 847/434-8000
www.aap.org

Information about obtaining continuing medical education and continuing education credit for book study may be obtained by visiting www.cmevillage.com.

Several different approaches to specific perinatal problems may be acceptable. The PCEP books have been written to present specific recommendations rather than to include all currently acceptable options. The recommendations in these books should not be considered the only accepted standard of care. We encourage development of local standards in consultation with your regional perinatal center staff.

The American Academy of Pediatrics is an organization of 67,000 primary care pediatricians, pediatric medical subspecialists, and pediatric surgical specialists dedicated to the health, safety, and well-being of all infants, children, adolescents, and young adults.

While every effort has been made to ensure the accuracy of this publication, the American Academy of Pediatrics does not guarantee that it is accurate, complete, or without error.

The recommendations in this publication do not indicate an exclusive course of treatment or serve as a standard of medical care. Variations, taking into account individual circumstances, may be appropriate.

Statements and opinions expressed are those of the authors and not necessarily those of the American Academy of Pediatrics.

Any websites, brand names, products, or manufacturers are mentioned for informational and identification purposes only and do not imply an endorsement by the American Academy of Pediatrics (AAP). The AAP is not responsible for the content of external resources. Information was current at the time of publication.

The publishers have made every effort to trace the copyright holders for borrowed materials. If they have inadvertently overlooked any, they will be pleased to make the necessary arrangements at the first opportunity.

This publication has been developed by the American Academy of Pediatrics. The contributors are expert authorities in the field of pediatrics. No commercial involvement of any kind has been solicited or accepted in the development of the content of this publication.

Every effort has been made to ensure that the drug selection and dosages set forth in this publication are in accordance with the current recommendations and practice at the time of publication. It is the responsibility of the health care professional to check the package insert of each drug for any change in indications or dosage and for added warnings and precautions.

Every effort is made to keep *Perinatal Continuing Education Program* consistent with the most recent advice and information available from the American Academy of Pediatrics.

Please visit www.aap.org/errata for an up-to-date list of any applicable errata for this publication.

Special discounts are available for bulk purchases of this publication. Email Special Sales at nationalaccounts@aap.org for more information.

© 2022 University of Virginia Patent Foundation

All rights reserved. No part of this publication may be reproduced, stored in a retrieval system, or transmitted in any form or by any means—electronic, mechanical, photocopying, recording, or otherwise—without prior permission from the publisher (locate title at https://ebooks.aappublications.org and click on © Get permissions; you may also fax the permissions editor at 847/434-8780 or email permissions@aap.org). First American Academy of Pediatrics edition published 2007; second, 2012; third, 2017. Original edition © 1978 University of Virginia.

Printed in the United States of America

5-314/0721   1 2 3 4 5 6 7 8 9 10

PC0027

ISBN: 978-1-61002-496-9

eBook: 978-1-61002-497-6

Cover design by Peg Mulcahy

Publication design by Peg Mulcahy

Library of Congress Control Number: 2020943714

Perinatal Continuing Education Program (PCEP), 4th Edition
Textbook Editorial Board

Editors

Editor in Chief, Neonatology
Robert A. Sinkin, MD, MPH, FAAP
Charles Fuller Professor of Neonatology
Department of Pediatrics
University of Virginia Children's Hospital
Vice Chair for Academic Affairs
Division Head, Neonatology
Charlottesville, VA

Editor in Chief, Obstetrics
Christian A. Chisholm, MD, FACOG
Medical Director for Outpatient Clinics, Labor, and Delivery
Vice Chair for Medical Education
Professor of Obstetrics and Gynecology
Division of Maternal-Fetal Medicine
Department of Obstetrics and Gynecology
University of Virginia School of Medicine
Charlottesville, VA

PCEP Editorial Board Members

Melissa F. Carmen, MD
Associate Professor of Pediatrics
Division of Neonatology
University of Rochester
Rochester, NY

Susan B. Clarke, MS, NPD-BC, RNC-NIC, CNS
NRP Instructor Mentor
Master Trainer, Helping Babies Survive
Affiliate Faculty, Center for Global Health
Colorado School of Public Health
University of Colorado Anschutz Medical Campus
Aurora, CO

Robert R. Fuller, MD, PhD
Associate Professor
Division of Maternal-Fetal Medicine
Department of Obstetrics and Gynecology
University of Virginia School of Medicine
Charlottesville, VA

Ann Kellams, MD, FAAP
Professor, Department of Pediatrics
Vice Chair for Clinical Affairs and Director of Breastfeeding Medicine Services
University of Virginia
Charlottesville, VA

Sarah Lepore, MSN, APRN, NNP-BC
University of Virginia Children's Hospital
Neonatal Intensive Care Unit
Charlottesville, VA

Peter D. Murray, MD, MSM, FAAP
Assistant Professor of Pediatrics
Division of Neonatology
University of Virginia Children's Hospital
Charlottesville, VA

Susan Niermeyer, MD, MPH, FAAP
Professor of Pediatrics
Section of Neonatology
University of Colorado School of Medicine
Colorado School of Public Health
Aurora, CO

Barbara O'Brien, MS, RN
Director, Oklahoma Perinatal Quality Improvement Collaborative
University of Oklahoma Health Sciences Center
Oklahoma City, OK

Chad Michael Smith, MD, FACOG
Medical Director, Oklahoma Perinatal Quality Improvement Collaborative
Vice President, Medical Affairs, Mercy Hospital Oklahoma City
Oklahoma City, OK

Jonathan R. Swanson, MD, MSc, FAAP
Professor of Pediatrics
Chief Quality Officer for Children's Services
Medical Director, Neonatal Intensive Care Unit
University of Virginia Children's Hospital
Charlottesville, VA

Sharon Veith, MSN, RN
Assistant Professor of Nursing
School of Nursing
University of Virginia
Charlottesville, VA

Santina Zanelli, MD
Associate Professor of Pediatrics
Division of Neonatology
University of Virginia Children's Hospital
Charlottesville, VA

Continuing Education Credit

Accreditation and Designation Statements

In support of improving patient care, this activity has been planned and implemented by the American Academy of Pediatrics and the University of Virginia School of Medicine and School of Nursing, which is jointly accredited by the Accreditation Council for Continuing Medical Education (ACCME), the Accreditation Council for Pharmacy Education (ACPE), and the American Nurses Credentialing Center (ANCC) to provide continuing education for the health care team.

AMA PRA Category 1 Credit

The University of Virginia School of Medicine and School of Nursing designates this enduring material (PI CME) for a maximum of *56.5 AMA PRA Category 1 Credits.*™ Physicians should claim only the credit commensurate with the extent of their participation in the activity.

ANCC Contact Hours

The University of Virginia School of Medicine and School of Nursing awards 56.5 contact hours for nurses who participate in this educational activity and complete the post-activity evaluation.

AAPA Category 1 CME Credit

This activity is designated for 56.5 AAPA Category 1 CME credits. Approval is valid for 3 years. PAs should only claim credit commensurate with the extent of their participation.

Credit is awarded upon passing book exams, not individual educational unit posttests. Possible credits: Book 1, 14.5; Book 2, 16; Book 3, 17; Book 4, 9. To obtain credit, register online at www.cmevillage.com, choose Courses & Programs, then E-Learning, and scroll down to the PCEP program. Click on the PCEP program link and navigate to https://med.virginia.edu/cme/learning/pcep/pcep-book-exam-certificate/ and pass the book exams.

Disclosure of Faculty Financial Affiliations

The University of Virginia School of Medicine and School of Nursing as a Joint Accreditation Provider adheres to the ACCME *Standards for Integrity and Independence in Accredited Continuing Education*, released in December 2020, as well as Commonwealth of Virginia statutes, University of Virginia policies and procedures, and associated federal and private regulations and guidelines. As the accredited provider for this CE/IPCE activity, we are responsible for ensuring that health care professionals have access to professional development activities that are based on best practices and scientific integrity that ultimately supports the care of patients and the public.

All individuals involved in the development and delivery of content for an accredited CE/IPCE activity are expected to disclose relevant financial relationships with ineligible companies occurring within the past 24 months (such as grants or research support, employee, consultant, stock holder, member of speakers bureau, etc). The University of Virginia School of Medicine and School of Nursing employ appropriate mechanisms to resolve potential conflicts of interest and ensure the educational design reflects content validity, scientific rigor, and balance for participants. Questions about specific strategies can be directed to the University of Virginia

School of Medicine and School of Nursing of the University of Virginia, Charlottesville, Virginia.

The faculty, staff, and planning committee engaged in the development of this CE/IPCE activity in the Joint Accreditation CE Office of the School of Medicine and School of Nursing have no financial affiliations to disclose.

Disclosure of Discussion of Non-FDA-Approved Uses for Pharmaceutical Products and/or Medical Devices

As a Joint Accreditation provider, the University of Virginia School of Medicine and School of Nursing, requires that all faculty presenters identify and disclose any off-label or experimental uses for pharmaceutical and medical device products.

It is recommended that each clinician fully review all the available data on new products or procedures prior to clinical use.

BOOK 2: Maternal and Fetal Care

UNIT 1:	Hypertension in Pregnancy	1
UNIT 2:	Obstetric Hemorrhage	37
UNIT 3:	Infectious Diseases in Pregnancy	83
UNIT 4:	Other Medical Risk Factors in Pregnancy	151
UNIT 5:	Obstetric Risk Factors: Prior or Current Pregnancy	177
UNIT 6:	Psychosocial Risk Factors in Pregnancy	209
UNIT 7:	Gestational Diabetes	231
UNIT 8:	Prelabor Rupture of Membranes and Intra-amniotic Infection	249
	Skill Unit: Sterile Speculum Examination	
	Skill Unit: Tests for Suspected or Proven Rupture of Membranes	
UNIT 9:	Preterm Labor	285
UNIT 10:	Inducing and Augmenting Labor	315
UNIT 11:	Abnormal Labor Progress and Difficult Deliveries	345
UNIT 12:	Imminent Delivery and Preparation for Maternal/Fetal Transport	403
PRETEST ANSWER KEY		423
GLOSSARY		429
INDEX		461

For more information, see the other books in the Perinatal Continuing Education Program (PCEP) series

Book 1. Maternal and Fetal Evaluation and Immediate Newborn Care

Unit 1: Is the Mother Sick? Is the Fetus Sick?
    Skill Unit: Determining Fetal Presentation With Leopold Maneuvers
Unit 2: Fetal Age, Growth, and Maturity
Unit 3: Fetal Well-being
    Skill Unit: Electronic Fetal Monitoring
Unit 4: Is the Baby Sick? Recognizing and Preventing Problems in the Newborn
    Skill Unit: Electronic Cardiorespiratory Monitoring
    Skill Unit: Pulse Oximetry
Unit 5: Resuscitating the Newborn
    Skill Unit: Suctioning
    Skill Unit: Management of Oxygen in the Delivery Setting
    Skill Unit: Free-Flow Oxygen and Positive-Pressure Ventilation
    Skill Unit: Endotracheal Intubation
    Skill Unit: Chest Compressions
    Skill Unit: Emergency Medications
    Skill Unit: Apgar Score
Unit 6: Gestational Age and Size and Associated Risk Factors
    Skill Unit: Estimating Gestational Age by Examination of a Newborn
Unit 7: Thermal Environment
    Skill Unit: Radiant Warmers
    Skill Unit: Incubators and Neutral Thermal Environment
Unit 8: Hypoglycemia
    Skill Unit: Blood Glucose Screenings
Pretest Answer Key
Glossary
Index

Book 3. Neonatal Care

Unit 1: Oxygen
    Skill Unit: Administering Oxygen
        Measuring Oxygen Concentration
        Blending Oxygen and Compressed Air
        Heating and Humidifying an Oxygen/Air Mixture
    Skill Unit: Monitoring Oxygen
        Peripheral Arterial Blood Gas Sampling
Unit 2: Respiratory Distress
    Skill Unit: Detecting a Pneumothorax
        Transillumination
        Chest Radiography
    Skill Unit: Treating a Pneumothorax
        Needle Aspiration
        Chest Tube Insertion
Unit 3: Umbilical Catheters
    Skill Unit: Inserting and Managing Umbilical Catheters
Unit 4: Low Blood Pressure (Hypotension)
    Skill Unit: Measuring Blood Pressure
Unit 5: Intravenous Therapy
    Skill Unit: Peripheral Intravenous Infusions
        Inserting and Managing Peripheral Intravenous Infusions
Unit 6: Feeding
    Part 1: Feeding Principles
    Part 2: Tube Feeding
    Skill Unit: Nasogastric Tube Feedings
Unit 7: Hyperbilirubinemia
    Appendix: Identification and Treatment of Jaundice During the First Week After Birth
Unit 8: Infections
Unit 9: Identifying and Caring for Sick and At-Risk Babies
    Subsection: Vital Signs and Observations
    Subsection: Tests and Results
Unit 10: Preparation for Neonatal Transport
    Subsection: Caring for Parents of Transported Babies
Unit 11: Neonatal Abstinence Syndrome (Neonatal Opioid Withdrawal Syndrome)
Pretest Answer Key
Glossary
Index

Book 4. Specialized Newborn Care

Unit 1: Direct Blood Pressure Measurement
    Skill Unit: Transducer Blood Pressure Monitoring
Unit 2: Exchange, Reduction, and Direct Transfusions
    Skill Unit: Exchange Transfusions
Unit 3: Continuous Positive Airway Pressure
    Skill Unit: Delivery of Continuous Positive Airway Pressure
Unit 4: Assisted Ventilation With Mechanical Ventilators
    Skill Unit: Endotracheal Tubes
Unit 5: Surfactant Therapy
    Skill Unit: Surfactant Administration
Unit 6: Therapeutic Hypothermia for Neonatal Hypoxic-Ischemic Encephalopathy
    Skill Unit: Passive Cooling
Unit 7: Continuing Care for At-Risk Babies
Unit 8: Biomedical Ethics and Perinatology
Pretest Answer Key
Glossary
Index

Unit 1: Hypertension in Pregnancy

Objectives 2

1. What are the risks of hypertension during pregnancy? 5
2. How is hypertension in pregnancy classified? 5
3. How is chronic hypertension managed during pregnancy? 11
4. Which women are at increased risk for development of hypertensive disorders of pregnancy? 15
5. What are the management guidelines for gestational hypertension? 16
6. What are the management guidelines for preeclampsia and eclampsia? 17
7. What measures should every hospital implement to ensure prompt management of hypertension in pregnancy? 19
8. How do you manage the labor of a woman with preeclampsia and stabilize a woman with worsening preeclampsia or eclampsia? 22
9. What should you do when a seizure occurs? 26
10. How do you know when a woman with eclampsia or worsening preeclampsia has been stabilized? 27
11. What should be done after the maternal condition has been stabilized? 27
12. How should women with HELLP syndrome be managed? 29
13. What are the risks from hypertension after delivery? 29

Tables, Figure, and Box

    Table 1.1. Hypertension in Pregnancy: Types and Characteristic Findings 7

    Table 1.2. Antihypertensive Medication During Pregnancy 13

    Figure 1.1. The Alliance for Innovation on Maternal Health Hypertension Bundle 20

    Box 1.1. Antihypertensive Medications for Acute Reduction in Blood Pressure During Labor for Women With Preeclampsia or to Stabilize Women With Worsening Preeclampsia or Eclampsia 24

Recommended Routines 31

Objectives

In this unit you will learn

A. The risks hypertension poses to the pregnant woman and fetus

B. How to identify chronic hypertension and hypertensive disorders of pregnancy and how to define the various types of hypertension during pregnancy

C. How to manage chronic hypertension during pregnancy and which fetal surveillance measures to use

D. How to manage hypertensive disorders of pregnancy and which fetal surveillance measures to use

E. When to seek help for the care of a woman with hypertension

F. How to stabilize a woman who has worsening preeclampsia or eclampsia

G. Which anticonvulsant and antihypertensive drugs to use and how to administer them, and which antihypertensive drugs to avoid

H. How to manage chronic hypertension during labor and delivery and what to anticipate for the care of the baby

I. How to manage hypertensive disorders of pregnancy during labor and delivery and what to anticipate for the care of the baby

J. How to manage hypertension during the postpartum period

Unit 1 Pretest

Before reading the unit, please answer the following questions. Select the *one best* answer to each question (unless otherwise instructed). Record your answers on the test and check them with the answers at the end of the book.

1. A woman with chronic hypertension is at increased risk during pregnancy for all of the following conditions, except:
   A. Post-term pregnancy
   B. A growth-restricted baby
   C. Compromised renal function
   D. Preeclampsia

2. True False A blood pressure of 160/110 mm Hg in a pregnant woman with proteinuria and persistent headache represents preeclampsia with severe features.

3. True False Magnesium sulfate is used for the acute reduction of blood pressure in women who have preeclampsia with severe features.

4. True False If gestational hypertension occurred in one pregnancy, there is an increased risk of it occurring in subsequent pregnancies.

5. True False Slowing of the fetal growth rate may occur before preeclampsia is evident.

6. True False In cases of preeclampsia with severe features, early delivery for the health of the pregnant woman or the baby may be necessary.

7. True False Women with hypertension during pregnancy are at increased risk for placenta previa.

8. True False When thrombocytopenia is present, epidural anesthesia is the preferred method of pain relief during labor.

9. All of the following conditions are possible maternal complications of hypertension during pregnancy, except:
   A. Intracranial hemorrhage
   B. Renal failure
   C. Pulmonary edema
   D. Diabetes mellitus

10. Which of the following actions should be taken first if a woman with preeclampsia has a seizure?
    A. Administer an intravenous bolus of magnesium sulfate.
    B. Protect the woman from injury and protect her airway.
    C. Page anesthesia personnel so a cesarean delivery can begin immediately.
    D. Administer intravenous diazepam.

11. Which of the following conditions is most likely to be present at birth in a newborn whose mother received large amounts of magnesium sulfate?
    A. Low blood sodium level
    B. High blood pressure
    C. Poor urine output
    D. Poor respiratory effort

(continued)

Unit 1 Pretest (continued)

12. Which of the following conditions is least likely to be present in a woman with HELLP syndrome?
    A. Increased hepatic transaminase levels
    B. Increased serum bilirubin levels
    C. Polyhydramnios
    D. Thrombocytopenia (low platelet count)

13. In women with severe hypertension, lowering blood pressure below 140/90 mm Hg should be avoided because blood pressure below that level is likely to result in
    A. Increased maternal cardiac output
    B. Decreased placental perfusion
    C. Venous stasis and thrombosis formation
    D. Inadequate blood flow to the lungs

14. Which of the following conditions should a woman with hypertension report immediately to her health professional?

Yes	No	
___	___	Decreased fetal movement
___	___	Significant peripheral edema
___	___	Persistent headache
___	___	Right upper abdominal pain
___	___	Blurred vision
___	___	Uterine contractions

15. Which of the following actions are appropriate measures for a woman with controlled chronic hypertension?

Yes	No	
___	___	Assess fetal growth by undergoing serial ultrasonographic examinations.
___	___	Check hepatic transaminase levels monthly, starting at 28 weeks of gestation.
___	___	Check creatinine clearance and total urine protein monthly, starting at 28 weeks of gestation.
___	___	Use narcotic analgesia preferentially for pain during labor.
___	___	Consult with a maternal-fetal medicine specialist if preeclampsia develops.
___	___	Plan for cesarean delivery.

16. Which of the following actions are appropriate postpartum care measures for a woman who had preeclampsia with severe features?

Yes	No	
___	___	Provide invasive cardiac output monitoring for 1 to 2 days.
___	___	Continue magnesium sulfate infusion for 12 to 24 hours.
___	___	Arrange for home blood pressure monitoring for 1 to 2 weeks.
___	___	Continue hospitalization and bed rest for 1 to 2 weeks.

1. What are the risks of hypertension during pregnancy?

High blood pressure during pregnancy may be caused by

- Chronic hypertension that was present before pregnancy
- An increase in blood pressure that occurs only with pregnancy (hypertensive disorders of pregnancy)
- A hypertensive disorder of pregnancy superimposed on chronic hypertension

Regardless of the cause, hypertension during pregnancy poses a potentially serious threat to the health of a pregnant woman and her fetus. In the United States and worldwide, hypertension is a major cause of maternal morbidity, is directly implicated in approximately 10% of maternal deaths, and adversely affects fetal and neonatal health.

High blood pressure increases the risk for each of the following complications:

A. Maternal risks
- Intracranial hemorrhage
- Stroke
- Seizures
- Congestive heart failure
- Pulmonary edema
- Renal failure
- Liver failure
- Placental abruption
- Death

B. Fetal/neonatal risks
- Impaired placental blood flow and function
- Fetal growth restriction (this is a frequent finding in hypertension during pregnancy but is not a factor in the diagnosis or classification of hypertensive disorders of pregnancy)
- Oligohydramnios
- Abnormal antepartum fetal surveillance
- Medically indicated preterm birth due to deteriorating maternal or fetal health
- Perinatal death

2. How is hypertension in pregnancy classified?

An important goal of frequent screening during prenatal care is the early identification and treatment of hypertension before it threatens the health of a woman or fetus. The management of hypertension in a pregnant woman will be determined by her diagnosis, gestational age of the fetus, severity of hypertension, coexisting medical conditions, and fetal status. Hypertension in pregnancy is classified as follows:

- Chronic hypertension
- Hypertensive disorders of pregnancy
    — Gestational hypertension
    — Preeclampsia (*mild preeclampsia* is an outdated term that is no longer used)
    — Preeclampsia with severe features
    — Eclampsia
    — HELLP (*H*emolysis, *E*levated *L*iver enzyme levels, and *L*ow *P*latelet count) syndrome
- Superimposed preeclampsia (preeclampsia in a woman with preexisting chronic hypertension)

A. Chronic hypertension
   Women with chronic hypertension may be identified in 2 ways.
   1. Documented history of chronic hypertension before pregnancy, regardless of whether the hypertension required treatment with medication (identified according to the medical history obtained during the initial visit)
   2. Persistent increase of blood pressure to 140/90 mm Hg or higher *before* 20 weeks of gestation or *after* 12 weeks postpartum. The American Heart Association has recently redefined hypertension as blood pressure higher than 130/80 mm Hg. If this classification is used, many more pregnant women will be classified as having chronic hypertension. To date, the effects of blood pressure between 130/80 and 140/90 mm Hg on pregnancy outcomes have not been studied in depth.

   Chronic hypertension may occur in isolation or may coexist with another condition, such as renal dysfunction, cardiac disease, or thyroid disorders. Women with chronic hypertension, regardless of the cause, are at increased risk for developing superimposed preeclampsia.

B. Hypertensive disorders of pregnancy
   The cause of hypertensive disorders of pregnancy is unknown. These conditions are temporally limited to pregnancy, with the onset of blood pressure increase first noted *after* 20 weeks of gestation.

   New-onset hypertension may develop during pregnancy. Hypertensive disorders of pregnancy may progress in severity, and this progression may be slow or rapid. The time course of progression cannot always be predicted. For some women, the initial presentation will include evidence of advanced illness or an atypical presentation. The extent of risk to the mother and fetus is in part related to the severity and progression of hypertension.

   Hypertensive disorders of pregnancy generally resolve within a few days after delivery but may take 6 to 12 weeks to resolve completely. Infrequently, symptoms worsen after delivery. In rare cases, preeclampsia may not become evident until as late as 10 days after birth. Table 1.1 summarizes the clinical and laboratory characteristics of hypertensive disorders of pregnancy.

Prompt detection and frequent surveillance of hypertensive disorders of pregnancy are important in reducing maternal and perinatal mortality and morbidity.

UNIT 1: HYPERTENSION IN PREGNANCY

Table 1.1. Hypertension in Pregnancy: Types and Characteristic Findings

Signs and Symptoms	Gestational Hypertension	Preeclampsia	Preeclampsia With Severe Features *Findings of preeclampsia, plus one or more of the following criteria:*	Eclampsia	HELLP Syndrome
Maternal Factors					
Blood pressure	>140/90 mm Hg	140–159 mm Hg systolic or 90–109 mm Hg diastolic	≥160 mm Hg systolic and/or >110 mm Hg diastolic	Usually increased	Usually increased
New-onset proteinuria	None (<300 mg/24 h, or urine protein to creatinine ratio <0.3)	>300 mg in 24 h, or spot protein to creatinine ratio >0.3	>300 mg in 24 h, or spot protein to creatinine ratio >0.3	>300 mg in 24 h, or spot protein to creatinine ratio >0.3	Usually present
Neurological changes	None	None	Cerebral disturbances (headache), visual disturbances (blurred vision, scotomata); clonus or hyperreflexia may be present but are not required for the diagnosis.	Seizure(s) or coma[a]	May be present
Urine output	Within reference range	Within reference range	May be decreased (decreased <0.5 mL/kg/h)	Usually decreased	Usually decreased
Serum creatinine	Within reference range	Within reference range	Serum creatinine level >1.1 mg/dL or 50% increase over baseline	Usually increased	Variable
Epigastric or right upper quadrant abdominal pain	None	None	May be present	May be present	Persistent pain
Hepatic transaminase levels	Within reference range	Within reference range	AST and ALT levels more than 2 times the upper limit of reference range.	AST and ALT levels may be increased.	AST and ALT levels increased (>2 times the upper limit of reference range)

(*continued*)

Table 1.1. Hypertension in Pregnancy: Types and Characteristic Findings (continued)						
Signs and Symptoms	Gestational Hypertension	Preeclampsia	Preeclampsia With Severe Features	Eclampsia	HELLP Syndrome
Maternal Factors (continued)					
Pulmonary edema	None	None	May be present	May be present	May be present
Platelets	Within reference range	Within reference range	Not all women will have thrombocytopenia. Platelet count <100,000/mm³ is a criterion for severe features	Variable	<100,000/mm³
Fetal Factors					
Fetal growth	May be restricted	May be restricted	May be restricted; while fetal growth restriction may coexist with a hypertensive disorder of pregnancy, it is not considered a diagnostic criterion for preeclampsia with severe features.	May be restricted	May be restricted

Abbreviations: ALT, alanine aminotransferase; AST, aspartate aminotransferase; HELLP, hemolysis, elevated liver enzyme levels, and low platelet count occurring in association with preeclampsia.

[a] The occurrence of a seizure or the onset of coma differentiates eclampsia from preeclampsia.

1. Gestational hypertension

   Gestational hypertension is defined as
   - Blood pressure of 140/90 mm Hg after 20 weeks of gestation in a woman who had blood pressure within reference range before 20 weeks of gestation
   - Absence of proteinuria
     The term is only used during pregnancy. After delivery and the postpartum period, a specific diagnosis can be established.
   - Additional signs and symptoms may develop during pregnancy, identifying the condition as preeclampsia, eclampsia, or HELLP syndrome.

   or
   - Preeclampsia does not develop, and blood pressure returns to reference range by 12 weeks after birth, allowing confirmation of the diagnosis of gestational hypertension.

   or
   - Blood pressure remains increased after birth, confirming the diagnosis of chronic hypertension.

2. Preeclampsia

   Preeclampsia is defined as
   - Blood pressure of 140 to 159 mm Hg systolic or 90 to 109 mm Hg diastolic in 2 readings obtained 4 hours apart

   plus
   - Proteinuria greater than 300 mg in 24 hours or a protein to creatinine ratio greater than 0.3 mg/mg in a voided, untimed urine specimen

3. Preeclampsia with severe features
   Preeclampsia with severe features includes changes that define preeclampsia plus one or more of the following findings:
   - Blood pressure of 160/110 mm Hg on 2 occasions at least 4 hours apart. A physician may elect to assign the diagnosis of preeclampsia with severe features and initiate treatment based on a single blood pressure measurement exceeding 160 mm Hg systolic and/or 110 mm Hg diastolic without waiting 4 hours for a second increased reading.
   - Cerebral or visual disturbances (persistent headache in particular)
   - Thrombocytopenia (platelet count <100,000/mm^3)
   - Pulmonary edema
   - Renal dysfunction (serum creatinine level >1.1 mg/dL or a 50% increase over baseline value)
   - Hepatic dysfunction (increased aspartate aminotransferase [AST] level and alanine aminotransferase [ALT] level >2 times the upper limit of reference range or severe and persistent epigastric or right upper-quadrant pain)

   Only *one* of these findings needs to be present for the diagnosis of preeclampsia with severe features to be established. Additionally, the presence of one of these features can be considered diagnostic of preeclampsia with severe features, even in the absence of proteinuria.

4. Eclampsia
   Eclampsia is defined by the occurrence of a grand mal seizure or onset of coma, with no other known cause, in a woman with preeclampsia.

5. HELLP syndrome
   HELLP syndrome is a form of preeclampsia that can be difficult to identify. While it most commonly occurs in the setting of other symptoms of preeclampsia, the woman may not develop hypertension or proteinuria until after she has other symptoms. Initial signs and symptoms of HELLP syndrome can mimic those of gastroenteritis or gall bladder disease and typically include
   - Nausea
   - Vomiting
   - Abdominal pain

   Mild jaundice is often detectable. Examine the woman carefully and obtain serum liver enzyme concentrations if nausea, vomiting, abdominal pain, or jaundice is found. Laboratory abnormalities include
   - AST and ALT levels of twice the upper limit of reference range or higher
   - Increased serum bilirubin level
   - Platelet count below 100,000/mm^3
   - Hemolysis (increased lactate dehydrogenase [LDH] level >600 and decreased haptoglobin level; abnormal blood smear result showing schistocytes and spherocytes)

C. Superimposed preeclampsia
   The onset of preeclampsia in a woman with chronic hypertension increases the risk of serious complications for the woman and her fetus. Superimposed preeclampsia occurs in 20% to 50% of women with chronic hypertension.

   The condition may be difficult to diagnose but includes
   - New-onset proteinuria (more than 300 mg in a 24-hour urine specimen) in a woman with hypertension present before 20 weeks of gestation and no prior evidence of proteinuria

- Sudden increase in proteinuria if it is already present
- Sudden increase in blood pressure in a woman whose hypertension has been well controlled
- Thrombocytopenia (platelets <100,000/mm^3)
- Increase in ALT or AST level to more than 2 times the upper limit of reference range

Development of persistent headache, scotomata, or epigastric pain may also indicate superimposed preeclampsia in a woman with chronic hypertension.

Self-test A

Now answer these questions to test yourself on the information in the last section.

A1. What blood pressure changes define gestational hypertension?

A2. What is the difference between gestational hypertension and preeclampsia?

A3. What is the difference between preeclampsia and eclampsia?

A4. Which of the following findings are observed in HELLP syndrome?

Yes	No	
___	___	Nausea and vomiting
___	___	Jaundice
___	___	Increased blood glucose level
___	___	Increased platelet count
___	___	Increased liver transaminase levels

A5. True False The diagnosis of preeclampsia is established when a pregnant woman develops a blood pressure of 140/90 mm Hg or higher and proteinuria.

A6. True False In women who develop HELLP syndrome, hypertension is always present.

A7. True False During pregnancy, a woman with any variety of hypertension is at higher risk for complications than a woman with blood pressure within reference range.

A8. Which of the following risks are increased when maternal hypertension is present?

Yes	No	
___	___	Preterm birth
___	___	Placental abruption
___	___	Maternal congestive heart failure
___	___	Placenta previa
___	___	Fetal growth restriction
___	___	Nonreactive nonstress test
___	___	Congenital anomalies
___	___	Maternal seizures
___	___	Maternal stroke

Check your answers with the list that follows the Recommended Routines. Correct any incorrect answers and review the appropriate section in the unit.

3. How is chronic hypertension managed during pregnancy?

Women with uncomplicated hypertension generally tolerate pregnancy well. Preconception control of blood pressure is important for optimal outcomes.

Because of the decrease in vascular resistance that normally occurs in pregnancy, many women with chronic hypertension have a decrease in blood pressure during the second trimester. This may influence whether antihypertensive medication is needed. Occasionally, women with chronic hypertension worsen in early pregnancy, which may jeopardize maternal or fetal health.

Management largely depends on whether complications of chronic hypertension, such as impaired renal function, or other comorbid medical conditions are present. If complications are present or develop during pregnancy, the risk to maternal or fetal health is significantly increased. Management can be complicated.

  A. Initial evaluation

    1. At the first prenatal visit, look for factors that may be associated with or may further complicate chronic hypertension.
- Previous pregnancy with preeclampsia, fetal growth restriction, or stillbirth.
- Increase in blood pressure above the woman's usual (nonpregnant) level.
- Other disorders that have a vascular component (eg, systemic lupus erythematosus, antiphospholipid syndrome, diabetes mellitus, chronic renal disease).

Assess maternal baseline health status related to hypertension.
- Assess maternal renal function, in particular, urine protein excretion (urine protein to creatinine ratio or 24-hour urine total protein level)
- Serum blood urea nitrogen and creatinine levels
- Serum electrolyte levels, including potassium
- Serum AST and ALT levels
- Retinal examination to assess for hypertensive changes
- Consider echocardiography and/or electrocardiography, especially in women with long-standing or complicated chronic hypertension

    2. Serious complications and/or superimposed preeclampsia

Serious complications and/or superimposed preeclampsia are more likely to develop if any of the following conditions are found:
- Uncontrolled blood pressure (inability to maintain pressure below 150–160 mm Hg systolic or 100–110 mm Hg diastolic)
- Need for more than one medication
- Presence of other vascular diseases (eg, diabetes mellitus, systemic lupus erythematosus, renal disease)
- Retinopathy
- Cardiomyopathy

Serious complications are also more common among Black women and women who smoke cigarettes.

Women with complicated hypertension can become seriously ill during pregnancy, sometimes suddenly. If complications are present or if superimposed preeclampsia develops, referral of the patient to maternal-fetal medicine specialists for ongoing care and delivery is strongly recommended.

B. Prenatal management
For women with uncomplicated chronic hypertension, assess maternal and fetal health frequently. If complications develop, it is essential to detect them early.
1. Instruct the woman to
   - Measure and record her blood pressure frequently, preferably at least once per day.
   - Report any change in blood pressure.
   - Begin taking 81 mg of aspirin daily by 16 weeks of gestation and continue until delivery to reduce the risk of preeclampsia.
2. Prescribe antihypertensive medication, as needed.
   Sustained systolic hypertension above 150 to 160 mm Hg is associated with an increased risk of complications, including stroke. Start antihypertensive medication to control the blood pressure to between 130 and 150 mm Hg systolic/80 and 100 mm Hg diastolic.
   a. *Women not being treated with antihypertensive medication before pregnancy*
      - Blood pressure may decline to reference-range levels and remain there throughout pregnancy.
      - Even for these women, the risk of developing preeclampsia and/or fetal growth restriction is increased.
   b. *Women being treated with antihypertensive medication before pregnancy*
      - Because of the normal decrease in blood pressure, antihypertensive medication may not be needed during part or all of the pregnancy.
      - Persistent hypertension of 150/100 mm Hg and higher or the presence of end-organ disease warrant the administration of antihypertensive medication. Some common antihypertensive drugs should be avoided during pregnancy (Table 1.2).
      - Diuretic therapy is generally not newly initiated in pregnant women. Diuretics can potentiate the antihypertensive effects of other medications, resulting in improved blood pressure control. The associated plasma volume reduction may have adverse effects on the fetus, especially when placental perfusion is already reduced, as it may be in maternal hypertension. Women whose blood pressure is well controlled prior to conception by taking a low dose of oral diuretic may usually continue this treatment during the pregnancy. Consultation with regional perinatal center specialists is recommended.
3. Schedule frequent prenatal visits
   Visit frequency should be individualized but may take place as often as every 2 weeks until approximately 28 to 32 weeks of gestation. After 28 to 32 weeks, consider increasing prenatal visits to every week until delivery.
4. Periodically reassess maternal urine protein excretion
   In women with preexisting proteinuria, a sudden increase in the amount of urine protein may signal the development of superimposed preeclampsia. Consider periodically checking for urine protein level throughout the pregnancy. Urine dipstick tests for protein are less sensitive than urine protein to creatinine ratio or 24-hour urine total protein level.
5. Assess fetal growth and well-being. Methods include
   - Ultrasonography (US) for evaluation of fetal anatomy at 18 to 20 weeks, followed by assessment of fetal growth at 28 to 32 weeks. Additional US may be performed at monthly intervals until delivery, as clinically indicated by fundal height measurements, maternal blood pressure trends, prior US assessment of fetal growth, and the presence of additional risk factors for abnormal fetal growth.

Table 1.2. Antihypertensive Medication During Pregnancy		
A. Drugs for Ongoing Control of *Chronic* Hypertension During Pregnancy		
Medication	**Administration**	**Comments and Cautions**
Labetalol hydrochloride	*Total daily dose:* 200–2,400 mg/d *Dose:* starting: 100 mg usual: 200–400 mg *Schedule:* 2–3 times/d *Route:* oral	Considered by most to be the first-line agent in pregnancy. Does not reduce uterine blood flow.
Nifedipine	*Usual daily dose:* 30–90 mg once daily extended-release tablet	Use caution when administering magnesium sulfate, which may potentiate the antihypertensive effect.
Methyldopa	*Total daily dose:* 500–2,000 mg *Dose:* 250–500 mg *Schedule:* 2–4 times/d *Route:* oral	Well-established safety profile in pregnancy but often not effective when taken < 3 times a day.
Hydrochlorothiazide	*Usual daily dose:* 12.5–25.0 mg once daily	May be continued if the woman is taking this medication before conception; not usually started as a new medication in pregnancy. Small risk of thrombocytopenia in newborn.
B. Antihypertensive Drugs That Should Be *Avoided* During Pregnancy		
Medication	**Comments and Cautions**	
Angiotensin-converting enzyme inhibitors (eg, captopril) and angiotensin II receptor antagonists (eg, losartan potassium)	1. Associated with birth defects and impaired fetal renal function. 2. Not recommended for use during pregnancy.	
Atenolol (β_1-adrenergic blocking agent)	1. Associated with fetal growth restriction. 2. Avoid use in early pregnancy; use with caution in late pregnancy.	

- All women should be advised to maintain a general awareness of fetal activity each day and to report decreased fetal movement promptly. Current evidence suggests that general awareness is as reliable as formal "kick counting."
- Tests of fetal well-being (eg, nonstress test, biophysical profile) are typically initiated at 32 to 34 weeks of gestation and performed once weekly. In women with complicated hypertension, coexisting medical conditions, fetal growth restriction, or oligohydramnios, testing may be initiated earlier in the pregnancy and may be performed twice weekly—or, rarely, more than twice weekly.

6. Induction of labor

   If spontaneous labor does not occur, schedule induction of labor according to the following guidelines:
   - Chronic hypertension controlled with no medications: $38^{0/7}$ to $39^{6/7}$ weeks
   - Chronic hypertension controlled with medications: $37^{0/7}$ to $39^{6/7}$ weeks
   - Chronic hypertension, uncontrolled or difficult to control: $36^{0/7}$ to $37^{6/7}$ weeks

Each patient's specific recommended timing of delivery should be individualized within these ranges, based on her particular risk factors; delivery early within these ranges is not automatically preferable.

 If a woman with chronic hypertension develops increased blood pressure and proteinuria or declining creatinine clearance, hospitalization may be necessary. Consult with regional perinatal center maternal-fetal medicine specialists.

C. Intrapartum management
   1. Provide pain control
      Provide pain control according to any of the following means:
      - Narcotic analgesia
      - Nitrous oxide
      - Epidural anesthesia (risk of epidural hematoma is increased in preeclampsia with thrombocytopenia < 70,000–100,000/mm^3)
   2. Further increase in blood pressure
      During labor, further increase in blood pressure may occur from normal hemodynamic changes, maternal fear or anxiety, pain, or superimposed preeclampsia. Because it may not be possible to determine the cause of an increase in blood pressure, all women who develop blood pressure increase and proteinuria during labor should be assessed for superimposed preeclampsia, and their blood pressure should be treated according to established guidelines.
   3. Placental function may be impaired and fetal heart rate abnormalities may occur during labor.
      Anticipate the possible need for emergency cesarean delivery and/or neonatal resuscitation.
   4. Be aware that the risk of placental abruption is increased.

D. Postdelivery management
   1. Maternal
      - Methylergonovine maleate may cause vasospasm and increase blood pressure. Administration of this drug for the management of postpartum hemorrhage is *contraindicated* in women with symptomatic heart disease or hypertension.
      - Women with chronic hypertension can develop encephalopathy, pulmonary edema, and heart failure or renal failure postpartum. Close blood pressure and laboratory monitoring should continue until the findings are stable.
   2. Neonatal
      - If resuscitation is needed, monitor for possible post-resuscitation complications (see Book 1: Maternal and Fetal Evaluation and Immediate Newborn Care, Unit 5, Resuscitating the Newborn).
      - Screen for hypoglycemia (see Book 1: Maternal and Fetal Evaluation and Immediate Newborn Care, Unit 8, Hypoglycemia).
      - Perform blood tests, as indicated.
        — Hydrochlorothiazide given to the mother may cause a transient decrease in platelets in the newborn, as well as fetal hemoconcentration.
        — Women with hypertension that develops during pregnancy—particularly women with HELLP syndrome—frequently have babies with thrombocytopenia and neutropenia.

Self-test B

Now answer these questions to test yourself on the information in the last section.

B1. True False Angiotensin-converting enzyme inhibitor antihypertensive medications are the drugs of choice for the treatment of chronic hypertension during pregnancy.

B2. True False Women with uncomplicated chronic hypertension usually tolerate pregnancy well.

B3. True False In women with chronic hypertension, blood pressure rarely declines during pregnancy.

B4. True False Women who require antihypertensive medication before pregnancy will always need such medication during pregnancy.

B5. Which of the following factors increase(s) the risk of complications associated with chronic hypertension during pregnancy?

Yes	No	
___	___	Walking 2 miles a day
___	___	Multiple sclerosis
___	___	Creatinine clearance below 100 mL/min
___	___	Diabetes mellitus
___	___	Development of gestational hypertension
___	___	Lupus erythematosus

B6. Which of the following actions are appropriate measures for a pregnant woman with uncomplicated chronic hypertension?

Yes	No	
___	___	Await 41 weeks of gestation before recommending delivery.
___	___	Use narcotic analgesia during labor.
___	___	Treat the woman for preeclampsia if blood pressure increases and proteinuria develops.
___	___	Plan for cesarean delivery instead of labor.

Check your answers with the list that follows the Recommended Routines. Correct any incorrect answers and review the appropriate section in the unit.

4. Which women are at increased risk for development of hypertensive disorders of pregnancy?

If a woman develops new-onset hypertension prior to 20 weeks of gestation, suspect a hydatidiform mole, triploidy, or fetal hydrops. Consult with specialists for diagnosis and treatment. Any woman may develop a hypertensive disorder of pregnancy. Monitoring for the development of hypertension is part of routine prenatal care for all women. Women with any of the following risk factors are at an increased risk of developing hypertension during the second half of pregnancy:

High-risk factors

- Hypertensive disorder in a previous pregnancy
- Multifetal gestation
- Chronic hypertension
- Renal disease

- Autoimmune disease (systemic lupus erythematosus or antiphospholipid antibody syndrome)
- Type 1 or type 2 diabetes

Moderate-risk factors

- Nulliparity
- Obesity (body mass index > 30 kg/m^2)
- Maternal age of 35 years and older
- Low socioeconomic status
- African American heritage
- Family history of preeclampsia (mother or sister)
- Prior low-birth-weight or small-for-gestational-age baby, prior adverse pregnancy outcome, interval longer than 10 years since last pregnancy

Women with one high-risk factor or more than one moderate-risk factor should be advised to start a low dose of aspirin (81 mg daily) by 16 weeks of gestation and should continue to take daily aspirin until delivery, to reduce the risk of hypertensive disorders of pregnancy.

While some women are at increased risk for hypertensive disorders of pregnancy, this condition can occur in any woman. All women should be monitored for possible onset of hypertension.

5. What are the management guidelines for gestational hypertension?

Close monitoring is needed if gestational hypertension is diagnosed before 37 weeks of gestation. A woman with gestational hypertension may develop preeclampsia.

A. Home care
   Carefully review the following care measures with the woman. Determine if each can realistically be achieved in the home. Modify the regimen or make arrangements for home care to be provided as needed.
   - Frequent blood pressure and weight measurement
   - Daily fetal activity determinations
   - Instructions for the woman to report promptly *any* of the following occurrences:
     — Increase in blood pressure
     — Persistent headache
     — Abdominal pain
     — Visual changes
     — Rapid weight gain
     — Decrease in fetal movement
     — Uterine contractions

B. Prenatal care
   - Provide prenatal visits once to twice a week (office, clinic, or patient's home), in addition to the monitoring measures being taken daily in the home.
   - Perform baseline laboratory tests at the time of diagnosis of gestational hypertension, including hematocrit value, hemoglobin level, platelet count, serum creatinine level, liver enzyme levels (AST and ALT), LDH level, and 24-hour urine protein level or spot urine protein to creatinine ratio. Comparison to test results obtained later will help establish an early diagnosis of preeclampsia, if it develops.

- Develop a plan for antenatal surveillance.
- Assess fetal growth with US. Maternal hypertension is associated with an increased risk of fetal growth restriction. Fetal growth restriction is a risk to fetal well-being and requires monitoring (see Book 1: Maternal and Fetal Evaluation and Immediate Newborn Care, Unit 2, Fetal Age, Growth, and Maturity). The onset of fetal growth restriction in a woman with gestational hypertension may be an indicator of the later diagnosis of preeclampsia.
- If spontaneous onset of labor does not occur by 37 weeks, plan induction of labor or cesarean delivery as appropriate, based on the usual obstetric considerations.
- If preeclampsia develops, hospitalization and/or delivery may be necessary. Consultation with regional center maternal-fetal medicine specialists is recommended.

C. Intrapartum care

Provide routine labor care. Women with gestational hypertension may develop preeclampsia during labor. Monitor closely for
- Increase in blood pressure
- Onset of symptoms of preeclampsia
- Decrease in urine output

6. What are the management guidelines for preeclampsia and eclampsia?

A. Preeclampsia (blood pressure of 140–159 mm Hg systolic or 90–109 mm Hg diastolic with proteinuria)

When hypertension is present, the onset of proteinuria often precedes a sudden worsening of the disease. The earlier in pregnancy preeclampsia is diagnosed, the greater the likelihood of maternal or fetal complications and the need for preterm birth. As soon as evidence of preeclampsia is detected, evaluation in a hospital is needed for adequate assessment of maternal condition.

Preeclampsia is a serious illness that requires careful evaluation and treatment, often in the hospital. Multiple organ systems may be affected.

Increase in blood pressure is not the only important finding. In some women with serious illness, the blood pressure increase may be minimal, but other signs of disease will be clinically significant.

1. Evaluate/monitor maternal-fetal condition
   a. *Check the blood pressure at least hourly*
      Ensure treatment occurs within 60 minutes if the blood pressure exceeds 160 mm Hg systolic or 110 mm Hg diastolic.
   b. *Physical examination*
      A physical examination should be performed every 4 to 8 hours, including
      - Reflexes: Achilles, patellar, and/or antecubital reflexes, including assessment for the presence of clonus
      - Central nervous system involvement, including headache, visual disturbances, decreased level of consciousness, or disorientation
      - Epigastric pain and/or right upper-quadrant tenderness

c. *Blood tests*
   - Complete blood cell count
   - Serum LDH level
   - AST and ALT levels
   - Serum creatinine level
d. *Urine tests*
   - Urine protein to creatinine ratio or timed (eg, 24-hour) urine collection for total protein and creatinine clearance
   - Monitor urine output
e. *Evaluate fetal well-being, growth, and amniotic fluid volume*
   Do this when preeclampsia is first diagnosed. If results are within reference ranges, conduct a nonstress test or biophysical profile twice weekly, assess amniotic fluid weekly, and assess fetal growth with US every 3 to 4 weeks.

2. Respond to patient condition
   After several hours of observation, her condition will either be
   a. *Improved or not worsened*
      Test results for fetal well-being are within reference range, and maternal blood pressure is stable or decreased.
      - If gestational age is 37 weeks or beyond, delivery is recommended.
      - If gestational age is less than 37 weeks and severe features are not present, consider a return to outpatient management with close surveillance of maternal and fetal condition.

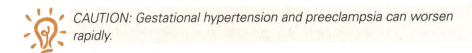

CAUTION: Gestational hypertension and preeclampsia can worsen rapidly.

   b. *Worsened*
      The blood pressure worsens (but does not meet the criteria for preeclampsia with severe features), or fetal test results are not normal. At a minimum, hospitalization for continued observation is appropriate, and delivery may be indicated if stabilization is not achieved.

B. Preeclampsia with severe features (preeclampsia, plus one or more of the findings listed in Section 2, How is hypertension in pregnancy classified? and in Table 1.1)

The risk of eclampsia, placental abruption, maternal intracranial hemorrhage, and fetal death is significantly increased in women with preeclampsia with severe features. Hospitalize the patient and stabilize her condition (see Section 8, How do you manage the labor of a woman with preeclampsia and stabilize a woman with worsening preeclampsia or eclampsia?). Transfer of the woman to a regional perinatal center should be considered. Delivery is recommended at no later than 34 weeks of gestation, but if the woman is less than 34 weeks of gestation and if she and the fetus are stable, delay of delivery for administration of corticosteroids may be considered.

Preeclampsia with severe features may necessitate delivery, regardless of fetal age, size, or maturity. Delivery may be necessary to preserve the health of the woman, the baby, or both.

C. Eclampsia (preeclampsia plus seizure[s] or development of coma)
If convulsions or coma develop, the risk of maternal or fetal death increases dramatically.

 Regardless of blood pressure or proteinuria, any woman pregnant beyond 20 weeks who has a seizure or develops coma should be assumed to have eclampsia and treated accordingly. Other causes for the seizure or coma should be considered while treatment is underway.

Self-test C

Now answer these questions to test yourself on the information in the last section.

C1. List at least 3 signs and symptoms a woman with gestational hypertension should be taught to report promptly to her health professional.
_____
_____
_____

C2. Of the following conditions, which are known to increase the likelihood a woman will develop a hypertensive disorder of pregnancy?

Yes	No	
____	____	Age 35 years and older
____	____	Twins
____	____	Renal disease
____	____	Short stature
____	____	Obesity
____	____	First pregnancy
____	____	Chronic hypertension

C3. True False Women with preeclampsia should be evaluated carefully in a hospital before deciding on a plan of care.

C4. True False Any pregnant woman may develop hypertension.

C5. True False If preeclampsia with severe features develops, maternal condition will not improve until the baby is delivered.

C6. True False Delivery may be necessary for a woman who develops preeclampsia with severe features or eclampsia, regardless of fetal gestational age.

Check your answers with the list that follows the Recommended Routines. Correct any incorrect answers and review the appropriate section in the unit.

7. What measures should every hospital implement to ensure prompt management of hypertension in pregnancy?

All hospitals providing labor and delivery care should be prepared to manage the complications of hypertension in pregnancy. The Alliance for Innovation on Maternal Health (AIM) has developed and disseminated evidence-based safety bundles to guide hospitals on the implementation of safety measures to identify and rapidly treat major maternal complications. Each bundle consists of Readiness, Recognition and Prevention, Response, and Reporting/Systems Learning components. The AIM Hypertension bundle is shown in Figure 1.1 and is available

PCEP BOOK 2: MATERNAL AND FETAL CARE

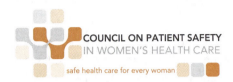

PATIENT SAFETY BUNDLE
Hypertension

 READINESS

Every Unit
- Standards for early warning signs, diagnostic criteria, monitoring and treatment of severe preeclampsia/eclampsia (include order sets and algorithms)
- Unit education on protocols, unit-based drills (with post-drill debriefs)
- Process for timely triage and evaluation of pregnant and postpartum women with hypertension including ED and outpatient areas
- Rapid access to medications used for severe hypertension/eclampsia: Medications should be stocked and immediately available on L&D and in other areas where patients may be treated. Include brief guide for administration and dosage.
- System plan for escalation, obtaining appropriate consultation, and maternal transport, as needed

 RECOGNITION & PREVENTION

Every Patient
- Standard protocol for measurement and assessment of BP and urine protein for all pregnant and postpartum women
- Standard response to maternal early warning signs including listening to and investigating patient symptoms and assessment of labs (e.g. CBC with platelets, AST and ALT)
- Facility-wide standards for educating prenatal and postpartum women on signs and symptoms of hypertension and preeclampsia

© 2015 American College of Obstetricians and Gynecologists

May 2015
(continued)

UNIT 1: HYPERTENSION IN PREGNANCY

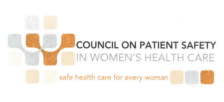

RESPONSE

Every case of severe hypertension/preeclampsia

- Facility-wide standard protocols with checklists and escalation policies for management and treatment of:
  - Severe hypertension
  - Eclampsia, seizure prophylaxis, and magnesium over-dosage
  - Postpartum presentation of severe hypertension/preeclampsia
- Minimum requirements for protocol:
  - Notification of physician or primary care provider if systolic BP =/> 160 or diastolic BP =/> 110 for two measurements within 15 minutes
  - After the second elevated reading, treatment should be initiated ASAP (preferably within 60 minutes of verification)
  - Includes onset and duration of magnesium sulfate therapy
  - Includes escalation measures for those unresponsive to standard treatment
  - Describes manner and verification of follow-up within 7 to 14 days postpartum
  - Describe postpartum patient education for women with preeclampsia
- Support plan for patients, families, and staff for ICU admissions and serious complications of severe hypertension

REPORTING/SYSTEMS LEARNING

Every unit

- Establish a culture of huddles for high risk patients and post-event debriefs to identify successes and opportunities
- Multidisciplinary review of all severe hypertension/eclampsia cases admitted to ICU for systems issues
- Monitor outcomes and process metrics

Note: "Facility-wide" indicates all areas where pregnant or postpartum women receive care. (E.g. L&D, postpartum critical care, emergency department, and others depending on the facility).

PATIENT SAFETY BUNDLE

Hypertension

© 2015 American College of Obstetricians and Gynecologists. Permission is hereby granted for duplication and distribution of this document, in its entirety and without modification, for solely non-commercial activities that are for educational, quality improvement, and patient safety purposes. All other uses require written permission from ACOG.

Standardization of health care processes and reduced variation has been shown to improve outcomes and quality of care. The Council on Patient Safety in Women's Health Care disseminates patient safety bundles to help facilitate the standardization process. This bundle reflects emerging clinical, scientific, and patient safety advances as of the date issued and is subject to change. The information should not be construed as dictating an exclusive course of treatment or procedure to be followed. Although the components of a particular bundle may be adapted to local resources, standardization within an institution is strongly encouraged.

The Council on Patient Safety in Women's Health Care is a broad consortium of organizations across the spectrum of women's health for the promotion of safe health care for every woman.

May 2015

For more information visit the Council's website at www.safehealthcareforeverywoman.org

Figure 1.1. The Alliance for Innovation on Maternal Health Hypertension Bundle
Available at https://safehealthcareforeverywoman.org/wp-content/uploads/2017/11/Severe-Hypertension-Bundle.pdf. Accessed May 20, 2020.

at https://safehealthcareforeverywoman.org/wp-content/uploads/2017/11/Severe-Hypertension-Bundle.pdf. Most states in the United States have a statewide initiative to implement AIM through their perinatal quality collaborative or other group.

8. How do you manage the labor of a woman with preeclampsia and stabilize a woman with worsening preeclampsia or eclampsia?

The clinical course of preeclampsia may be unpredictable. Each woman needs a monitoring plan to identify changes in her condition early and to allow timely intervention to maintain maternal and fetal health. Women with worsening preeclampsia or eclampsia need to be treated aggressively to prevent further deterioration of maternal condition and fetal status, regardless of whether they are in labor.

A. Prevent seizures from occurring or recurring
   1. Administer magnesium sulfate

   Magnesium sulfate is used to prevent and treat convulsions caused by preeclampsia with severe features or eclampsia, but it has little direct effect on blood pressure. Use an intravenous (IV) infusion of magnesium sulfate
   - During initial evaluation if preeclampsia with severe features is suspected.
   - During transportation of a stable patient to a tertiary care center.
   - During delivery, whether spontaneous labor, induced labor, or cesarean, if severe features are present.
   - After delivery, until stable after birth (which may be 24 hours or longer).

   Currently, magnesium sulfate is not recommended for use during labor when severe features are not present, because of the low likelihood of eclampsia in these women. Severe features may develop for the first time during labor; therefore, it is important to remain vigilant for them and initiate administration of magnesium sulfate if they occur.

   A loading dose of 4 to 6 g of magnesium sulfate is administered over 20 minutes, followed by continuous infusion of 2 g/h. *Continue* administration of magnesium sulfate throughout labor and for 24 hours, or longer if necessary, after delivery. Magnesium sulfate is discontinued after delivery when symptoms have resolved, blood pressure has stabilized, urine output is adequate (usually >100 mL/h), and abnormal laboratory values have begun to improve.

   Note: *Myasthenia gravis, heart block, and recent myocardial infarction are absolute contraindications for the use of magnesium sulfate. Magnesium sulfate is especially risky to use in women with renal failure. The usual loading dose may be administered, but maintenance doses should be reduced and may not be needed at all. Therapy should be guided by serum magnesium levels, which should be checked regularly.*

   2. Monitor magnesium levels

   Consider checking the serum magnesium level 4 to 6 hours after therapy is started, and periodically thereafter, depending on the woman's clinical status. Adjust the dosage as necessary to maintain the serum level between 4 and 8 mEq/L (4.8 and 9.6 mg/dL). Often the magnesium level can be gauged clinically by finding depressed, but not absent, deep tendon reflexes (DTRs).

Check the vital signs and DTRs every hour.
- If DTRs disappear, stop the magnesium sulfate infusion and check the serum magnesium levels.
- In the rare event that respirations become depressed or absent as a result of magnesium toxicity, **stop the magnesium infusion**. Perform endotracheal intubation, ventilate the woman as necessary, and administer calcium gluconate (1 g) via *slow* IV push.

Monitor oxygen saturation. Repeat calcium gluconate administration as necessary until spontaneous respirations return.

Signs of magnesium sulfate toxicity include loss of DTRs, depressed respiration, cardiac arrest, and visual symptoms. Blurred vision may be a symptom of worsening preeclampsia or of magnesium toxicity.

Magnesium level in serum
- Greater than 7 mEq/L (>9 mg/dL): associated with loss of DTRs
- Greater than 10 mEq/L (>12 mg/dL): associated with respiratory depression
- Greater than 25 mEq/L (>30 mg/dL): associated with cardiac arrest

3. If a seizure occurs while a patient is receiving magnesium sulfate

   Rarely, a woman may continue to have seizures despite having a magnesium level in the therapeutic range (4–8 mEq/L). Under such circumstances, administer diazepam (Valium), 5 to 10 mg, intravenously, over 5 to 10 minutes. This anticonvulsant stops eclamptic seizures quickly, but IV administration may cause respiratory arrest. Be prepared with personnel and equipment (eg, endotracheal tubes, laryngoscope, ventilation bag) to intubate and provide assisted ventilation. Diazepam readily crosses the placenta and can depress fetal respirations, necessitating resuscitation and prolonged ventilatory support for some newborns.

4. If magnesium sulfate and diazepam both fail

   Amobarbital sodium or thiopental sodium may be administered intravenously. It is advisable that this be done by a health professional who is skilled in the use of these drugs, such as an anesthesiologist or anesthetist.

   Patients who do not improve with anticonvulsant therapy may have intracranial bleeding or other pathology as the cause of their seizures. Consultation with regional center specialists or a local neurologist is recommended.

B. Control hypertension

   Hypertension needs to be controlled to
   - Prevent a dangerous blood pressure increase during labor in women with preeclampsia.
   - Provide acute blood pressure reduction in women with worsening preeclampsia or eclampsia.

   In either case, a blood pressure higher than 160/110 mm Hg needs to be lowered promptly, to the range of 130–150/80–100 mm Hg. This lower blood pressure reduces the risk of intracranial hemorrhage and stroke but does not cure the preeclampsia or eclampsia. Pressure lowered too far, however, may compromise placental blood flow.

Blood pressure should be lowered promptly to the goal range; treatment should be initiated within 15 minutes of confirming an increased blood pressure over 160 mm Hg systolic or 110 mm Hg diastolic. Avoid bringing it below 130/80 mm Hg to minimize the risk of impaired placental perfusion and fetal heart rate abnormalities.

Guidelines for the administration of medications (Box 1.1) for the acute reduction of blood pressure are as follows:

1. Check the maternal blood pressure every 5 to 10 minutes (maximal effect usually occurs within 5 minutes of injection for the drugs listed).
2. Repeat the dose every 10 to 30 minutes, until the desired blood pressure is achieved.
3. The goal is stable blood pressure of 140–150/90–100 mm Hg.
4. Assess the woman for postural hypotension because it may occur with tachycardia, headaches, nausea, or difficulty sitting or standing.
5. Hydralazine or labetalol may be used as a first-line agent. Nifedipine may be used as a first-line agent for a woman who does not have IV access.

Box 1.1. Antihypertensive Medications for Acute Reduction in Blood Pressure During Labor for Women With Preeclampsia or to Stabilize Women With Worsening Preeclampsia or Eclampsia

Hydralazine hydrochloride

- Initial dose, 5 mg or 10 mg; administered in an IV bolus over 2 minutes.
- 20 minutes later, if BP remains increased over 160/110 mm Hg, administer 10 mg in an IV bolus over 2 minutes.
- If the desired effect is not achieved after 2 doses, change to labetalol.
- Labetalol is preferred for women with baseline pulse rate >120 beats/min or who develop tachycardia during treatment with hydralazine.

Labetalol hydrochloride

- Initial dose, 20 mg; administered in an IV bolus over 2 minutes.
- If BP is not reduced appropriately in 20 minutes, increase dose to 40 mg.
- If BP is not reduced appropriately in another 20 minutes, increase dose to 80 mg; may repeat once in 20 minutes if blood pressure remains >160/110 mm Hg.
- If BP is not reduced appropriately in another 20 minutes, change to hydralazine.
- Hydralazine is preferred in women with a baseline pulse rate of <60 beats/min or who develop bradycardia during treatment with labetalol.
- Avoid use in women with asthma or congestive heart failure.

Immediate-release nifedipine

Initial dose, 10 mg given orally for acute blood pressure control, followed by 20 mg if blood pressure is not controlled after 20 minutes; the 20-mg dose may be repeated once for a total dose of 50 mg over 1 hour. Nifedipine is the agent of first choice in a woman with severe hypertension and no IV access.

Abbreviations: BP, blood pressure; IV, intravenous.

Note: See Table 1.2 for drugs that should be avoided.

C. Monitor fetal well-being and maternal health
1. Be sure to evaluate all aspects of maternal and fetal health
   As you stabilize the maternal condition in preparation for delivery, be sure to evaluate all aspects of maternal and fetal health. Other complications, related or unrelated to hypertension, can also occur (eg, maternal infection, cord prolapse, placental abruption). While appropriate treatment of hypertension is critical to maternal and fetal health, be careful not to focus exclusively on it.
2. Record fluid intake and output
   Beginning at the time of hospital admission and continuing through 24 hours after delivery, record the woman's fluid intake and output. Fluid balance is often altered with preeclampsia, particularly during labor and if oxytocin is administered. Fluid overload with pulmonary edema may occur. If evidence of pulmonary edema or oliguria (urine output of <20 mL/h) develops, consultation with regional perinatal center staff is recommended.

Self-test D

Now answer these questions to test yourself on the information in the last section.

D1. When eclampsia is present, _____ is generally used to prevent recurrence of maternal seizures.

D2. Which of the following is a sign of magnesium toxicity?

Yes	No	
___	___	Exaggerated reflexes
___	___	High serum sodium level
___	___	Slow respiratory rate
___	___	Loss of deep tendon reflexes
___	___	Decreased urine output

D3. True   False   When the maternal blood pressure is 160/110 mm Hg or higher, it should be lowered to below 130/80 mm Hg.

D4. True   False   Diazepam (Valium) may be used if magnesium sulfate fails to control seizures in a woman with eclampsia.

D5. True   False   For women with severe preeclampsia, the goal of antihypertensive treatment is to achieve a blood pressure of 90/60 mm Hg.

D6. True   False   If magnesium sulfate is administered during labor, it should be stopped as soon as the baby is delivered.

D7. What can happen if the maternal blood pressure is lowered too far?
_____
_____

D8. If magnesium sulfate fails to stop seizures in a woman with eclampsia, what should be done?

Yes	No	
___	___	Consult a neurologist or regional perinatal center specialists.
___	___	Administer diazepam (Valium) intravenously.
___	___	Be prepared to provide assisted ventilation to the woman.
___	___	Perform cesarean delivery immediately.
___	___	Consider that intracranial hemorrhage may have occurred.
___	___	Be prepared to assist the baby's respirations.

Check your answers with the list that follows the Recommended Routines. Correct any incorrect answers and review the appropriate section in the unit.

9. What should you do when a seizure occurs?

A seizure is a dramatic event. You need to react immediately but *calmly*. Stay focused on what needs to be done to help the woman, not on the seizure itself. A team response should be as practiced and as planned as it is for cardiopulmonary resuscitation.

A. Initial response
1. Place the woman in the lateral decubitus position to maximize uterine perfusion and prevent aspiration.
   Protect her from injury, such as a fall or striking her head against a bed rail. Wait for the seizure to subside, which may take 60 to 90 seconds.
2. Administer oxygen via mask.
   Be sure the mask fits tightly, and use a flow rate of 6 to 10 L/min to keep the oxygen saturation level above 90%.
3. Apply a pulse oximeter to allow continuous monitoring of the oxygen saturation level.
4. Insert an oral airway or perform endotracheal intubation if the woman cannot maintain adequate oxygenation.
   Suction excess secretions or vomitus from her mouth.
5. Check the maternal blood pressure.
   If it is higher than 160/110 mm Hg, administer hydralazine, 10 mg, via IV bolus, or labetalol, 20 mg, via IV bolus, over 2 minutes. Recheck the blood pressure every 10 to 20 minutes and follow the stabilization protocol in Section 8, How do you manage the labor of a woman with preeclampsia and stabilize a woman with worsening preeclampsia or eclampsia? in this unit.
6. Administer magnesium sulfate.
   - Use a loading dose of 4 to 6 g, administered intravenously over 20 minutes, of a magnesium sulfate solution containing 40 g of magnesium per 1,000 mL of sterile water; follow this with a continuous infusion of 2 g/h. (See the stabilization protocol in Section 8, How do you manage the labor of a woman with preeclampsia and stabilize a woman with worsening preeclampsia or eclampsia? A1. Administer magnesium sulfate.)
   - If the infusion of magnesium sulfate is already started, DTRs are present (check the patellar reflex), and the patient is breathing spontaneously, administer another 4-g IV bolus of magnesium sulfate over 20 minutes.
   - If an eclamptic seizure occurs in a woman with no IV access, a total dose of 10 g of magnesium sulfate may be administered intramuscularly, 5 g in each buttock.
7. Check and monitor fetal heart rate.
   Fetal bradycardia often occurs during and soon after a maternal seizure. The woman may be cyanotic, with slow and deep respirations. The woman will recover spontaneously, given an open airway (in rare cases, assisted ventilation may be needed), oxygen, and time. As the woman recovers her oxygenation, fetal heart rate and condition will also recover.

UNIT 1: HYPERTENSION IN PREGNANCY

 This is the time when a woman is in the most danger from overzealous drug therapy, anesthesia, and surgery. The first actions you should take are to stabilize the woman's condition. Once fully stabilized, delivery should be conducted promptly.

Performing cesarean delivery before maternal stabilization is dangerous. Even if fetal bradycardia is present, the woman's condition should be stabilized before delivery is undertaken.

B. Post-seizure care
Follow the stabilization protocol in Section 8, How do you manage the labor of a woman with preeclampsia and stabilize a woman with worsening preeclampsia or eclampsia? in this unit. Consult with maternal-fetal medicine specialists. Arrange for patient transfer and delivery, as appropriate.

10. How do you know when a woman with eclampsia or worsening preeclampsia has been stabilized?

A. The woman is awake and aware.
A stable patient knows where she is, can answer questions appropriately, can carry on a conversation, and can cooperate with her care.

B. Her blood pressure is stable.
Her blood pressure has not required acute treatment for 4 to 6 hours.

C. There are no findings that indicate worsening conditions.
A woman whose condition is stable will have *none* of the following findings:
- Oliguria (urine output <25 mL/h)
- Persistent headache
- Blurred vision, "spots before the eyes"
- Epigastric or abdominal pain
- Shortness of breath, cyanosis, or pulmonary edema

11. What should be done after the maternal condition has been stabilized?

A. Consult with regional perinatal center experts
A thorough assessment of maternal and fetal condition is required for optimal outcomes for women with preeclampsia who have severe features, eclampsia, or HELLP syndrome. The management may be complicated, and occasionally intensive care is needed. Even if stabilized initially, maternal or fetal condition may become unstable and deteriorate further, requiring reassessment and rapid intervention. Decisions about location, timing, and route of delivery require careful weighing of fetal condition, maternal condition, and gestational age.
Consultation with maternal-fetal medicine and neonatal intensive care specialists is recommended, whether or not you plan to transfer the woman to a regional perinatal center.

B. Transfer the woman to a regional perinatal center
Women with preeclampsia with severe features, eclampsia, or HELLP syndrome may become extremely ill. Central hemodynamic monitoring, while uncommonly used in pregnancy, may be necessary during labor. Intensive care of the baby may be needed after delivery. Transfer of the pregnant woman to a regional perinatal center may be indicated, even for a term pregnancy. Transport should generally not be undertaken until a woman's condition is stabilized; however, once the woman's condition is stabilized, transport should be accomplished without delay, *unless* she is in labor.

C. Prepare for delivery
If the woman is in active labor or if transfer to a regional perinatal center is not advisable for other reasons, proceed with plans for delivery. Consult pediatric specialists to prepare for the delivery room and neonatal care of the baby.
1. Consider administration of corticosteroids
For gestational ages between 23 and 37 weeks, administration of corticosteroids is generally recommended to promote fetal lung maturity, even if delivery is expected to occur in less than 24 hours. See Unit 9, Preterm Labor, in this book or consult with regional perinatal center maternal-fetal medicine specialists.
2. Induce labor
- Women with eclampsia or worsening preeclampsia should be delivered in a timely manner, often within 24 hours of their condition being stabilized.
- Epidural or spinal anesthesia may be administered if the platelet count is higher than 70,000/mm^3. General anesthesia has particularly high risks for these women, making vaginal delivery safer than cesarean delivery.
- Provide routine care and pain management. Opioids and/or nitrous oxide may be used on the basis of patient preference or if regional anesthesia is contraindicated.
- Cervical ripening with a cervical balloon catheter, misoprostol, or dinoprostone may be used (see Unit 10, Inducing and Augmenting Labor, in this book).
- Induction of labor may be successful, even if the cervix is not ripe and the pregnancy is far from term.
- If placental function is diminished because of hypertension, the fetus is more likely to have a category II or III fetal heart rate tracing during labor. Anticipate the need for emergency cesarean delivery or neonatal resuscitation.
3. Cesarean delivery
If induction of labor is contraindicated or is not successful, cesarean delivery is indicated. The timing and location of delivery should be based on maternal and fetal condition. If cesarean delivery becomes necessary, anesthesia considerations are complex, and consultation with regional center experts is recommended.
4. Prepare for care of the baby
- Be prepared for a hypotonic baby with poor respiratory effort if the mother received prolonged administration of magnesium sulfate or received diazepam or other benzodiazepines for seizures.
- Feed the baby early and screen for hypoglycemia. (See Book 1: Maternal and Fetal Evaluation and Immediate Newborn Care, Unit 8, Hypoglycemia.)
- If resuscitation is needed, monitor the baby for possible post-resuscitation complications. (See Book 1: Maternal and Fetal Evaluation and Immediate Newborn Care, Unit 5, Resuscitating the Newborn.)

12. How should women with HELLP syndrome be managed?

Women with HELLP syndrome are at increased risk for serious maternal complications, including disseminated intravascular coagulation, hepatic hematoma or necrosis, and death. The risk for fetal complications, including intrauterine death, is also increased. Once the diagnosis of HELLP syndrome is established, delivery is a short-term goal and transfer to a regional perinatal center is strongly recommended. Cesarean delivery is often indicated. Consultation with maternal-fetal medicine specialists on therapy and pre-transport stabilization is also recommended.

If a woman is in labor when HELLP syndrome is diagnosed and labor is too far advanced or the woman's condition too unstable for safe transfer, provide management as outlined previously for severe preeclampsia and eclampsia.

13. What are the risks from hypertension after delivery?

Careful monitoring of a woman's condition is needed until discharge from the hospital. If magnesium sulfate therapy is administered before delivery, it is generally continued after birth for 24 hours or longer. The duration of magnesium therapy after delivery is determined by the severity of maternal illness and the evidence of preeclampsia resolution.

While gestational hypertension will resolve completely after delivery, it may not do so immediately. Occasionally, the condition of women with hypertensive disorders of pregnancy worsens during the postpartum period before it begins to resolve. Women may become seriously ill with preeclampsia with severe features or eclampsia. The highest risk period for development of eclampsia is the first 24 hours after birth. Worsening hypertension and seizures develop most commonly within 1 or 2 days after delivery but, in rare cases, may not occur until 10 days after birth.

Chronic hypertension may also be unstable after delivery. Continued use or readjustment of antihypertensive medication may be needed during this time. Some patients may continue to be hypertensive. For these women, antihypertensive therapy is required and is continued for 2 to 4 weeks or longer after discharge from the hospital.

A woman's blood pressure should be within reference range, or have declined to safer levels, before hospital discharge, and she should have evidence of sustained diuresis.

Home monitoring for 1 to 2 weeks after birth may be considered for women whose pregnancies were complicated by chronic hypertension, preeclampsia, or eclampsia. Assessment includes

- Frequent blood pressure measurement
- Prompt reporting of any of the following signs or symptoms:
  — Increase in blood pressure
  — Persistent headache
  — Epigastric/abdominal pain
  — Blurred vision or other visual disturbances

Early follow-up in the outpatient setting, within 10 days after delivery, is recommended. Signs and symptoms of pregnancy-related hypertension can be expected to resolve by the time of the 6-week postpartum examination. If they have not, the woman should be reexamined 12 weeks after giving birth.

Self-test E

Now answer these questions to test yourself on the information in the last section.

E1. True False In general, women who have preeclampsia with severe features, eclampsia, or HELLP syndrome should be stabilized and then transferred for delivery at a regional perinatal center.

E2. True False Cesarean delivery is usually safer than vaginal delivery for a woman with hypertension.

E3. True False Hypertension can worsen after birth, causing serious illness in the mother.

E4. True False If fetal bradycardia is present in a woman experiencing an eclamptic seizure, an emergency cesarean delivery should be done immediately, regardless of maternal condition.

E5. Which of the following actions is appropriate for post-discharge postpartum care for a woman who had severe preeclampsia?

Yes	No	
___	___	Blood pressure monitoring at home for 1 to 2 weeks
___	___	Complete bed rest
___	___	Daily dipstick check of urine for protein level
___	___	Low-salt diet

E6. You see a woman with preeclampsia begin to have a seizure. What would you do?

Immediately	Within Several Minutes	Not Indicated	
___	___	___	Check her blood pressure
___	___	___	Check her serum potassium level
___	___	___	Apply a pulse oximeter
___	___	___	Protect the woman from soft-tissue and skeletal injury
___	___	___	Administer magnesium sulfate
___	___	___	Prepare for cesarean delivery within 30 minutes
___	___	___	Administer oxygen via mask

Check your answers with the list that follows the Recommended Routines. Correct any incorrect answers and review the appropriate section in the unit.

UNIT 1: HYPERTENSION IN PREGNANCY

HYPERTENSION IN PREGNANCY
Recommended Routines

All the routines listed below are based on the principles of perinatal care presented in the unit you have just finished. They are recommended as part of routine perinatal care.
Read each routine carefully and decide whether it is standard operating procedure in your hospital. Check the appropriate blank next to each routine.

Procedure Standard in My Hospital	Needs Discussion by Our Staff	Recommended Routine
_____	_____	1. Establish guidelines for the consistent classification, and reclassification if the condition changes during pregnancy, of pregnant women with hypertension as having • Chronic hypertension • Hypertensive disorders of pregnancy, including — Gestational hypertension or transient hypertension of pregnancy — Preeclampsia — Preeclampsia with severe features — Eclampsia — HELLP syndrome • Preeclampsia superimposed on chronic hypertension
_____	_____	2. Establish written instructions for the home care of women who develop hypertension during pregnancy, including a list of findings to report to their health professional.
_____	_____	3. Establish guidelines for the assessment of women admitted to the hospital for evaluation of preeclampsia.
_____	_____	4. Establish guidelines for the immediate stabilization of a woman who has rapidly worsening preeclampsia or eclampsia.
_____	_____	5. Establish a protocol for response to maternal seizure(s) due to eclampsia.
_____	_____	6. Establish guidelines for intravenous infusion of • Magnesium sulfate • Antihypertensive medication
_____	_____	7. Establish guidelines for the postpartum assessment of every woman whose pregnancy was complicated by hypertension.

Self-test Answers

These are the answers to the Self-test questions. Please check them with the answers you gave and review the information in the unit wherever necessary.

Self-test A

A1. Increase in blood pressure to 140/90 mm Hg after 20 weeks of gestation

A2. Proteinuria is present with preeclampsia but not with gestational hypertension.

A3. Preeclampsia becomes eclampsia when a pregnant woman has a grand mal seizure or becomes comatose and no other cause is known.

A4.
Yes	No	
X	___	Nausea and vomiting
X	___	Jaundice
___	X	Increased blood glucose level
___	X	Increased platelet count
X	___	Increased liver transaminase levels

A5. True

A6. False *Reason:* Initially, blood pressure may not be increased in women with HELLP syndrome. In this form of severe preeclampsia, other symptoms, which may at first suggest gastroenteritis or gall bladder disease, are sometimes present before hypertension and proteinuria develop. Even when the diagnosis is established, hypertension may not be severe.

A7. True

A8.
Yes	No	
X	___	Preterm birth
X	___	Placental abruption
X	___	Maternal congestive heart failure
___	X	Placenta previa
X	___	Fetal growth restriction
X	___	Nonreactive nonstress test
___	X	Congenital anomalies
X	___	Maternal seizures
X	___	Maternal stroke

Self-test B

B1. False *Reason:* Angiotensin-converting enzyme inhibitors, such as captopril, can cause fetal deformity or renal failure, as well as severely reduce placental perfusion. These drugs should not be used during pregnancy.

B2. True

B3. False *Reason:* In women with chronic hypertension, blood pressure often declines during pregnancy because of the decrease in vascular resistance that normally occurs in all women when they are pregnant.

B4. False *Reason:* Women with chronic hypertension who needed antihypertensive medication before pregnancy may not need it during pregnancy. (See question B3.)

UNIT 1: HYPERTENSION IN PREGNANCY

B5. | Yes | No |
| --- | --- |
| ____ | _X_ | Walking 2 miles a day
| ____ | _X_ | Multiple sclerosis
| _X_ | ____ | Creatinine clearance below 100 mL/min
| _X_ | ____ | Diabetes mellitus
| _X_ | ____ | Development of gestational hypertension
| _X_ | ____ | Lupus erythematosus

B6. | Yes | No |
| ____ | _X_ | Await 41 weeks of gestation before recommending delivery.
| _X_ | ____ | Use narcotic analgesia during labor.
| _X_ | ____ | Treat the woman for preeclampsia if blood pressure increases and proteinuria develops.
| ____ | _X_ | Plan for cesarean delivery instead of labor.

Self-test C

C1. Any 3 of the following signs and symptoms:
- Persistent headache
- Visual disturbance
- Epigastric pain
- Weight gain of more than 2 lb in 1 day
- Protein in the woman's urine
- Blood pressure increase
- Fetal movement decrease
- Uterine contractions

C2. | Yes | No |
| _X_ | ____ | Age 35 years and older
| _X_ | ____ | Twins
| _X_ | ____ | Renal disease
| ____ | _X_ | Short stature
| _X_ | ____ | Obesity
| _X_ | ____ | First pregnancy
| _X_ | ____ | Chronic hypertension

C3. True

C4. True

C5. True

C6. True

Self-test D

D1. When eclampsia is present, *magnesium sulfate* is generally used to prevent recurrence of maternal seizures.

D2. | Yes | No |
| ____ | _X_ | Exaggerated reflexes
| ____ | _X_ | High serum sodium level
| _X_ | ____ | Slow respiratory rate
| _X_ | ____ | Loss of deep tendon reflexes
| ____ | _X_ | Decreased urine output

D3. False *Reason:* When maternal blood pressure is 160/110 mm Hg or higher, it should be lowered as quickly as possible, but care should be taken to avoid dropping the blood pressure below 140/90 mm Hg because, below that pressure, placental perfusion may be reduced, resulting in fetal distress.

D4. True

D5. False *Reason:* The treatment goal is to keep the blood pressure no lower than 140/90 mm Hg and no higher than 160/105 mm Hg.

D6. False *Reason:* If magnesium sulfate is administered during labor, the infusion is continued for 12 to 48 hours, or longer, after delivery.

D7. Placental perfusion may decrease, which can, in turn, lead to fetal distress.

D8.
Yes	No	
X		Consult a neurologist or regional perinatal center specialists.
X		Administer diazepam (Valium) intravenously.
X		Be prepared to provide assisted ventilation to the woman.
	X	Perform cesarean delivery immediately.
X		Consider that intracranial hemorrhage may have occurred.
X		Be prepared to assist the baby's respirations.

Self-test E

E1. True

E2. False *Reason:* Anesthesia and surgery nearly always carry more risks than vaginal delivery.

E3. True

E4. False *Reason:* If the condition of a woman who has had an eclamptic seizure is unstable, a cesarean delivery should not be done, even if the fetus appears to be in distress. The risk of maternal death from surgery and anesthesia is high. Surgery should not be undertaken until the woman's condition has been stabilized. The fetus, however, usually recovers from the stress brought on by the mother's convulsion.

E5.
Yes	No	
X		Blood pressure monitoring at home for 1 to 2 weeks
	X	Complete bed rest
X		Daily dipstick check of urine for protein level
	X	Low-salt diet

E6.
Immediately	Within Several Minutes	Not Indicated	
	X		Check her blood pressure
		X	Check her serum potassium level
	X		Apply a pulse oximeter
X			Protect the woman from soft-tissue and skeletal injury
	X		Administer magnesium sulfate
		X	Prepare for cesarean delivery within 30 minutes
	X		Administer oxygen via mask

Note: If an intravenous line is in place, magnesium sulfate can also be started immediately. All of the "within several minutes" responses should be performed as soon as the seizure stops.

Unit 1 Posttest

After completion of each unit there is a free online posttest available at www.cmevillage.com to test your understanding. Navigate to the PCEP pages on www.cmevillage.com and register to take the free posttests.

Once registered on the website and after completing all the unit posttests, pay the book exam fee ($15) and pass the test at 80% or greater to earn continuing education credits. Only start the PCEP book exam if you have time to complete it. If you take the book exam and are not connected to a printer, either print your certificate to a .pdf file and save it to print later or come back to www.cmevillage.com at any time and print a copy of your educational transcript.

Credits are only available by book, not by individual unit within the books. Available credits for completion of each book exam are as follows: Book 1: 14.5 credits; Book 2: 16 credits; Book 3: 17 credits; Book 4: 9 credits.

For more details, navigate to the PCEP webpages at www.cmevillage.com.

Unit 2: Obstetric Hemorrhage

Objectives 38

1. What is obstetric hemorrhage? 41
2. What does your hospital need to manage obstetric hemorrhage? 42
3. What emergency care should you give a pregnant woman who presents with life-threatening hemorrhage from an unknown cause? 42
4. What are the causes of bleeding in early pregnancy? 46
5. What are the causes of bleeding in late pregnancy? 48
6. How do you determine the cause of late-pregnancy bleeding? 53
7. How do you manage placenta previa and placental abruption? 56
8. How do you recognize and treat disseminated intravascular coagulation? 59
9. What care should you anticipate for the newborn? 62
10. What additional care do you need to provide to Rh(D)-negative women? 62
11. What is postpartum hemorrhage? 65
12. What are the causes of postpartum hemorrhage? 65
13. What should you do *routinely* to prevent or reduce postpartum hemorrhage? 66
14. How is postpartum hemorrhage treated? 67
15. How is uterine inversion managed? 72
16. What needs to be documented? 75

Tables and Figures

   Table 2.1. Usual Characteristics of Placenta Previa Versus Placental Abruption 48
   Table 2.2. Placental Abruption: Grades of Placental Separation 50
   Figure 2.1. Alliance for Innovation on Maternal Health Obstetric Hemorrhage Bundle 43
   Figure 2.2. Types of Low Placental Implantation 49
   Figure 2.3. Manual Compression of the Uterus 69
   Figure 2.4. Uterine Inversion 69

Recommended Routines 76

Objectives

In this unit you will learn

A. The risk obstetric hemorrhage carries for a woman and her fetus

B. How to respond to life-threatening obstetric hemorrhage when the cause is unknown

C. How to identify and manage the causes of early pregnancy bleeding

D. How to identify and treat the causes of late-pregnancy bleeding

E. How to determine the difference between placenta previa and placental abruption

F. How to recognize and provide emergency treatment for disseminated intravascular coagulation

G. What care to anticipate for a baby born to a woman with obstetric hemorrhage

H. Which women should receive Rh immunoglobulin and when it should be administered

I. What routine measures are needed to prevent or reduce postpartum hemorrhage

J. How to recognize postpartum hemorrhage and identify its causes

K. How to treat postpartum hemorrhage

L. What every hospital needs to respond to obstetric hemorrhage

Unit 2 Pretest

Before reading the unit, please answer the following questions. Select the *one best* answer to each question (unless otherwise instructed). Record your answers on the test and check them with the answers at the end of the book.

1. **True / False** — In a woman being treated for obstetric hemorrhage, decreasing urine output suggests blood is being lost from her vascular system.

2. **True / False** — Cesarean delivery is the recommended route of delivery when a placenta previa is present, even if no bleeding has occurred.

3. **True / False** — A woman who had a placental abruption with one pregnancy has an increased risk for having another placental abruption with a subsequent pregnancy.

4. **True / False** — Even with fetal death, in severe cases of placental abruption cesarean delivery of the dead fetus may be necessary to reduce maternal morbidity.

5. **True / False** — Placenta accreta is more common with placenta previa.

6. **True / False** — The most common cause of postpartum hemorrhage is disseminated intravascular coagulation.

7. **True / False** — Placental abruption can usually be prevented.

8. **True / False** — Steady, slow, persistent bleeding postpartum suggests uterine atony.

9. Placental abruption
   A. Is usually caused by a perinatal infection
   B. May be associated with disseminated intravascular coagulation
   C. Most often occurs in women who use heroin
   D. Is always accompanied by visible bleeding

10. When late-pregnancy placental bleeding occurs
    A. The fetus will almost always go into severe shock.
    B. The degree of fetal blood loss correlates closely with the degree of maternal bleeding.
    C. Maternal blood, but not fetal blood, is lost.
    D. Fetal health may be compromised by decreased placental perfusion.

11. Which of the following parameters would be especially important to check in a baby whose mother had a bleeding placenta previa?

Yes	No	
—	—	Hematocrit value
—	—	Serum creatinine level
—	—	Bilirubin level
—	—	Blood pressure level
—	—	Blood culture

(*continued*)

Unit 2 Pretest (continued)

12. **True / False** — Maternal tachycardia and decreasing blood pressure are early signs of placental abruption.

13. **True / False** — With certain types of obstetric hemorrhage, blood loss may occur internally and is not externally visible.

14. **True / False** — Any bleeding during pregnancy requires investigation.

15. **True / False** — Disseminated intravascular coagulation can develop with placental abruption or HELLP (*h*emolysis, *e*levated *l*iver enzyme levels, and *l*ow *p*latelet count) syndrome.

16. **True / False** — An Rh(D)-negative woman had an episode of significant bleeding at 10 weeks of gestation and received Rh immunoglobulin at that time. At 25 weeks of gestation, she has another episode of bleeding. She should receive Rh immunoglobulin again, within 72 hours of the bleeding.

17. Which of the following is most likely to be associated with postpartum hemorrhage?
    A. Primigravid state
    B. Preterm delivery
    C. Post-term delivery
    D. High parity

18. All of the following statements about ectopic pregnancy are accurate, except
    A. Surgical removal or chemotherapy may be used to treat ectopic pregnancy.
    B. Clinically significant maternal internal bleeding may occur.
    C. The implantation site is most often in a fallopian tube.
    D. Symptoms rarely occur before 12 to 14 weeks of gestation.

19. All of the following findings are generally an indication of placental abruption, except
    A. Sudden increase in fundal height
    B. Bright red, painless bleeding
    C. Uterus that is tender when palpated
    D. Increased uterine tone

20. Which of the following actions should you take first when postpartum hemorrhage is detected?
    A. Prepare for immediate surgery.
    B. Check clotting studies.
    C. Palpate the uterus.
    D. Administer an intravenous bolus of 40 U oxytocin.

21. All of the following conditions increase the risk for placenta previa, except
    A. Maternal hypertension
    B. Multifetal gestation
    C. High parity
    D. Previous cesarean delivery

1. What is obstetric hemorrhage?

A. Definition
Obstetric hemorrhage is clinically significant bleeding from the reproductive tract (vagina, cervix, placenta, or uterus). It may occur before, during, or after birth. The etiologic origin varies, according to the timing. Approximately 5% of deliveries are complicated by postpartum hemorrhage, defined as the loss of more than 1,000 mL of blood in the first 24 hours after delivery.

B. Maternal versus fetal blood loss
When the placenta is the source of the bleeding, primarily maternal blood is lost, but fetal blood loss may also occur. Because of the relatively small blood volume of the fetus, even a small amount of fetal blood loss can be life-threatening.

Fetal health may be severely compromised by the loss of fetal blood or decreased placental perfusion from maternal blood loss.

C. Necessity for prompt evaluation
Postpartum hemorrhage is a major cause of maternal death in low- and middle-income countries and is the cause of approximately 10% of maternal deaths in the United States. Antepartum hemorrhage may also be fatal for the woman or fetus. Regardless of the source of the bleeding, maternal blood loss may be minor or may rapidly progress to severe hemorrhage. When bleeding first starts, it is difficult to predict how severe it may become.

Any bleeding during pregnancy should be reported and evaluated without delay in a clinic, emergency department, or labor and delivery unit.

D. Estimation of blood loss
Most young, pregnant women have expanded blood volume and efficient autonomic vascular reflexes, so that clinically significant blood loss may occur in the initial absence of the usual signs of shock (eg, tachycardia, hypotension). The visible amount of blood loss may be misleading. In women who experience obstetric hemorrhage from placental abruption or uterine rupture, clinically significant bleeding can occur either behind the placenta or into the woman's abdomen; this is sometimes called a *concealed hemorrhage*. The amount of blood being lost via the vagina may only be a small portion of the total volume of blood lost from a woman's vascular system.

Renal blood flow is particularly sensitive to changes in blood volume. Diminishing urine output suggests that renal perfusion is decreased, because blood is being lost from the circulatory system. In women who experience or are suspected of having obstetric hemorrhage, monitor urine output each hour. Crystalloid or colloid solutions should be administered intravenously to maintain urine output of 30 mL/h or more.

Visual estimation of blood loss has been shown to be inaccurate and may lead to under-estimation of blood loss by as much as 50%. Systems used to quantify blood loss will result in a more accurate determination of cumulative blood loss and a more timely response to hemorrhage. These systems consist of a method to

- Account for blood loss on lap sponges, drapes, and sheets by weighing them (1 mL of blood weighs approximately 1 g)

- Measure liquid blood loss in suction canisters or drapes placed under the woman's buttocks

More information on quantification of blood loss is available at https://awhonn.org/postpartum-hemorrhage-pph/.

2. What does your hospital need to manage obstetric hemorrhage?

Although certain conditions are known to increase the risk for obstetric hemorrhage, clinically significant bleeding can also occur suddenly and without warning in any woman. All hospitals that provide labor and delivery care should be prepared to manage obstetric hemorrhage. The Alliance for Innovation on Maternal Health (AIM) has developed and disseminated evidence-based safety bundles that guide hospitals in the implementation of safety measures to identify and rapidly treat major maternal complications. Each bundle consists of Readiness, Recognition and Prevention, Response, and Reporting/Systems Learning components. The AIM Obstetric Hemorrhage bundle is shown in Figure 2.1. Most states in the United States have a statewide initiative to implement AIM through their perinatal quality collaborative or other group.

All obstetric units should have

1. A prepared and practiced care team that conducts emergency drills to rehearse key skills
2. Access to adequate blood products for emergency transfusion
3. Capability for emergency cesarean delivery and other surgical interventions

3. What emergency care should you give a pregnant woman who presents with life-threatening hemorrhage from an unknown cause?

Occasionally, a woman will come into a hospital with sudden onset of heavy vaginal bleeding and no history of placenta previa or other easily identified reason for the bleeding. Your immediate actions should be directed at stabilizing the woman's condition while simultaneously assessing for the cause of the hemorrhage.

Your intervention on behalf of a woman with obstetric hemorrhage needs to be prompt and aggressive.

Your intervention on behalf of a fetus, even if the fetal condition is concerning, should usually wait until the maternal condition has been stabilized. Until the woman's condition is stabilized, the life of the woman and fetus may be in serious jeopardy. In some circumstances (placental abruption, placenta previa), it will be recognized that surgical intervention may be needed early in the treatment course to resolve the bleeding.

UNIT 2: OBSTETRIC HEMORRHAGE

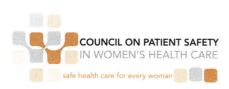

PATIENT SAFETY BUNDLE

Obstetric Hemorrhage

READINESS

Every unit

- Hemorrhage cart with supplies, checklist, and instruction cards for intrauterine balloons and compressions stitches
- Immediate access to hemorrhage medications (kit or equivalent)
- Establish a response team - who to call when help is needed (blood bank, advanced gynecologic surgery, other support and tertiary services)
- Establish massive and emergency release transfusion protocols (type-O negative/uncrossmatched)
- Unit education on protocols, unit-based drills (with post-drill debriefs)

RECOGNITION & PREVENTION

Every patient

- Assessment of hemorrhage risk (prenatal, on admission, and at other appropriate times)
- Measurement of cumulative blood loss (formal, as quantitative as possible)
- Active management of the 3rd stage of labor (department-wide protocol)

RESPONSE

Every hemorrhage

- Unit-standard, stage-based, obstetric hemorrhage emergency management plan with checklists
- Support program for patients, families, and staff for all significant hemorrhages

REPORTING/SYSTEMS LEARNING

Every unit

- Establish a culture of huddles for high risk patients and post-event debriefs to identify successes and opportunities
- Multidisciplinary review of serious hemorrhages for systems issues
- Monitor outcomes and process metrics in perinatal quality improvement (QI) committee

© 2015 American College of Obstetricians and Gynecologists. Permission is hereby granted for duplication and distribution of this document, in its entirety and without modification, for solely non-commercial activities that are for educational, quality improvement, and patient safety purposes. All other uses require written permission from ACOG.

Standardization of health care processes and reduced variation has been shown to improve outcomes and quality of care. The Council on Patient Safety in Women's Health Care disseminates patient safety bundles to help facilitate the standardization process. This bundle reflects emerging clinical, scientific, and patient safety advances as of the date issued and is subject to change. The information should not be construed as dictating an exclusive course of treatment or procedure to be followed. Although the components of a particular bundle may be adapted to local resources, standardization within an institution is strongly encouraged.

The Council on Patient Safety in Women's Health Care is a broad consortium of organizations across the spectrum of women's health for the promotion of safe health care for every woman.

May 2015

For more information visit the Council's website at www.safehealthcareforeverywoman.org

Figure 2.1. Alliance for Innovation on Maternal Health Obstetric Hemorrhage Bundle
From https://safehealthcareforeverywoman.org/wp-content/uploads/2017/11/Obstetric-Hemorrhage-Bundle.pdf.

A. Get help
Many actions need to be taken concurrently with speed and skill. Often, 2 physicians and several experienced nurses are needed to provide the care that a pregnant woman needs during obstetric hemorrhage. Emergency surgery may be needed, so all surgical support and blood bank services also need to be mobilized immediately. Pediatric practitioners should be notified of a woman's status so that preparations for delivery room and nursery care of the baby can be made.

B. Administer volume expansion and stabilize the woman's condition
It is much more effective to prevent shock than treat it.

Whenever possible, replacement therapy for obstetric hemorrhage should begin before the woman develops signs of shock.

If the visible volume of blood lost constitutes a life-threatening amount, you suspect a large amount of internal bleeding, or the woman shows signs of shock, institute general life support measures **immediately**, without taking time for invasive diagnostic examinations. These measures include

- *Insertion of 2 large-bore intravenous (IV) lines* (18 gauge or larger): Massive hemorrhage can deplete blood volume so quickly that several IV lines may be needed to replace fluids in a woman with sufficient speed.
- *Rapid infusion of isotonic solutions such as saline or lactated Ringer's injection.*
- *Infusion of blood products as soon as possible:* Under the circumstance of massive hemorrhage, the use of a massive transfusion protocol with transfusion of uncrossmatched (type O Rh-negative) blood is advised to avoid delays in treatment while obtaining crossmatched blood.

Severe preexisting anemia can dramatically worsen the effects of blood loss. When a woman has preexisting anemia, she has less physiological reserve to tolerate blood loss. The loss of additional blood may lead to compromised delivery of oxygen to body tissues, leading to lactic acidosis and coagulopathy. Death may result from inadequate perfusion of vital organs with oxygenated blood and from the effects of coagulopathy.

C. Evaluate fetal well-being and gestational age
Fetal status may influence the timing and type of intervention used. Determine if the fetus is alive. This can be done simply by finding a fetal heartbeat with a handheld fetal Doppler device or a fetoscope.

If the fetus is alive, estimation of fetal gestational age may be important. This can be done by asking the woman or checking her records (if available) or by conducting a clinical or ultrasonographic (US) examination. In the most critical cases, however, surgical intervention may be needed to save the woman's life, regardless of fetal gestational age.

Intrauterine resuscitation measures, such as turning the woman onto her side and giving her oxygen by mask, may be appropriate and may benefit fetal health, as long as they do not interfere with the resuscitation or life support measures needed for the woman.

D. Perform maternal blood tests
   1. Send blood samples
      - Type and crossmatch (at least 4 units of packed red blood cells)—use the massive transfusion protocol for immediate needs
      - Determine the availability of platelets and fresh frozen plasma (FFP)
      - Complete blood cell count
      - Prothrombin time and partial thromboplastin time (PTT)
      - Platelet count
      - Fibrinogen level
      - Blood chemistry or electrolyte panel
   2. Collect a 5-mL red-top tube of blood and tape it to the patient's bed
      The tube should be free of anticoagulant. If a clot does not form within 8 to 10 minutes, disseminated intravascular coagulation (DIC) is probably present.

E. Deliver the baby promptly
   If the *bleeding does not stop,* delivery should be accomplished as soon as the woman is stable enough. Factors to consider when deciding on a vaginal birth or a cesarean delivery include the ability to stabilize the woman and maintain stable vital signs, the amount of ongoing vaginal bleeding, the gestational age of the pregnancy, the presence of any signs of labor, and the presence or absence of placenta previa. If US is not readily available to assess whether placenta previa is present, consider performing a double-setup examination, which is described in section 6 later in this unit.

F. Determine the cause of the bleeding
   If the *bleeding stops,* the woman's condition is stable, and the results of fetal heart rate monitoring are reassuring, proceed with testing to identify the source of the bleeding (described in the sections that follow).

PCEP BOOK 2: MATERNAL AND FETAL CARE

Self-test A

Now answer these questions to test yourself on the information in the last section.

A1. What preparations should every hospital make to manage obstetric hemorrhage?
_____
_____
_____
_____
_____
_____
_____

A2. Obstetric hemorrhage is bleeding from the _____ during pregnancy or postpartum.

A3. Blood loss with obstetric hemorrhage may be visible or _____.

A4. With obstetric hemorrhage, clinically significant blood loss may occur before signs of _____ appear in the woman.

A5. True   False   When the source of the bleeding is the placenta (eg, placenta previa, placental abruption), both the woman and the fetus may experience blood loss.

A6. Which actions should you take as soon as a woman is admitted with late-pregnancy obstetric hemorrhage from an unknown source?

Yes	No	
___	___	Get help immediately.
___	___	Check her blood pressure.
___	___	Insert large-bore intravenous lines.
___	___	Begin infusion of saline solutions.
___	___	Type and crossmatch blood.
___	___	Obtain a tube of blood; tape it to the patient's bed.
___	___	Give oxygen by mask to the pregnant woman.

A7. What amount of bleeding during pregnancy requires investigation?
_____
_____

Check your answers with the list that follows the Recommended Routines. Correct any incorrect answers and review the appropriate section in the unit.

4. What are the causes of bleeding in early pregnancy?

When any woman in the reproductive years (approximately 12–50 years of age) misses a menstrual period and then has vaginal bleeding or lower abdominal pain, early pregnancy loss or ectopic pregnancy should be suspected.

Confirm pregnancy with a qualitative human chorionic gonadotropin (hCG) test of serum or urine. If the result is positive, a quantitative serum β-hCG titer may help differentiate a normal intrauterine pregnancy from spontaneous abortion and ectopic pregnancy. Interpret the results as follows:

- *Negative* serum β-hCG result: The woman is not pregnant but may have a gynecological cause of the bleeding.
- *Positive* serum β-hCG result: If it is 5 to 6 weeks or longer since a woman's last menstrual period or the β-hCG value is higher than 1,500 to 2,000 mIU/mL, an intrauterine pregnancy should be identifiable within the uterus with transvaginal US.

1. If there is *evidence of an intrauterine pregnancy* (a gestational sac, with or without a yolk sac, an embryo/fetus, or fetal cardiac activity), the possible diagnoses are
   a. Threatened miscarriage: The cervical os is closed at examination.
   b. Inevitable miscarriage: The cervical os is open at examination.
2. If the *uterus appears empty,* the possible diagnoses include
   a. Ectopic pregnancy: pregnancy implanted outside the uterus, most commonly in a fallopian tube
   b. Complete early pregnancy loss
   c. An early intrauterine pregnancy with a gestational sac too small to be visualized with US
   Of these possibilities, tubal ectopic pregnancy is the most potentially serious and should be investigated further.
3. If a *pregnancy cannot be detected in the uterus or a fallopian tube* with US and the woman is stable, wait 48 to 72 hours and repeat the serum β-hCG titer. The hCG level usually doubles within 72 hours in a normal early pregnancy.
   - If pain and bleeding continue and the β-hCG titer is decreasing, this indicates a nonviable pregnancy, which may be intrauterine or ectopic.
   - If the bleeding stops or the serum β-hCG titer continues to increase, the pregnancy may be normal and intrauterine. When the serum β-hCG level is 1,500 mIU/mL or higher, perform another transvaginal US examination to determine whether the pregnancy is intrauterine. Ectopic pregnancies cannot always be visualized with US.

A. Early pregnancy loss (spontaneous miscarriage)
Of all recognized pregnancies, approximately 10% to 15% end in miscarriage. More than 60% of early pregnancy losses are caused by abnormal development of the fetus or placenta and usually occur within the first 5 to 10 weeks of pregnancy.

Vaginal bleeding in early pregnancy is not always associated with progression to miscarriage. US examination may demonstrate an intact gestational sac and fetal cardiac activity. In these cases, the bleeding usually resolves, and the pregnancy continues.

Vaginal bleeding in early pregnancy may increase in amount and be accompanied by uterine cramps and even passage of tissue. If tissue is passed, the pregnancy will not continue. Up to 80% of early pregnancy losses will be completed without medical intervention, but this may be difficult to determine at clinical examination. In many cases, transvaginal US examination, together with physical examination, can be used to distinguish between incomplete and complete miscarriage. Surgical evacuation of the uterus (referred to as *dilation and curettage* or *dilation and evacuation*) may be necessary to be sure all fetal and placental tissues are removed so the bleeding will stop.

B. Ectopic pregnancy
An ectopic pregnancy is one that has implanted somewhere other than inside the uterus. The most common location of an ectopic pregnancy is the fallopian tube, but an ectopic pregnancy may also implant in the cervix or ovary, within a cesarean scar in the uterus, or in the abdominal cavity. Women with prior tubal surgery, a prior ectopic pregnancy, an intrauterine device in place, or a history of pelvic inflammatory disease are at increased risk, but an ectopic pregnancy can occur in any woman.

A pregnancy implanted in the tube may initially grow and even demonstrate development of an embryo with cardiac activity, but growth usually stops after a few weeks because the tissues on which the placenta is implanted cannot provide adequate support for continued growth. Abdominal-pelvic pain is the most common initial symptom of ectopic pregnancy and may be accompanied by vaginal bleeding. The source of vaginal bleeding is breakdown of the uterine decidua as the pregnancy ceases progression. More serious, and potentially life-threatening, is internal bleeding, which may occur with placental separation from the implantation site or from rupture of the fallopian tube by the growing gestational sac. The internal blood loss may not be clinically evident until signs of early shock are present.

Depending on the woman's condition, immediate intervention may be needed to stop internal bleeding. Surgery is often necessary to locate and remove an ectopic pregnancy.

If the woman is stable, consultation with specialists who are skilled in the management of ectopic pregnancy is recommended. Referral to a regional center for therapy may be indicated, especially if the woman desires preservation of future fertility. Treatment options include laparoscopic removal of the ectopic pregnancy, with or without preservation of the fallopian tube. Chemotherapy with methotrexate may be used for nonsurgical treatment in stable women with lower hCG concentrations and smaller ectopic pregnancies.

5. What are the causes of bleeding in late pregnancy?

A. Bloody show
Discharge of a mixture of blood and mucus from the vagina is a normal occurrence in early labor. The quantity of bloody show is usually not more than menstrual flow and will not result in clinically significant blood loss.

Other causes of late pregnancy bleeding, however, often progress to serious hemorrhage. In general, *any* bleeding should be considered abnormal and investigated in a hospital.

B. Placental bleeding
The 2 main causes of late pregnancy bleeding are placenta previa and placental abruption. These clinical conditions and their presentation are described in this section and summarized in Table 2.1.

Table 2.1. Usual Characteristics of Placenta Previa Versus Placental Abruption		
Finding	**Placenta Previa**	**Placental Abruption**
Maternal		
Blood color	Bright red	Dark red, clots
Pain	Painless (unless in labor)	Painful (constant uterine pain)
Uterine tenderness	Absent	Usually present
Uterine tone	Normal	Increased, may feel tense, hard, or rigid on palpation
Shock	Uncommon	Frequent, especially with severe grades
Disseminated intravascular coagulation	Uncommon	Frequent, especially with severe grades
Ultrasonography	Can almost always demonstrate the location of placenta	In about half of abruptions, a retroplacental clot may be seen with ultrasonography.
Fetal		
Fetal well-being	The fetal heart rate pattern is usually normal, unless maternal shock or clinically significant fetal blood loss are present.	Fetal heart rate abnormalities are common, especially with more severe degrees of abruption.

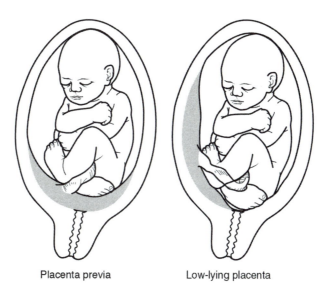

Figure 2.2. Types of Low Placental Implantation

1. Placenta previa

   Placenta previa is defined as a placental implantation that at least partially covers the cervical os. The terms *complete, partial,* and *marginal* placenta previa are no longer used. Placenta previa is differentiated from low-lying placenta, which is defined as a placental implantation that is within 2 cm of the cervical os but does not cover the cervix (Figure 2.2).

   Sometimes, a US examination performed early in pregnancy shows what appears to be a placenta previa. A placenta that appears to cover the internal cervical os in early pregnancy very often, however, does not cover it at term. In most cases, the development of the lower uterine segment in late pregnancy will "move" the placenta away from the internal os. Women with the appearance of a placenta previa at US performed before 20 weeks of gestation usually do not require special management, unless bleeding ensues.

   Placenta previa should be considered as a possible cause of new-onset vaginal bleeding after 20 weeks of gestation. Most commonly, bleeding from a placenta previa is bright red and is not associated with abdominal pain. Clinically significant bleeding can occur with placenta previa.

   Placenta previa is more likely to occur
   - With multifetal gestation
   - In women who have undergone a previous cesarean delivery
   - In women with high parity
   - In women with large or numerous uterine fibroids
   - If it occurred in a previous pregnancy

   Women with placenta previa are more likely to have an abnormal fetal presentation (the fetal position may be influenced by the location of the placenta).

   Bleeding from placenta previa will always be visible externally. Initial bleeding may not be heavy and may be characterized by intermittent but persistent spotting. Alternatively, clinically significant blood loss may occur with the first episode of bleeding. Sometimes, placenta previa is not recognized until labor begins, when cervical

Table 2.2. Placental Abruption: Grades of Placental Separation			
Finding	**Grade 1**	**Grade 2**	**Grade 3**
General			
Amount of placenta separated from the uterine wall	10%–25%	25%–50%	>50%
Diagnostic criteria	Vaginal bleeding and maternal signs clearly indicate an abruption.	Fetal compromise is present (see Book 1: Maternal and Fetal Evaluation and Immediate Newborn Care, Unit 3, Fetal Well-being).	Fetal death
Maternal Signs			
Maternal bleeding (may be concealed)	Present, usually visible externally; rarely progresses	Present, with a high risk that abruption will progress (worsen)	Present and continues, often concealed
Need for blood transfusion	Usually not	May be needed	Usually needed
Shock	No	May develop	Present
DIC	No	May develop	Likely to develop
Uterus	Tender, may be tense	Tender, firm	Tender, hard
Life-threatening	No	Rarely	Yes
Labor	Usually normal	Fetal death unless delivered promptly	The uterus may be contracting strongly, but progress is often poor
Delivery	Usually vaginally	Emergency cesarean delivery is usually required for fetal health	If DIC is present, cesarean delivery may be needed to stop the process
Fetal Signs			
Fetal heart rate abnormalities	Not present at the time of observation; continually reassess the fetal status.	Present	By definition of grade 3, the fetus is dead.

Abbreviation: DIC, disseminated intravascular coagulation.

changes cause the onset of bleeding for the first time. Placenta previa is usually only diagnosed this late in pregnancy in women who have not undergone any prior US examinations. Cervical dilation, uterine contractions, or digital examination may cause the bleeding to worsen dramatically. Digital vaginal examinations are contraindicated in patients with placenta previa.

2. Placental abruption

Placental abruption is a premature separation of a normally implanted placenta from the uterine wall, caused by rupture of maternal vessels in the placental bed and subsequent hemorrhage (Table 2.2).

Placental abruption is unpredictable and can occur at any time during pregnancy. Most late pregnancy abruptions begin before the onset of labor. The woman will report the onset of vaginal bleeding and abdominal pain, which may be severe. Signs of abruption include increasing uterine resting tone and sudden vaginal bleeding. Bleeding is usually accompanied by uterine cramps, tenderness, and firmness on palpation. The blood may be bright red but is more commonly dark red with clots. Bleeding may be visible vaginally but may also be completely concealed behind the placenta. If the upper margin or center of the placenta separates but the lower margin remains normally attached, much of the bleeding will remain in the uterus. Even if completely concealed, the volume of blood lost during placental abruption can still be high.

Abruption accounts for approximately one-third of antepartum bleeding. Although most abruptions occur spontaneously with no known cause, the risk is increased with
- *History of an abruption in a previous pregnancy* (risk of recurrence ≥ 5%–6%)
- *Acute abdominal trauma* (eg, traffic accident, intimate partner violence, maternal fall)
- *Maternal hypertension* (especially severe acute hypertension)
- *Smoking* (vasoconstrictive effects of smoking are known to limit placental perfusion and may foster premature separation of the placenta)
- *Sudden uterine decompression* (particularly if the uterus was overdistended)
  — Multifetal gestation (eg, abruption of Twin B's placenta may occur after Twin A is delivered)
  — Rupture of membranes (especially if polyhydramnios was present)
  — After amniocentesis (uncommon)
- *High parity*
- *Uterine fibroids* or *malformations* (thought to create an inadequate site for placental growth and adherence of the anchoring villi)
- *Cocaine use* (the vasoactive effects of acute cocaine use can result in rupture of decidual vessels and placental abruption)
- *Preterm prelabor rupture of membranes* (placental abruption affects approximately 10% of women with premature rupture of membranes)

In addition to the risks posed by hemorrhage, a woman with placental abruption is also at risk for the development of DIC, which is a life-threatening complication.

C. Cervical bleeding

Clinically significant bleeding from the cervix itself is unusual. The most common cause is chronic cervicitis. Other causes include cervical polyps and, rarely, cervical carcinoma. An even more unusual but serious cause of cervical bleeding that can appear early in gestation is cervical ectopic pregnancy. Signs and symptoms of this, as well as evaluation, are similar to those for ectopic pregnancy, but the hemorrhage is likely to be much greater and to manifest vaginally.

D. Obstetric bleeding of unknown cause

It is not always possible to definitively determine the cause of antepartum bleeding. Even if a cause cannot be identified, late-pregnancy bleeding makes it more likely that the pregnancy will experience additional problems. In some cases, women mistake bleeding hemorrhoids or hemorrhagic cystitis as blood coming from the vagina.

Self-test B

Now answer these questions to test yourself on the information in the last section.

B1. **True / False** — The initial signs and symptoms of ectopic pregnancy and threatened abortion are similar.

B2. **True / False** — More than half the time, the cause of late-pregnancy bleeding cannot be identified.

B3. **True / False** — Women with placenta previa are at high risk for disseminated intravascular coagulation.

B4. **True / False** — Much of the bleeding that accompanies ectopic pregnancy may be internal, into the woman's abdominal cavity.

B5. **True / False** — Women with placenta previa may present with sudden onset of profuse bleeding or with persistent, intermittent spotting.

B6. **True / False** — Undetected cancer of the cervix is the most common cause of cervical bleeding during pregnancy.

B7. **True / False** — Bloody show is a mixture of blood and mucus that is normally passed vaginally during early labor.

B8. List at least 3 causes of abnormal late-pregnancy bleeding.
_____
_____
_____

B9. Identify whether the following factors are associated with placenta previa, placental abruption, both, or neither.

	Placenta Previa	Placental Abruption	Neither
Multifetal gestation	_____	_____	_____
Acute abdominal trauma	_____	_____	_____
Maternal cocaine use	_____	_____	_____
Maternal diabetes mellitus	_____	_____	_____
Uterine fibroids	_____	_____	_____
Multiparous woman	_____	_____	_____
Occurred in a previous pregnancy	_____	_____	_____
Previous cesarean delivery	_____	_____	_____
Maternal hypertension	_____	_____	_____
Abnormal fetal presentation	_____	_____	_____
First pregnancy	_____	_____	_____
Short umbilical cord	_____	_____	_____
Maternal smoking	_____	_____	_____
Polyhydramnios	_____	_____	_____

Check your answers with the list that follows the Recommended Routines. Correct any incorrect answers and review the appropriate section in the unit.

6. How do you determine the cause of late-pregnancy bleeding?

Emergency management of severe obstetric hemorrhage, prior to identification of the bleeding source, was described earlier in this unit. Most women who experience late-pregnancy bleeding, however, will *not* have life-threatening hemorrhage when admitted to the hospital. Take the following steps to identify the source of the bleeding:

A. Obtain a history
  1. Estimate blood loss
     Ask the woman about her bleeding.
     - How does this compare to your normal menstrual flow?
     - When did the bleeding start?
     - What color has the blood been?
     - How many pads have you saturated?
     - Have there been cramps, contractions, or abdominal pain?
  2. Review prenatal care
     If the prenatal record is not available, obtain a full history from the patient.

B. Examine the woman
  1. Physical examination
     a. Check her vital signs
     b. Measure the fundal height
        Mark the height with ink on the woman's abdomen for comparison with subsequent measurements, and measure hourly. An increasing fundal height suggests placental abruption with ongoing bleeding concealed behind the placenta.
     c. Assess uterine tenderness, contractions, and baseline tone
        With placental abruption (usually not with placenta previa), the uterus will be tender with increased tone. An external monitor may not indicate these changes as well as palpation by an experienced perinatal care practitioner.
     d. Vaginal examination
        A digital vaginal examination should not be done in patients who have bleeding during late pregnancy, unless you are *certain* a placenta previa is *not* present.
  2. Laboratory tests
     a. For all women with late-pregnancy bleeding, obtain
        - Type and crossmatch, so blood will be immediately available if the need for it arises (request at least 4 units of packed red blood cells)
        - Complete blood cell count
     b. If placental abruption is suspected, investigate the possibility of DIC and obtain
        - Prothrombin time and PTT
        - Platelet count
        - Fibrinogen level
        - Fibrin degradation products, fibrin split products, or dimerized plasmin fragment D (D-dimer)
  3. US examination
     a. US is used to determine whether placenta previa is present.
        If placenta previa is suspected but not yet confirmed, first perform a transabdominal US scan to attempt to identify placenta previa. However, in women with obesity or if the urinary bladder is empty, transabdominal imaging may be suboptimal. In such cases, transvaginal US may be performed with caution if additional clinical

information is needed. The transvaginal probe should remain 1 to 2 cm from the cervix for optimal image quality.

b. US may aid in the assessment of suspected placental abruption.
In the setting of an acute abruption, there may not be evidence of an organized hematoma behind the placenta. With a chronic abruption, this finding is more likely. An apparent mass between the placenta and the uterine wall should be differentiated from a uterine fibroid or a focal uterine contraction. Ultimately, the clinical evaluation of a patient suspected of having abruption is more informative than a US examination.

Placenta previa can be identified reliably with US examination.

Placental abruption cannot reliably be identified with US examination, and US results may be misleading.

4. Double-setup vaginal examination (a pelvic examination performed in an operating room, with simultaneous readiness to initiate a cesarean delivery immediately)
Placenta previa is most readily diagnosed with US, making a double-setup examination rarely necessary. If US is unavailable and placenta previa is suspected, a double-setup examination may be performed. The term "double setup" describes a pelvic examination that is performed in an operating room, in which all preparations and personnel necessary to perform an immediate cesarean delivery are in place. A digital cervical examination is performed to attempt to palpate the internal cervical os for the presence or absence of placental tissue. If placenta is present at the cervix, palpating it digitally may precipitate substantial bleeding and may require the team to perform an emergency cesarean delivery.

5. Assess the fetus
   a. Estimate or reconfirm fetal age
      If gestational age was not established previously, use US to measure biparietal diameter, head circumference, abdominal circumference, and femur length to be able to estimate it.
   b. Evaluate fetal well-being
      Use continuous electronic fetal monitoring or a biophysical profile. Do *not* attempt to insert a fetal scalp electrode or an intrauterine pressure catheter.

Use continuous external fetal heart rate monitoring whenever there is an episode of bleeding.

Self-test C

Now answer these questions to test yourself on the information in the last section.

C1. List the classic characteristics of placenta previa and placental abruption.

Finding	Placenta Previa	Placental Abruption
Blood color	_____	_____
Pain	_____	_____
Uterine tenderness	_____	_____
Uterine tone	_____	_____
Shock	_____	_____
Disseminated intravascular coagulation	_____	_____

C2. What is the reason a digital vaginal examination should not be done when third-trimester bleeding from an unknown source is present?
_____
_____
_____
_____

C3. When late-pregnancy bleeding from an unknown source is present, what is the likely explanation for a sudden increase in fundal height?
_____
_____

C4. True False When late-pregnancy bleeding occurs, ultrasonography is used to locate the placenta.

C5. True False Continuous external fetal monitoring should be used during any episode of bleeding.

C6. True False Whenever a woman is admitted with late-pregnancy bleeding, her blood should be typed and crossmatched, with at least 4 units of packed red blood cells readied for possible transfusion.

C7. True False Uterine tenderness is usually present with placenta previa but rarely with placental abruption.

C8. Which of the following blood tests should be performed when placental abruption is suspected?

Yes	No	
____	____	Prothrombin time and partial thromboplastin time
____	____	Complete blood cell count
____	____	Serum electrolytes
____	____	Platelet count
____	____	Blood urea nitrogen and creatinine concentration
____	____	Fibrinogen concentration

Check your answers with the list that follows the Recommended Routines. Correct any incorrect answers and review the appropriate section in the unit.

7. How do you manage placenta previa and placental abruption?

A. Placenta previa
  1. Confirm the presence of placenta previa
     Repeat a US examination in the early third trimester to confirm the continued presence of a placenta that covered the cervical os earlier in pregnancy. If placenta previa is still present, a final repeat US examination at 34 to 36 weeks of gestation may be helpful, to be certain the placental edge still covers the cervix.
  2. Manage according to maternal condition and fetal gestational age

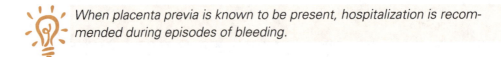

When placenta previa is known to be present, hospitalization is recommended during episodes of bleeding.

Some women may be monitored at home, during stable periods when there is no bleeding. Patients with minimal, intermittent bleeding may be followed up expectantly. Blood transfusion may be necessary to maintain a stable maternal hematocrit value, which provides a margin of reserve in the event of major bleeding episodes. Instruct the woman that *any* episode of vaginal bleeding should be reported promptly and treated as an emergency.

Small amounts of bleeding can suddenly become heavy. The pattern of bleeding or spotting with placenta previa can vary widely. Some women will have intermittent bleeding with relatively little blood loss. Other women may have one minor episode of bleeding, followed by no spotting or bleeding until later in pregnancy or when labor begins. Massive hemorrhage may then occur, without warning.

For some women, hospitalization is necessary until the pregnancy reaches term, severe bleeding occurs, or labor begins. Hospitalization at a regional center equipped to care for preterm or sick babies is advisable because life-threatening hemorrhage can occur at any time and without any warning. Transfer of the woman to another hospital, however, should not be undertaken until she is stable and bleeding has stabilized.

Assess fetal well-being frequently with a nonstress test or biophysical profile. Use continuous external fetal heart rate monitoring during any episode of bleeding.

Unless uncontrollable bleeding necessitates emergency intervention, plan for a cesarean delivery between $36^{0/7}$ and $37^{6/7}$ weeks of gestation, although earlier delivery is often necessary for women who have experienced recurrent episodes of bleeding.

Clinically significant bleeding can occur even after delivery. Because a placenta previa is implanted in an area of the uterus that may not contract well, postpartum hemorrhage is more common and can be difficult to control.

Discuss with the pregnant woman the possibility of *placenta accreta,* which is defined as abnormal placental attachment onto or invasion into the uterine muscle, making separation of the placenta difficult or impossible. Most often, hysterectomy is required as the only means to control bleeding. Placenta accreta is more common with placenta previa, especially in women who have undergone a previous cesarean delivery.

B. Placental abruption
   1. Clinical findings
      Placental separation may be partial or complete. In general, the condition of the woman and the fetus depends on the amount of placental surface separated from the uterine wall.
   2. Management
      In cases of partial placental abruption when the maternal vital signs and fetal monitoring are stable, and the fetus is preterm, hospitalization is recommended for observation and administration of antenatal corticosteroids to accelerate fetal maturity. Close observation is necessary because a woman with placental abruption may experience the sudden onset of additional bleeding and require emergency delivery. When maternal vital signs or fetal heart monitoring findings are abnormal, or when the pregnancy is at or near term, delivery is indicated. Specific management depends on the severity of the abruption, maternal hemodynamic stability (including evidence of shock or DIC), the fetal heart rate pattern, or, alternatively, the occurrence of fetal death.

 Regardless of the degree of abruption, blood products need to be available at all times, in case they are required. An abruption can worsen suddenly and dramatically at any time.

Self-test D

Now answer these questions to test yourself on the information in the last section.

D1. True / False — Placental abruption may be complete or partial.

D2. True / False — Regardless of the degree of abruption, cesarean delivery is always required.

D3. True / False — A placenta that covers the internal cervical os before 16 weeks at US examination will remain a placenta previa at term.

D4. True / False — An increasing platelet count and fibrinogen level signal the onset of disseminated intravascular coagulation in a woman with a placental abruption.

D5. True / False — When placental abruption occurs, disseminated intravascular coagulation may develop and result in ongoing blood loss.

D6. Which of the following risks apply to a woman with placenta previa diagnosed at 34 weeks of gestation?

Yes	No	
___	___	Preterm delivery may be necessary.
___	___	Placenta accreta may be present and may necessitate a hysterectomy after delivery.
___	___	Preeclampsia is likely to occur.
___	___	If bleeding occurs, the woman and fetus can lose large amounts of blood.
___	___	Postpartum hemorrhage is more likely to occur.
___	___	Disseminated intravascular coagulation is likely to develop.

D7. A placenta previa is diagnosed at 32 weeks of gestation. Bleeding has stopped, maternal vital signs and laboratory values are stable, and tests of fetal well-being have reassuring results. What should you do?

  A. Begin administration of steroids to the woman and deliver the baby by cesarean delivery 24 hours later.
  B. Hospitalize the woman and continue observation until fetal maturity is achieved, unless bleeding or labor ensues and necessitates cesarean delivery.
  C. Perform cesarean delivery within the next several hours, before the placenta begins to bleed again.
  D. Give the woman a blood transfusion and deliver the baby by cesarean delivery within the next 24 hours.

Check your answers with the list that follows the Recommended Routines. Correct any incorrect answers and review the appropriate section in the unit.

8. How do you recognize and treat disseminated intravascular coagulation?

A. What is DIC?

DIC occurs when an event triggers the release of a surplus amount of thromboplastins into the bloodstream. Thromboplastic substances normally cause or accelerate clot formation, but the overstimulation of the clotting system results in clots being formed more rapidly than the thromboplastins can be replaced. Rather than one large clot forming, numerous microscopic clots appear throughout the vascular system. Because these tiny clots are so numerous, they consume the factors required for clotting. Because the microscopic clots have "tied up" all the plasma coagulation (clotting) factors, the remaining blood cannot clot. If bleeding is present for any reason, it will worsen significantly because of the lack of available plasma coagulation factors. Overwhelming hemorrhage can result.

Whenever possible, women with disseminated intravascular coagulation should be treated in a regional perinatal medical center; however, do not transfer a woman who is in unstable condition.

B. Who is at risk for DIC?

A variety of conditions can lead to DIC. In severe infections, thromboplastins produced by bacteria (in particular, *Escherichia coli*) can cause septic shock and DIC. When a fetus dies but is not delivered for several weeks, DIC may develop slowly, over a period of 4 to 8 weeks. With placental abruption or amniotic fluid embolism, DIC can develop rapidly. Pregnant women at risk for DIC include those with

- Placental abruption (the most common cause of DIC in pregnant women)
- Amniotic fluid embolism
- Fetal death, with the dead fetus retained for 4 weeks or longer
- HELLP (*h*emolysis, *e*levated *l*iver enzyme levels, and *l*ow *p*latelet count occurring in association with preeclampsia) syndrome (a severe hypertensive disorder of pregnancy) (See Unit 1, Hypertension in Pregnancy, in this book.)

In addition, women with obstetric hemorrhage who are transfused with a massive amount of blood may develop clotting problems. Because the blood lost contained plasma coagulation factors, but packed red blood cells do not, transfusion of large volumes of blood dilutes the natural clotting proteins and may significantly reduce the capability of the blood to coagulate. To maintain normal coagulation of blood when a massive transfusion is underway for obstetric hemorrhage, both FFP and platelets should be transfused along with red blood cells to replace clotting factors and platelets. Each center should have its own protocol for massive transfusion, which will determine the ratio of red blood cells to FFP to platelets to be transfused. All obstetrics team members should know how to activate the massive transfusion protocol.

C. Which blood tests are important?

For some tests, it can take several hours to obtain results. While the tests should be performed, it may not be prudent to wait for the results before beginning therapy. For this reason, also collect 5 mL of the patient's blood in an anticoagulant-free tube. Tape the tube to her bedside. Check it every few minutes. If a clot does not form within 8 to 10 minutes, DIC is probably present.

If disseminated intravascular coagulation is strongly suspected, do not delay therapy while awaiting laboratory test results. Proceed with treatment, according to the woman's clinical condition.

Perform the following tests and recheck frequently, until the patient is stable:
- Prothrombin time and PTT: If these are prolonged but the platelet count and fibrinogen level are within reference range, it suggests the patient does not have DIC but may have another coagulation problem.
- Platelet count: A low platelet count is <50,000/mm^3.
- Fibrinogen level: A low fibrinogen level (<150 mg/dL) indicates DIC.

D. How is DIC treated?

Overall, treatment of a pregnant woman with DIC has 3 goals.
- Replace blood components to maintain adequate plasma coagulation factors.
- Stabilize the woman.
- Deliver the baby.

A woman with placental abruption and DIC may be critically ill, with a fetus that is dead or in serious jeopardy, and may require complex management, including critical care resources and personnel. Treatment will depend, in part, on whether the woman is bleeding heavily.

The management plans that follow are designed as a guide for emergency therapy when the patient is too unstable for safe transport to a regional perinatal center.

Consultation with maternal-fetal medicine specialists at a regional perinatal center is recommended as soon as disseminated intravascular coagulation is suspected.

1. Coagulation factor replacement

    Administration of FFP, cryoprecipitate, and platelets are directed at restoring normal coagulation but are not intended to restore blood volume. If large amounts of plasma coagulation factors are needed, such as in the treatment of DIC, cryoprecipitate can deliver these factors in a smaller volume than FFP, which may help to prevent volume overload.

    a. Cryoprecipitate
       - Contains clotting proteins, including fibrinogen, factor VIII, and factor XIII, in a volume of 20 to 50 mL

    b. FFP
       - Contains all of the clotting proteins of the original unit of whole blood from which it is derived, in a usual volume of 250 mL

    c. Platelets
       - Administration of one pack of platelets, which includes pooled platelets from 4 to 6 donated units, will raise the platelet count by approximately 30,000/μL.

If these blood components are not kept in your hospital, know where and how to obtain them quickly, 24 hours a day, 7 days a week.

2. Treatment of women *without* severe hemorrhage is aimed at restoring clotting profile and/or platelet count to a specific goal.
    a. Perform frequent monitoring
       Frequently monitor fetal heart rate and the woman's blood pressure and other vital signs.
    b. Provide clotting factors via IV infusion
       Use cryoprecipitate or FFP to bring the fibrinogen level above 100 mg/dL.
    c. Recheck
       - Serum fibrinogen level every 4 hours
       - Platelet count every 4 hours
       - Complete blood cell count every 4 hours
    d. Consider administering platelets
       Transfusion of platelets may be indicated, depending on the platelet level and the route of delivery.
       - *Vaginal delivery:* Consider platelet transfusion if the count is less than 20,000/mm³ and if there is evidence of poor clot formation despite an adequate fibrinogen level (>100 mg/dL).
       - *Cesarean delivery:* Consider platelet transfusion if the count is less than 50,000/mm³; if possible, delay surgery until the level reaches 50,000/mm³.
    e. Assess the progress of labor
       If vaginal delivery seems possible, it may be safer for the woman than cesarean delivery. If labor is not expected to progress, however, cesarean delivery should be performed as soon as the serum fibrinogen level is above 100 mg/dL and the platelet count is above 50,000/mm³.
3. Management of women *with* severe hemorrhage
   Management of a woman with DIC and bleeding crisis should be conducted in an area equipped for intensive care. Multiple, large-bore IV lines are needed. Monitor the patient's blood pressure and other vital signs continuously. Provide life-support measures, as needed.

 For a patient in shock with disseminated intravascular coagulation, stabilizing treatment should be initiated in the original hospital; the patient should not be transported in unstable condition.

   a. Administer blood components and fluid volume
      - Packed red blood cells through one IV line.
      - Cryoprecipitate or FFP through a second IV line.
      - Platelets or saline through a third IV line.
      - Common transfusion ratios for red blood cells to FFP to platelets are 1:1:1 and 6:4:1. Follow your hospital's specific protocol.

b. Recheck the serum fibrinogen level and platelet count
Check frequently until the patient is stable.
c. Perform emergency cesarean delivery
Perform emergency cesarean delivery as soon as the fibrinogen level exceeds 100 mg/dL and the platelet count is higher than 50,000/mm^3, whether or not the fetus is alive.

9. What care should you anticipate for the newborn?

Antepartum hemorrhage may result in fetal compromise related to abnormal placental gas exchange and may result in fetal blood loss, as well. The neonate may be anemic and require administration of fluids and transfusion of blood. The neonate may also demonstrate respiratory depression, decreased tone, or decreased reflex responsiveness and may need resuscitation. Complete placental abruption and bleeding from vasa previa may result in fetal death. At delivery, you should be prepared with personnel and equipment for resuscitation of the newborn (see Book 1: Maternal and Fetal Evaluation and Immediate Newborn Care, Unit 5, Resuscitating the Newborn). You should be able to assess the baby for signs of acute blood loss, check the baby's blood pressure, and provide blood volume replacement, if necessary, in the delivery room.

A central (not heel-stick) hematocrit level should be measured soon after delivery and other therapy provided as indicated by clinical and laboratory findings. (See Book 3: Neonatal Care, Unit 4, Low Blood Pressure [Hypotension], for neonatal hypovolemia [low blood volume] and hypotension [low blood pressure] management.)

10. What additional care do you need to provide to Rh(D)-negative women?

Women who are Rh(D) negative and have a negative Rh(D) antibody screening result may develop antibodies against Rh(D) during an episode of bleeding at any point during pregnancy. When obstetric bleeding occurs, fetal blood may enter the maternal circulation. If the fetus is Rh(D) positive, an Rh(D)-negative woman may develop antibodies in response; this process is known as *alloimmunization*. This rarely affects the current pregnancy. Future pregnancies will be at risk for fetal hemolytic anemia owing to passage of anti-Rh(D) antibodies across the placenta. Alloimmunization is prevented by the administration of Rh immunoglobulin (RhIg).

When vaginal bleeding occurs in pregnancy, RhIg should be administered within 72 hours of the onset of bleeding. Protection against alloimmunization lasts for approximately 12 weeks. Depending on the course of the pregnancy, subsequent doses may be needed.

A. Early pregnancy bleeding
Fetomaternal (from the fetus to the mother) transfusion may or may not occur with early pregnancy bleeding. To prevent alloimmunization, it is safest to administer RhIg with an episode of bleeding in early pregnancy, even if the amount of bleeding is small, as it is not possible to reliably determine if fetal blood has entered the maternal circulation. In the first trimester, 50 mcg is the recommended dose; however, this dosage is not always commercially available. If it is not stocked in your facility, use the standard 300-mcg dose. If a repeat episode(s) of bleeding occurs within the subsequent 12 weeks, repeat RhIg administration is not indicated.

B. Late-pregnancy bleeding
During late-pregnancy bleeding, the volume of fetomaternal transfusion is likely to be greater than earlier in pregnancy, both because the fetus has a larger blood volume and because placental abruption is more likely to cause fetomaternal transfusion. After the first trimester, the recommended dose of RhIg is 300 mcg.

When there has been clinically significant maternal bleeding, such as may occur with placenta previa or placental abruption, a Kleihauer-Betke (acid elution) test is used to estimate the amount of fetal blood that may have entered the maternal circulation. The volume of fetal red cells estimated with the Kleihauer-Betke test is divided by 15. This indicates the number of doses of 300 mcg of RhIg that are needed (each 300 mcg of RhIg is adequate for each 15 mL of fetal cells that entered the maternal circulation).

Administration of RhIg should be repeated if bleeding episodes are separated by 12 weeks or more.

C. During pregnancy for all Rh(D)-negative women
Even in pregnancies with no evidence of obstetric bleeding, fetomaternal transfusion may still occur. Nearly all Rh(D)-negative women who deliver an Rh(D)-positive baby will be protected from alloimmunization by the dose of RhIg administered after delivery. However, it is recommended that all Rh(D)-negative women receive RhIg at 28 weeks of gestation, unless they already have a positive antibody screening result for Rh(D) antibodies. This will prevent the small number of cases of antepartum alloimmunization in women who may have unrecognized fetomaternal bleeding during pregnancy. Because term delivery would be 12 weeks after this dose of RhIg, all women who received RhIg during pregnancy should also receive a dose after birth.

D. After birth
Fetomaternal transfusion can also occur during delivery of a healthy baby from an uncomplicated pregnancy. The recommended dose of RhIg after delivery of an Rh(D)-positive baby to an Rh(D)-negative woman is 300 mcg. Every Rh(D)-negative woman who has an Rh(D)-positive baby should receive a dose of RhIg after birth. A Kleihauer-Betke test is performed to assess whether the degree of fetomaternal transfusion exceeds the amount that would be protected against by a single dose of RhIg. This postpartum dose should be administered whether or not a dose was provided earlier in pregnancy.

Self-test E

Now answer these questions to test yourself on the information in the last section.

E1. True / False — Disseminated intravascular coagulation is a complicated, life-threatening condition that, whenever possible, should be treated at a regional perinatal medical center.

E2. True / False — When a woman has disseminated intravascular coagulation, whether her condition is stable or unstable, rapid transfer to a regional perinatal center is advisable.

E3. True / False — If a tube of blood drawn from a woman with placental abruption fails to clot within 6 minutes, disseminated intravascular coagulation is probably present.

E4. True / False — The need for resuscitation of the newborn cannot be predicted according to the amount of blood the woman has lost.

E5. What are the 3 main goals of treatment for a woman with disseminated intravascular coagulation?
_____
_____
_____

E6. Name 3 products that are used to replace plasma coagulation (clotting) factors.
_____
_____
_____

E7. A woman has a placental abruption with vaginal bleeding and disseminated intravascular coagulation. Cryoprecipitate, packed red blood cells, and saline solution are being infused rapidly to provide plasma coagulation factors and blood volume expansion. Maternal blood pressure is stable, but heavy vaginal bleeding continues. The fetus is dead. An oxytocin infusion has been started and membranes were ruptured, but labor does not progress well. What should you do?
  A. Perform cesarean delivery as soon as the platelet count is above 50,000/mm^3 and the fibrinogen level is above 100 mg/dL.
  B. Continue to provide plasma coagulation factors and increase the oxytocin infusion until vaginal delivery occurs.
  C. Perform immediate cesarean delivery.
  D. Transfer the woman immediately to a regional perinatal center.

E8. When a woman has obstetric hemorrhage, what should you be prepared to do for the baby at delivery?
_____
_____
_____
_____
_____
_____

Check your answers with the list that follows the Recommended Routines. Correct any incorrect answers and review the appropriate section in the unit.

11. What is postpartum hemorrhage?

Early postpartum hemorrhage is defined as cumulative blood loss of more than 1,000 mL during delivery and in the first 24 hours after birth. The clinical picture may include the sudden onset of heavy vaginal bleeding or, alternatively, persistent and prolonged vaginal bleeding of a more than normal amount. Sudden heavy bleeding suggests uterine atony, while persistent bleeding with normal uterine tone suggests a laceration. Postpartum hemorrhage occurs in approximately 5% of births and is responsible for approximately 10% of maternal deaths in the United States. Pregnant women have an increase in their blood volume by approximately 1,500 to 2,000 mL by term, which serves in part to minimize the effects of postpartum hemorrhage. Many women with postpartum hemorrhage do not require treatment beyond the routine prophylaxis that should be given to all women to minimize postpartum bleeding. Women who experience clinically significant blood loss at delivery or who have clinically significant ongoing blood loss may become physiologically unstable rapidly and require an aggressive response to prevent morbidity or death.

Note: Postpartum hemorrhage is not a specific diagnosis that explains the origin of the bleeding. Nearly 80% of postpartum hemorrhage is caused by uterine atony. While initiating treatment for blood loss, it is important to simultaneously seek and address the specific source of the bleeding.

12. What are the causes of postpartum hemorrhage?

Blood flow to the uterus increases as pregnancy nears term and comprises at least 700 mL per minute. After delivery of the placenta, bleeding from the placental site is normally controlled by uterine contractions that dramatically reduce the volume of blood flowing through the arteries and veins of the uterus. Life-threatening hemorrhage can occur in any of the following situations:

A. Uterine atony

   Uterine contractions are not strong enough or frequent enough to stop bleeding from the placental site. This is called *atony*. Atony accounts for 80% of the cases of postpartum hemorrhage and is more likely to occur in women
   - With high parity
   - With a previously overdistended uterus (polyhydramnios, multifetal gestation)
   - With uterine fibroids
   - After prolonged labor, especially if labor was augmented with oxytocin
   - After rapid labor
   - With intraamniotic infection
   - With a history of previous postpartum hemorrhage

B. Retained placental fragments

   When fragments of the placenta or membranes are retained, the uterus may not contract normally to be able to control bleeding from the placental site. Clinically significant hemorrhage can result, even if the retained placental fragment is small.

C. Lacerations

Lacerations anywhere in the genital tract (perineum, vagina, cervix) result in bleeding that will not be controlled with uterine contraction. Such lacerations account for 5% to 10% of the cases of postpartum hemorrhage and are more likely to occur
- With rapid labor
- With a very large baby
- After a forceps-assisted or vacuum extraction delivery
- When an episiotomy is performed

D. Uterine rupture

Although rare (<1% of cases of postpartum hemorrhage), uterine rupture occurs most often
- In patients who underwent previous uterine surgery (eg, cesarean delivery, hysterotomy)
- After rapid labor in multiparous women
- After difficult forceps-assisted or vacuum extraction delivery

E. Abnormal blood clotting

Coagulopathy accounts for less than 1% of postpartum hemorrhage. In the obstetric setting, coagulopathy is most often acquired (DIC) as a result of placental abruption, septic shock, fetal demise, or amniotic fluid embolism.

Inherited bleeding disorders, such as von Willebrand disease, result in abnormal coagulation via the absence or abnormal function of clotting proteins. Such conditions will almost always be known before pregnancy, and maternal-fetal medicine specialists or hematology experts should be involved in the woman's care throughout pregnancy.

F. Uterine inversion

This is a rare but potentially serious complication. It occurs when the uterine fundus delivers through the cervix into the vagina, and sometimes even protrudes externally through the vulva. The uterus is essentially turned "inside out." Uterine inversion may be caused by vigorous traction on the umbilical cord, especially when the placenta is implanted at the fundus. Pulling on the cord may pull the placenta, with the fundus still attached, into the lower uterus, through the cervix, and into the vagina, rather than separate the placenta from the uterine wall. The placenta may separate and be delivered just before the diagnosis of inversion is established or (especially in cases of inversion with placenta accreta) may remain attached to the inverted fundus.

There may be other, unexplained causes for uterine inversion. Whatever the cause, blood loss can be extremely heavy, and the woman may go into shock. With rapid diagnosis and treatment, hypovolemic shock can usually be prevented.

13. What should you do *routinely* to prevent or reduce postpartum hemorrhage?

A. Administer uterotonic medication

Oxytocin is used routinely to cause uterine contractions *after* delivery to prevent or reduce postpartum hemorrhage from uterine atony. Active management of the third stage of labor is recommended for all deliveries, to reduce the incidence of postpartum hemorrhage. This approach consists of the administration of oxytocin immediately after delivery of the anterior shoulder of the baby. Some protocols also call for continuous traction

on the umbilical cord, but this is not an essential component. Active management of the third stage of labor may be performed in conjunction with delayed cord clamping.
1. Oxytocin is administered intravenously or intramuscularly.
   a. For patients with an IV line in place a standardized dilute solution of 30 units of oxytocin in 500 mL of physiological (normal) saline or lactated Ringer's solution should be administered. A suggested initial infusion rate is 250 mL/h, although each obstetric unit may have its own specific protocol.
   b. For women without an IV line in place 10 units of oxytocin should be administered into the anterior thigh. Do not administer undiluted oxytocin intravenously, as it may cause severe hypotension.

 Do not administer an intravenous bolus of undiluted oxytocin, because hypotension and cardiac arrhythmia can result.

B. Inspect the placenta
Routinely inspect *every* placenta for missing segments (cotyledons). Do this by holding the placenta in your cupped hands, with the uterine side facing you. If the placental margin is irregular, it suggests that a fragment is retained in the uterus. Manually explore the uterus and retrieve any missing fragments of the placenta or membranes.

C. Examination for lacerations
After *every* delivery, visually examine the cervix, vagina, and perineum for lacerations.

D. Provide intensive surveillance for first postpartum hour
The first hour after delivery, a period sometimes called the "fourth stage" of labor, is when most postpartum hemorrhage occurs. Bleeding may be minimal immediately after delivery but may become massive 20 or 30 minutes later. Intensive monitoring of the maternal condition during this immediate postpartum period is recommended for *all* women.

14. How is postpartum hemorrhage treated?

Postpartum hemorrhage can occur in any pregnancy. Treatment requires prompt, coordinated actions of all health care team members to achieve optimal outcome. Precise documentation is also important. Every hospital, including those with relatively few deliveries, needs to be able to respond appropriately and efficiently to this crisis situation.

Adequate response is facilitated when

- A comprehensive but simple plan of action is established and is familiar to all team members.
- Clear, user-friendly documentation is used and familiar to all team members.

The plan outlined in this section begins with the most common cause of postpartum hemorrhage and proceeds to less common causes, which generally require more invasive intervention. Some actions will need to be taken simultaneously. Early identification of postpartum hemorrhage is an essential component of treatment. Typical signs of shock may develop so late in some women that death can occur despite emergency intervention and blood transfusion.

Simultaneously with beginning to determine the cause of the hemorrhage, steps must be taken to prevent the woman from becoming hypotensive. While beginning to investigate the cause of

obstetric hemorrhage, the care team must simultaneously implement clinical resuscitation measures to prevent hypotension and hemorrhagic shock and their potential complications.
- Establish IV access.
- Provide volume expansion, as needed. (See Section 3, What emergency care should you give a pregnant woman who presents with life-threatening hemorrhage from an unknown cause?)
- Send a blood sample for crossmatching.
- If appropriate, activate the massive transfusion protocol.

 Postpartum hemorrhage is an emergency. Begin treatment at the first evidence of hemorrhage, before rapid heart rate, hypotension, or other signs of shock develop.

A. Palpate the uterus
Uterine atony is the most common cause of postpartum hemorrhage and should therefore be investigated first.
1. Firm fundus
If the fundus is firm and round and located at or below the umbilicus, uterine atony is not the problem. Look for another cause, such as retained placental fragment(s) or birth canal laceration.
2. "Boggy" uterus
If the uterus is "boggy" with a soft fundus, easily indented by examining fingers, and well above the umbilicus, uterine atony is most likely the cause of the bleeding. Fundal massage will usually result in contraction of the uterus.
   a. First maneuver
   - *Stabilize the position of the uterus:* Slide one hand over the symphysis pubis and press your fingers into the lower abdomen, below the fundus; keep your fingers firmly pressed in this position to stabilize the uterus and prevent it from being pushed into the pelvis during massage. (Massage is much less effective if the fundus is compressed in the pelvis.)
   - *Massage the top of the fundus:* Use your other hand to massage the fundus to cause it to contract.
   b. Second maneuver
   If abdominal massage of the fundus does not result in firming and uterine contraction with marked reduction in bleeding, manual compression of the uterus may be needed.
   - *Continue to massage the fundus:* Keep your hand that is above the umbilicus and massaging the fundus in place. (See the first maneuver and Figure 2.3.)
   - *Insert your other hand into the vagina:* Form a fist with that hand.
   - *Compress the uterus against the vaginal fist:* Continue to massage the fundus.
3. If the fundus cannot be palpated
If the fundus cannot be palpated at abdominal examination, consider that uterine inversion may have occurred. Uterine inversion is diagnosed if a large, round mass, covered by the shaggy decidual lining of the uterus, is identified in the vagina.

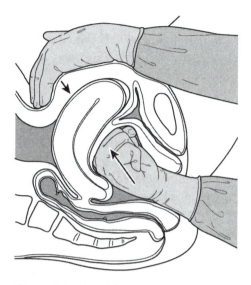

Figure 2.3. Manual Compression of the Uterus

Management of uterine inversion varies from the approach used for other forms of postpartum hemorrhage. Response to this uncommon emergency is described separately, at the end of this section.

Figure 2.4 shows incomplete inversion, comparable to stage 2 inversion in the inset of the figure.

The inset shows the progression as the uterus inverts completely. In stage 4, the uterus has prolapsed outside the woman's body.

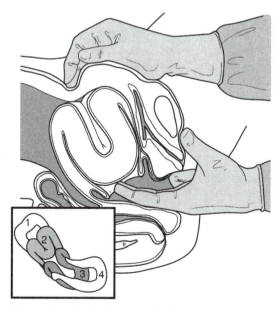

Figure 2.4. Uterine Inversion. The inset shows stages 1, 2, 3, and 4 of inversion.

B. Administer uterotonic medication
Drugs that cause contraction of uterine muscle should be administered. *Exception: Uterotonic medication should **not** be given to a woman with uterine inversion until the uterus is restored to its normal position.*
1. Begin infusion of dilute oxytocin
   - Oxytocin should be administered intravenously as a solution of standard concentration. The most common concentration is 30 units of oxytocin in 500 mL of fluid. The usual initial rate for active management of the third stage of labor is 250 mL/h; in the event of active postpartum hemorrhage, increase the rate to 500 mL/h while taking additional steps to correct uterine tone.
   - If an IV is not in place, administer an initial dose of 10 units of oxytocin intramuscularly into the thigh while an IV is being placed.
2. Administer methylergonovine maleate (Methergine)
   A 0.2-mg dose of methylergonovine maleate may be administered intramuscularly and may be repeated in 2 to 4 hours, if needed. Do *not*, however, administer this drug to a woman with hypertension (from any cause) or symptomatic heart disease. Methylergonovine maleate is a smooth muscle stimulant that leads to vasospasm and may cause serious adverse effects.
   - Venous vasospasm: Blood return to the heart and cardiac output are reduced, and severe hypotension and cardiac arrhythmias can result, which may be fatal for women with symptomatic heart disease.
   - Arterial vasospasm: May cause acute blood pressure increase and is contraindicated in women with hypertension.
3. Administer carboprost tromethamine (Hemabate)
   Administer 250 mcg of carboprost tromethamine intramuscularly or directly into uterine muscle (fundus). This dose may be repeated at 15-minute intervals for up to 8 doses. If uterine atony with heavy bleeding continues after several doses, however, a hysterectomy is usually necessary.
4. Administer misoprostol (Cytotec)
   Administer 800 to 1,000 mcg of misoprostol via the sublingual, buccal, or rectal route. Vaginal administration is not recommended; active vaginal bleeding may result in expulsion of the tablets before absorption. Misoprostol may be less effective for immediate control of uterine atony than other agents but may help to maintain normal uterine tone once it is established. It may be used in women with hypertension or asthma, for whom other agents are contraindicated.

C. Other interventions
If the previously described actions do not establish and maintain uterine tone and decrease uterine bleeding, prepare to go to the operating room to assess the patient for uterine rupture or lacerations of the cervix or vagina.
1. Administer 1,000 mg of tranexamic acid via slow IV push over 10 minutes. This agent inhibits fibrinolysis (the normal breakdown of fibrin clots) and will help control bleeding. It is usually administered when the blood loss exceeds 1,000 mL.
2. Prepare for surgery
   a. Continue to elevate the uterus out of the pelvis and to massage the fundus.
   b. Communicate patient needs to anesthesia staff and surgical personnel.

c. Ensure the patient has at least 2 working IVs. Large-bore (18-gauge and larger) IVs will allow for rapid infusion of additional fluids and blood products if bleeding continues.
d. Activate the massive transfusion protocol.
e. Send blood for crossmatching (if not already done).
Request at least 4 units of packed red blood cells be prepared.
f. Draw blood samples for the following tests:
- Complete blood cell count
- Platelet count
- Prothrombin time and PTT
- Fibrinogen level

Tape an anticoagulant-free tube to the patient's bedside and check for clot formation every few minutes. (If a clot does not form within 6 minutes, see the management of DIC in Section 8, How do you recognize and treat disseminated intravascular coagulation?)
g. Discuss the woman's status with her family (as soon as time permits).

3. Manual exploration

Most women will require anesthesia for uterine and upper vaginal exploration. Anesthesia personnel should be continuously available to provide intensive monitoring of vital signs and life-support measures.
a. Explore the vagina and cervix
Repair or pack lacerations as they are encountered.
b. Explore the uterus
If bleeding appears to be coming from the uterus
- *Explore the uterine cavity for retained placental fragments*: Bedside US may aid in the identification of retained placenta.
- *Examine the patient for uterine rupture*: If uterine rupture is found and is thought to be the source of the bleeding, a laparotomy will be necessary to repair or remove the uterus to stop the bleeding.

4. Perform laparotomy

If the uterus and vagina have been explored and no lacerations found, or if lacerations were found and repaired but uterine hemorrhage continues, a laparotomy may be necessary.
a. Explore the pelvis
Explore the pelvis thoroughly for evidence of uterine rupture or upward extension of cervical lacerations. Repair any lacerations that are identified. If vaginal bleeding persists, the source of the bleeding must be within the uterus. Under these circumstances, a prompt hysterectomy (total or subtotal) may be necessary.
b. Can fertility be preserved?
If there is a strong desire to preserve the woman's future fertility, procedures may be undertaken to control the bleeding and retain the uterus.
- Uterine artery ligation is performed by placing large figure-8 sutures through the broad ligament at the vesicouterine peritoneal fold and into the wall of the uterus. Care should be taken to avoid including the ureters in the suture.
- If necessary, the utero-ovarian and infundibulopelvic ligaments may also be ligated without sacrificing the ovaries or uterus. Ligating these vessels may diminish uterine blood flow sufficiently to slow blood loss and permit

replacement of blood and clotting factors. Sufficient uterine blood flow will be retained to allow for future pregnancies.
- Compressive suture techniques have been described to treat uterine atony, as well as localized sources of uterine bleeding from a focal placenta accreta. These techniques, which include the B-Lynch compression suture, allow the uterus to remain compressed while blood loss and coagulopathy are corrected; the sutures are ultimately absorbed.
- Bilateral ligation of the hypogastric (internal iliac) arteries has also been performed for the purpose of diminishing uterine blood flow in the treatment of postpartum hemorrhage. Ligation of these arteries is more technically difficult, more likely to result in complications—including ureteral injury—and less effective than uterine artery ligation.

c. Total or subtotal hysterectomy
In the most severe cases, a woman may remain in shock after vaginal bleeding has been stopped during the hysterectomy. In this situation, a subtotal hysterectomy may be quicker, with less blood loss, than a total hysterectomy. A subtotal hysterectomy involves removal of the fundus, above the point where the uterine arteries have been ligated, leaving the cervix in place.

d. Fallopian tubes and ovaries
If a hysterectomy is performed, the fallopian tubes may also be removed. The ovaries rarely need to be removed.

15. How is uterine inversion managed?

Uterine inversion is an emergency that requires an immediate, knowledgeable response. Follow the steps described below.

Do not administer uterotonic medication (oxytocin, methylergonovine, misoprostol, or carboprost) until after the uterus is restored to its proper position.

A. Prepare for surgery; begin blood volume expansion
Provide management, as outlined previously, for any type of postpartum hemorrhage. Laparotomy and/or hysterectomy may not be needed, but preparations and personnel should be in place in the event they become necessary. If the placenta is still attached, do not remove it until blood volume expansion fluids are being administered. Bleeding will likely worsen if the placenta detaches from the fundus and will continue until the uterus is replaced.

B. Uterine replacement
If the placenta has not separated, leave it in place until the uterus is replaced to prevent the fundus from contracting, which may prevent uterine replacement. Replace the uterus by placing your fingers in the center of the inverted fundus and pushing inward, trying to push the leading point of the fundus back through the cervix and restoring the uterus to its normal position.

If the cervix and lower uterine segment have contracted to form a tight, unyielding ring so the fundus cannot be pushed back through it, administer magnesium sulfate (4–6 g, intravenously, over 5–10 minutes), terbutaline (0.25 mg, intravenously), or nitroglycerine (1–2 metered sprays sublingually) for uterine relaxation.

C. If these maneuvers do not achieve replacement
   If initial attempts at uterine replacement fail, administer deep general anesthesia with an inhalational agent, such as sevoflurane, desflurane, or isoflurane, to obtain relaxation of the cervix. Attempt again to replace the uterus by pushing it back through the cervix.

D. If the uterus still cannot be replaced vaginally
   If all previous attempts, as outlined previously, fail, continue the anesthesia and proceed promptly to surgical intervention with a laparotomy. Various techniques have been described to aid in restoration of the uterus to normal position. These include using clamps to grasp the round ligaments and elevate the uterus or making an incision in the constriction ring to allow uterine replacement.

E. As soon as the uterus is replaced
   1. Administer uterotonic medications
      - Begin infusion of dilute oxytocin solution.
      and
      - Administer 0.2 mg of methylergonovine intramuscularly or 800 mcg of misoprostol rectally.
   2. Hold the fundus and compress the uterus until it begins to contract
      This will help prevent inversion from recurring, as well as help control the bleeding until uterine tone is regained. The technique used is the same as that shown earlier in the first maneuver for management of uterine atony. If this does not control the bleeding or keep the uterus from re-inverting, use the second maneuver. (See Section 14, How is postpartum hemorrhage treated?)

F. Perform vaginal and abdominal examinations
   1. Continue examinations for 4 to 6 hours, to be sure inversion does not recur.
   2. Reexamine the patient if postpartum vaginal bleeding occurs.

Self-test F

Now answer these questions to test yourself on the information in the last section.

F1. True / False — Uterine atony is the most common cause of postpartum hemorrhage.

F2. True / False — In an emergency, undiluted oxytocin may be administered via intravenous push to stop massive postpartum hemorrhage.

F3. True / False — After every delivery, the placenta should be inspected for missing segments.

F4. True / False — Early detection of postpartum hemorrhage is one of the most important components of treating it.

F5. True / False — If uterine inversion occurs with the placenta still attached, the placenta should be removed immediately.

F6. True / False — An oxytocin infusion should be started as soon as uterine inversion is recognized.

F7. What are 4 things that should be done routinely to help prevent postpartum hemorrhage?
_____
_____
_____
_____

F8. Methylergonovine should not be administered to women who have _____ or _____.

F9. A steady, slow, unrelenting flow of blood postpartum suggests _____ _____.

F10. List at least 3 causes of postpartum hemorrhage.
_____
_____
_____

F11. If uterine inversion occurs, should uterotonic medication be given *before* or *after* the uterus is restored to its normal position?

Check your answers with the list that follows the Recommended Routines. Correct any incorrect answers and review the appropriate section in the unit.

16. What needs to be documented?

The steps taken to diagnose and manage obstetric hemorrhage should be documented in detail in the medical record, noting the sequence of steps performed and the individuals who performed them. It is recommended that the team debrief after the hemorrhage event to review the management that was performed and to identify opportunities for improvement.

As with any response to a life-threatening crisis, your actions and those of other team members in your hospital need to be practiced and rehearsed. Obstetric emergency simulation drills are a recommended activity for all obstetric units, to practice and fine-tune the team response to emergencies. Role delineation (IV access, medications, documentation, activating emergency blood release) will assist the response by ensuring that all team members know their responsibility.

A documentation tool similar to a "code sheet" may be adopted to facilitate real-time recording of interventions for later documentation in the medical record; this may also exist in a flow sheet in the medical record. This tool may include

1. Delivery: time and date
2. Condition of the patient when the problem was first identified
3. Therapy
   - Medication(s): drug name/dosage/route/time given/response
   - Fluid(s)
     — *Crystalloid:* type/amount/time given/response
     — *Blood/blood components:* type/amount/time given/response
   - Laboratory: test(s)/time sent/result(s)
   - Vital signs: values/time/relation to therapy given
4. Periodic reassessment of patient condition or cause of the bleeding
5. Surgical intervention
   - Time decision made, anesthesia and other staff notified
   - Discussion with family
   - Time surgery started
   - Results of exploration: vagina/cervix/uterus
   - Lacerations repaired, placental fragment(s) retrieved, other surgical repair
6. Summary
   - Estimation of total blood loss
   - Urine output
   - Total fluids administered: crystalloid/blood/blood components
   - Patient condition: findings/therapy/response to therapy
   - Ongoing management plan

OBSTETRIC HEMORRHAGE
Recommended Routines

All the routines listed below are based on the principles of perinatal care presented in the unit you have just finished. They are recommended as part of routine perinatal care.

Read each routine carefully and decide whether it is standard operating procedure in your hospital. Check the appropriate blank next to each routine.

Procedure Standard in My Hospital	Needs Discussion by Our Staff	Recommended Routine
_____	_____	1. Develop a system whereby an emergency cesarean delivery can be started within 30 minutes from the time the decision to operate is made, at any time of day or night, any day of the week.
_____	_____	2. Develop a system whereby an emergency hysterectomy can be performed urgently, at any time of day or night, any day of the week.
_____	_____	3. Establish guidelines for the emergency treatment and stabilization of women with • Obstetric hemorrhage of unknown origin • Bleeding placenta previa • Placental abruption • Disseminated intravascular coagulation • Postpartum hemorrhage
_____	_____	4. Establish a routine to ensure the prevention or early detection of postpartum hemorrhage for *every* woman, including • Administration of uterotonic medication after placental delivery • Visual inspection of the placenta • Visual inspection of the birth canal • Intensive monitoring during the first postpartum hour
_____	_____	5. Establish written instructions for obtaining blood components quickly, 24 hours a day, 7 days a week. If your blood bank maintains all blood products in-house, develop a massive transfusion protocol.
_____	_____	6. Develop flow diagram(s) for quick and clear recording of events and actions during crisis management of • Severe antepartum obstetric hemorrhage • Disseminated intravascular coagulation • Severe postpartum hemorrhage

UNIT 2: OBSTETRIC HEMORRHAGE

Self-test Answers

These are the answers to the Self-test questions. Please check them with the answers you gave and review the information in the unit wherever necessary.

Self-test A

A1. Clear plan of action with staff trained in implementing it
Access to adequate blood supplies and technical personnel 24 hours a day, 7 days a week
Capability for emergency cesarean delivery or hysterectomy within 30 minutes, 24 hours a day, 7 days a week

A2. Obstetric hemorrhage is bleeding from the *reproductive tract (cervix, placenta, vagina, or uterus)* during pregnancy or postpartum.

A3. Blood loss with obstetric hemorrhage may be visible or *concealed*.

A4. With obstetric hemorrhage, clinically significant blood loss may occur before signs of *shock* appear in the woman.

A5. True

A6.
Yes	No	
X	___	Get help immediately.
X	___	Check her blood pressure.
X	___	Insert large-bore intravenous lines.
X	___	Begin infusion of saline solutions.
X	___	Type and crossmatch blood.
X	___	Obtain a tube of blood; tape it to the patient's bed.
X	___	Give oxygen by mask to the pregnant woman.

A7. Any bleeding during pregnancy should be investigated in a hospital, without delay.

Self-test B

B1. True

B2. False   *Reason:* Approximately one-third of the cases of clinically significant late-pregnancy bleeding never have a cause identified.

B3. False   *Reason:* Women with placental abruption are at high risk for disseminated intravascular coagulation. Disseminated intravascular coagulation rarely occurs with placenta previa.

B4. True

B5. True

B6. False   *Reason:* Undetected cancer of the cervix is a rare but important cause of cervical bleeding.

B7. True

B8. At least 3 of the following causes:
- Placental bleeding: placenta previa and placental abruption
- Cervical bleeding: chronic cervicitis; cervical polyps; rarely, cervical cancer; or, more rarely, cervical pregnancy
- Unknown causes

B9.

	Placenta Previa	Placental Abruption	Neither
Multifetal gestation	X	X (with second twin)	
Acute abdominal trauma		X	
Maternal cocaine use		X	
Maternal diabetes mellitus		X	X
Uterine fibroids	X	X	
Multiparous woman	X	X	
Occurred in a previous pregnancy	X	X	
Previous cesarean delivery	X		
Maternal hypertension		X	
Abnormal fetal presentation	X		
First pregnancy			X
Short umbilical cord		X	
Maternal smoking		X	
Polyhydramnios		X (with sudden decompression when membranes rupture)	

Self-test C

C1.

Finding	Placenta Previa	Placental Abruption
Blood color	Bright red	Dark red—old clots
Pain	Painless	Painful
Uterine tenderness	Absent	Present
Uterine tone	Normal	Increased—firm, hard, rigid
Shock	Uncommon	Frequent
Disseminated intravascular coagulation	Very rare	Frequent

Note: The findings for question C1 show the classic characteristics of these placental abnormalities. Findings, however, may vary for an individual woman.

C2. If placenta previa is present, the examining finger may disrupt the placental attachment to the lower uterine segment, which may start or worsen bleeding, sometimes with a dramatic increase in the volume of blood lost. A digital examination should not be done until you are certain a previa is not present.

C3. Placental abruption is present, with active bleeding and accumulation of blood concealed behind the placenta.

C4. True

C5. True

C6. True

C7. False *Reason:* Uterine tenderness is usually present with placental abruption but rarely with placenta previa.

C8.
Yes	No	
X	___	Prothrombin time and partial thromboplastin time
X	___	Complete blood cell count
___	X	Serum electrolytes
X	___	Platelet count
___	X	Blood urea nitrogen and creatinine concentration
X	___	Fibrinogen concentration

Self-test D

D1. True

D2. False *Reason:* Vaginal delivery is often possible with grade 1 abruptions and may be possible with grade 3 abruptions.

D3. False *Reason:* A placenta that covers the cervical os early in pregnancy usually does not cover the os at term.

D4. False *Reason:* A declining platelet count and fibrinogen level are hallmarks of disseminated intravascular coagulation with placental abruption.

D5. True

D6.
Yes	No	
X	___	Preterm delivery may be necessary.
X	___	Placenta accreta may be present and may necessitate a hysterectomy after delivery.
___	X	Preeclampsia is likely to occur.
X	___	If bleeding occurs, the woman and fetus can lose large amounts of blood.
X	___	Postpartum hemorrhage is more likely to occur.
___	X	Disseminated intravascular coagulation is likely to develop.

D7. B. Hospitalize the woman and continue observation until fetal maturity is achieved, unless bleeding or labor ensues and necessitates cesarean delivery.

Self-test E

E1. True

E2. False *Reason:* Any pregnant woman, especially one with disseminated intravascular coagulation, should not be transferred in unstable condition.

E3. True

E4. True

E5. Administer blood components to provide plasma coagulation (clotting) factors.
Stabilize the woman's condition.
Deliver the baby.

E6. Fresh frozen plasma
Cryoprecipitate
Platelets

E7. A. Perform cesarean delivery as soon as the platelet count is above 50,000/mm^3 and the fibrinogen level is above 100 mg/dL.

E8. Provide neonatal resuscitation, as needed.
Assess the baby for signs of acute blood loss.
Check the baby's blood pressure.
Provide blood volume replacement, if necessary.
Check the central (not heel-stick) hematocrit value soon after delivery.

Self-test F

F1. True

F2. False *Reason:* Intravenous injection of undiluted oxytocin can cause maternal cardiac arrhythmia and hypotension.

F3. True

F4. True

F5. False *Reason:* Bleeding is likely to worsen dramatically as soon as the placenta is removed. It should not be removed until just before you begin to try to re-invert the uterus.

F6. False *Reason:* Oxytocin (or any uterotonic medication) will make the uterus harder to manipulate and therefore should not be administered until the uterus has been re-inverted. As soon as the uterus is back in its normal position, begin the administration of uterotonic medications.

F7. Administer oxytocin and methylergonovine or provide misoprostol after delivery of the placenta.
Inspect the placenta for missing pieces.
Inspect the birth canal for tears.
Provide intensive monitoring during the first hour after delivery.

F8. Methylergonovine should not be administered to women who have *hypertension (from any cause)* or *symptomatic heart disease*.

F9. A steady, slow, unrelenting flow of blood postpartum suggests *there are retained placental fragments*.

F10. Any 3 of the following causes:
- Uterine atony
- Retained pieces of the placenta
- Birth canal tears
- Uterine rupture
- Abnormal maternal blood clotting
- Uterine inversion

F11. If uterine inversion occurs, uterotonic medication should be administered *after* the uterus is restored to its normal position.

Unit 2 Posttest

After completion of each unit there is a free online posttest available at www.cmevillage.com to test your understanding. Navigate to the PCEP pages on www.cmevillage.com and register to take the free posttests.

Once registered on the website and after completing all the unit posttests, pay the book exam fee ($15) and pass the test at 80% or greater to earn continuing education credits. Only start the PCEP book exam if you have time to complete it. If you take the book exam and are not connected to a printer, either print your certificate to a .pdf file and save it to print later or come back to www.cmevillage.com at any time and print a copy of your educational transcript.

Credits are only available by book, not by individual unit within the books. Available credits for completion of each book exam are as follows: Book 1: 14.5 credits; Book 2: 16 credits; Book 3: 17 credits; Book 4: 9 credits.

For more details, navigate to the PCEP webpages at www.cmevillage.com.

Unit 3: Infectious Diseases in Pregnancy

Objectives 85

1. What risks are associated with infectious diseases during pregnancy? 88
2. What factors determine how a perinatal infection will affect the fetus? 88
3. How are perinatal infections managed? 92
   - A. Sexually transmitted infections that may affect a fetus 92
     1. Chlamydia 92
     2. Gonorrhea 95
     3. Herpes simplex virus (HSV-1 or HSV-2) 96
     4. HIV 100
     5. Human papillomavirus 104
     6. Syphilis 105
   - B. Other maternal infections that may affect a fetus 110
     1. Cytomegalovirus 110
     2. Hepatitis A virus 115
     3. Hepatitis B virus 115
     4. Hepatitis C virus 117
     5. Listeriosis 118
     6. Parvovirus B19 (fifth disease or erythema infectiosum) 119
     7. Rubella (German measles) 120
     8. Group B streptococcus 123
     9. Toxoplasmosis 129
     10. Tuberculosis 130
     11. Varicella-zoster virus (chickenpox) 133
     12. Coronavirus disease 2019 (COVID-19) 135
   - C. Sites of maternal infection with a variety of causative organisms 137
     1. Bacterial vaginosis 137
     2. Urinary tract infection and acute pyelonephritis 137
     3. Intra-amniotic infection 139
     4. Puerperal endometritis 139
     5. Group A streptococcus 140
     6. Mastitis 141

Tables and Figures

Table 3.1. Antimicrobial Medications That Should Be Avoided or
Used With Caution During Pregnancy or Lactation 91

Table 3.2. Sexually Transmitted Infections That May Affect a Fetus 93

Table 3.3. Recommendations for Medication Management at Delivery and
Route of Delivery for Women With HIV Infection 103

Table 3.4. Penicillin Treatment of Syphilis During Pregnancy 107

Table 3.5. Other Maternal Infections That May Affect a Fetus 110

Figure 3.1. Algorithm for Screening for Group B Streptococcal (GBS)
Colonization and Use of Intrapartum Prophylaxis for
Women With Preterm Labor 126

Figure 3.2. Algorithm for Screening for Group B Streptococcal (GBS)
Colonization and Use of Intrapartum Prophylaxis for Women
With Preterm Rupture of Membranes 127

Figure 3.3. Intrapartum Antibiotic Prophylaxis Regimen for Women
Colonized with Group B Streptococcus (GBS) 128

Recommended Routines 143

UNIT 3: INFECTIOUS DISEASES IN PREGNANCY

Objectives

In this unit you will learn

A. Which infections are particularly important during pregnancy and after delivery

B. What factors govern the effects of infection on a woman and her fetus and newborn

C. What risks perinatal infections pose to a woman and her fetus and newborn

D. How perinatal infections are transmitted

E. How various perinatal infections are treated

F. Antimicrobial therapy that should, and should not, be used during pregnancy

G. What should be done for the woman, and for the newborn after delivery, if infection is suspected or identified

Note: This unit is a bit different from other units in this book. Unlike the other units, which provide information important in the day-to-day care of women and newborns, many of the infections presented herein are uncommon, and some are rare.

Information concerning these infections is important, however, because perinatal infections are responsible for a large portion of maternal, fetal, and neonatal mortality and morbidity. Nevertheless, a specific infection may be encountered infrequently, or never, by an individual perinatal care practitioner.

Material in this unit is intended to be consistent with American Academy of Pediatrics, American College of Obstetricians and Gynecologists. *Guidelines for Perinatal Care*. Kilpatrick SJ, Papile L, Macones GA, Watterberg KL, eds. 8th ed. American Academy of Pediatrics; 2017; American Academy of Pediatrics. *Red Book: 2021 Report of the Committee on Infectious Diseases*. Kimberlin DW, Barnett ED, Lynfield R, Sawyer MH, eds. 32nd ed. American Academy of Pediatrics; 2021; and various statements issued by the Centers for Disease Control and Prevention, American College of Obstetricians and Gynecologists, and American Academy of Pediatrics. However, you are also encouraged to consult the most recent version of those publications and documents for any specific infection.

Unit 3 Pretest

Before reading the unit, please answer the following questions. Select the *one best* answer to each question (unless otherwise instructed). Record your answers on the test and check them with the answers at the end of the book.

1. Which of the following babies should be isolated from other babies?

   Yes   No
   ___   ___   A baby with congenital rubella infection
   ___   ___   A baby with chlamydial conjunctivitis
   ___   ___   A baby whose mother has untreated gonorrhea at the time of delivery
   ___   ___   A baby with suspected herpes infection
   ___   ___   A baby with congenital cytomegalovirus infection

2. A 32-year-old primigravida woman has active genital herpes. Her membranes rupture at 38 weeks of gestation. Two hours later, she comes to the hospital, but she is not in labor. What should be done?
   A. Bed rest and antiviral therapy
   B. Cesarean delivery as soon as possible
   C. Induce labor with oxytocin
   D. Biophysical profile to assess fetal well-being

3. True False If a mother is a carrier of hepatitis B, the only neonatal treatment available is to isolate the baby from the mother.

4. True False Positive urine culture results, whether or not a pregnant woman has symptoms, should be treated with appropriate antibiotics.

5. True False A woman with gonorrhea is at increased risk for premature rupture of the amniotic membranes.

6. True False Transplacental infection of the fetus always causes congenital malformations.

7. True False Reinfection is the most common reason sexually transmitted infections recur in a person.

8. True False Erythromycin ophthalmic ointment will effectively treat chlamydial conjunctivitis in a newborn.

9. True False Penicillin is the drug of choice for treatment of gonorrhea.

10. True False If a woman has intra-amniotic infection, the baby is at risk for neonatal sepsis.

11. True False In general, women with puerperal mastitis may continue to breastfeed, as long as antibiotics have been started and an abscess has not formed.

12. All of the following statements about human papillomavirus are correct, except
    A. Women with papillomavirus infection are at increased risk for cervical dysplasia.
    B. Genital papillomas occasionally grow large enough to interfere with vaginal delivery.
    C. Babies born to women with human papillomavirus infection may develop laryngeal papillomas at several years of age.
    D. All genital papillomas should be surgically removed.

13. Which of the following statements about syphilis is true?
    A. Babies with congenital syphilis always have a characteristic facial appearance.
    B. Pregnant women with syphilis can pass the infection to their fetuses only during the primary stage of their infection.
    C. Penicillin is the only drug that reliably cures syphilis in the mother and fetus.
    D. Fetal infection in early pregnancy rarely results in permanent damage if proper treatment is started soon after birth.

14. Although most babies are born healthy, transplacental infection with parvovirus puts the fetus at risk for
    A. Developing severe anemia
    B. Developing congenital malformations
    C. Becoming a chronic carrier of the virus
    D. Developing thrombocytopenia

15. All of the following statements about colonization of the maternal genital tract with group B streptococcus are correct, except
    A. Neonatal illness is seldom life-threatening.
    B. Risk for postpartum endometritis is increased.
    C. Antibiotics administered intravenously to a woman during labor can significantly reduce the likelihood the baby will become infected.
    D. Many women have no symptoms.

16. **True   False**   If an acute toxoplasmosis infection is identified during pregnancy, maternal treatment may reduce transmission to the fetus.

17. **True   False**   Congenital rubella infection in the first trimester frequently causes severe, permanent damage to the fetus.

18. All of the following conditions increase the risk for puerperal endometritis, except
    A. Chlamydia infection
    B. Group B β-hemolytic streptococci colonization
    C. Chorioamnionitis
    D. Hepatitis B infection

19. Which of the following statements about HIV infection is true?
    A. All babies born to HIV-positive women will be infected with the virus.
    B. Drug therapy given to an HIV-positive woman during pregnancy and labor, and to the baby after birth, can reduce the number of babies who become infected with the virus.
    C. Women rarely become infected with HIV through injected drug use and sharing of needles.
    D. Cesarean delivery should be avoided in HIV-positive women.

1. What risks are associated with infectious diseases during pregnancy?

Perinatal infections may cause one or more of the following complications:

- Maternal illness
  — Permanent damage to one or more organ systems may occur.
  — Chronic disease may develop.
- Maternal death
- Fetal malformations
- Fetal growth restriction
- Fetal death
- Premature labor
- Life-threatening neonatal illness

Some infections important in the perinatal period may also cause serious illness in non-pregnant adults and children. Care should be taken to protect yourself, your coworkers, and other patients from transmission of infectious organisms.

Observe strict blood and secretion precautions for every delivery.

Standard precautions should be followed at all times, for all patients.

Notify all perinatal personnel (nursing, medical, and support staff) of any suspected or documented maternal infection as soon as it is identified. If the woman or baby will move to another care area after delivery, be sure personnel in that area(s) are aware of the infection before transfer of the mother or baby.

2. What factors determine how a perinatal infection will affect the fetus?

Fetal effects from maternally acquired infections can vary widely. The following factors work alone and in combination to influence the effect an infection has on a fetus or newborn:

- Transmission route
- Gestational age at the time of transmission
- Specific organism
- Individual maternal or neonatal immunity
- Degree of maternal illness
- Treatment administered

    A. Transmission route and timing

    1. Transmission route
       Some infectious agents can be passed from a woman to her fetus or newborn through only one mode of transmission. Other infections can be passed by more than one route. Routes of transmission are
       a. Transplacental
          Organisms in a woman's bloodstream infect the placenta and then enter the fetus's bloodstream. The organisms that have the capability of crossing the placenta and

infecting the fetus include viruses, parasites, and some bacteria, and these may have devastating effects in the fetus.

    b. Ascending
Organisms in a woman's lower genital tract cause infection of the amniotic cavity and uterus, most often after the membranes have ruptured, but occasionally through intact amniotic membranes. This can result in serious fetal and neonatal infection or postpartum uterine infection (endometritis).

    c. Vaginal delivery
Organisms in the birth canal come in direct contact with the baby and may enter through mucous membranes, breaks in the skin, or the umbilicus.

    d. Postpartum
Some organisms—most commonly viruses—may be passed from mother to baby in breast milk, and in these rare cases, breastfeeding is contraindicated. Infections may be transmitted from the mother or other caregivers by any of the ways that infections are passed from person to person (eg, droplet, direct contact).

2. Timing of transmission

The time during gestation at which infection occurs may influence the effects an organism has on a fetus or newborn. Infection by the same organism at different gestational ages may have different effects.

Early in pregnancy, when fetal organ systems are forming, transplacental infection may interfere with normal development and result in congenital malformations. Infection with the same organism during late pregnancy may have no effect at all on the fetus, effects that are much less severe, or effects that do not become apparent for months or years.

Infections acquired at or near the time of delivery (ascending, vaginal delivery, or postpartum transmission) will not cause deformities but may result in life-threatening neonatal sepsis. Neonatal infection in preterm babies is likely to be more severe than infection with the same organism in term babies.

B. Specific organism and host factors

1. Specific organism

Fetal or neonatal infection with a specific organism may have manifestations and outcomes that are different than with adult illness caused by the same organism. Some organisms (particularly viruses) cause mild illness in an adult but may cause congenital malformations and permanent damage to the brain and other organs in a fetus. Other pathogens may be present in a woman's genitourinary tract without causing her to have symptoms and will not affect fetal development but may cause life-threatening sepsis in a newborn.

2. Immune system protection

    a. Against specific organisms
During her lifetime, a woman will make antibodies to specific organisms to which she has been exposed. These antibodies may reduce the severity of or provide protection against subsequent (secondary) infections with the same organism and may therefore also protect the fetus if maternal antibodies cross the placenta in sufficient quantities.

A fetus is particularly at risk for adverse consequences from a primary (initial) maternal infection with an organism that can be passed transplacentally when this infection occurs in the first trimester. The woman will not have previously developed antibodies against the organism and, thus, her immune system can offer little protection to herself or her fetus. If fetal infection occurs, it may cause severe, permanent damage, but not all fetuses in this situation become infected. While it is not fully understood why some fetuses are not affected by primary maternal infection, various protective factors, including placental defenses, are thought to contribute.

b. Passed to the fetus

Most maternal antibodies cross the placenta in the second half of pregnancy, creating some degree of passive immunity for the fetus and newborn. The newborn immune system is not fully functional at birth, with preterm babies having a less effective system than term babies. Maternal antibodies that cross the placenta may help protect the baby from infections during the first 3 to 6 months after birth. By then, the baby's immune system is functioning as effectively as an adult immune system.

Because most maternal antibodies cross the placenta late in pregnancy, babies born before term will not have received maternal antibodies for the same length of time as babies born at term. For these and other reasons, preterm babies are at higher risk for neonatal infection than term babies (see Book 3: Neonatal Care, Unit 8, Infections).

C. Maternal illness

The effect an infection has on a fetus often does not correlate with how sick the pregnant woman is with the infection.

- Serious maternal illness may not affect the fetus, or it may cause indirect effects if the woman has a high fever, becomes dehydrated, or develops systemic complications.
- Mild or asymptomatic viral illness in a woman early in pregnancy may have profound, irreversible effects on the fetus.
- Systemic infection in a woman may cause premature labor, even if the infection does not involve the placenta, membranes, or fetus.

D. Treatment administered

Antimicrobial drug therapy is provided for several reasons.

- Treat and cure maternal illness.
- Reduce or prevent maternal signs and symptoms that may affect the fetus.
- Reduce or prevent exposure of the fetus to the infecting organism.
- Minimize effects of infection on the fetus.

Be aware that treatment is not available for all perinatal infections. For infections that can be treated, recommendations for specific medications accompany the description of each infection. Medication dosages given in this unit are for use during pregnancy and the immediate postpartum period.

Due to changes in metabolism and expanded blood volume, drug levels are generally lower in pregnant women than in non-pregnant women. All antibiotics cross the placenta to the fetus but in varying amounts, depending on fetal gestational age and the chemical structure of the drug.

Certain antimicrobial medications, or families of drugs, should be *avoided* during pregnancy or lactation, if possible. Use during pregnancy should have individualized consideration of the risks and benefits to the woman and fetus. Alternate medications that might provide needed therapy should also be explored. Drugs to avoid are listed in Table 3.1.

Table 3.1. Antimicrobial Medications That Should Be Avoided or Used With Caution During Pregnancy or Lactation		
	Possible Adverse Effects	
Drug	**During Pregnancy**	**During Lactation**
Amantadine	Association with cardiac defects if given during the first trimester	This agent is a dopamine agonist that may impair prolactin secretion; thus, use of this agent during breastfeeding is generally avoided.
Aminoglycosides (especially streptomycin and kanamycin)	May cause eighth cranial nerve damage in the fetus (hearing impairment in the baby)	Poor excretion into human (breast) milk. Neonatal intestinal absorption is poor. There are no known ototoxic effects. May affect neonatal GI flora.
Fluoroquinolones (eg, ciprofloxacin)	Cartilage and bone toxicity have been observed in animal studies	Insufficient data are available to make a recommendation
Isoniazid	Crosses the placenta but does not appear to increase the risk of birth defects.	Usually compatible with breastfeeding. Both isoniazid and acetylisoniazid are excreted into the breast milk, but no hepatotoxicity has been reported in babies. Some experts recommend pyridoxine HCl for the baby.
Metronidazole	In vitro mutagenic effects can occur, but this drug is considered safe during pregnancy.	Discontinue breastfeeding during maternal therapy and for 12–24 hours after single-dose therapy, to allow excretion of the drug.
Nitrofurantoin	Hemolysis can occur in a baby with G6PD deficiency	Usually compatible with breastfeeding; toxicity may be observed in preterm infants and those less than 1 month old.
Ribavirin	Teratogenic and embryotoxic	Has been used in neonates to treat RSV infections; the amount present in breast milk is expected to be lower but has not been studied.
Sulfonamides	The risk occurs mainly in the third trimester; the drug increases the risks of neonatal hyperbilirubinemia by interfering with the binding capacity of albumin, thus increasing the amount of unbound bilirubin (see Book 3: Neonatal Care, Unit 7, Hyperbilirubinemia).	Pass into the breast milk. There is low risk to healthy term newborns, but breastfeeding is not recommended for sick or preterm babies until maternal therapy has ended. Use caution with G6PD deficiency.
Tetracyclines	Nausea, vomiting, liver disease in the woman; impaired growth and (later) teeth stained yellow or brown in the child	There is no restriction to breastfeeding, with little or no absorption by the baby.

Abbreviations: GI, gastrointestinal; G6PD, glucose-6-phosphate dehydrogenase; HCl, hydrochloride; RSV, respiratory syncytial virus.

3. How are perinatal infections managed?

For sections A and B that follow, descriptions of specific infections are mostly listed in alphabetical order, according to the most common name of the illness or the infecting organism. Infections in section C are listed in chronological order of occurrence (ie, antepartum, intrapartum, postpartum).

  A. Sexually transmitted infections that may affect a fetus

    The U.S. Centers for Disease Control and Prevention (CDC) publishes recommendations for screening for sexually transmitted infections (STIs); in some states, testing may also be determined by state law or health department regulation. In populations with a high prevalence of STIs or risk factors for STIs, it may be reasonable to implement universal screening. Table 3.2 summarizes current CDC recommendations for STI screening. If an infection is present, maternal treatment may significantly influence neonatal outcome. Women who receive a diagnosis of an STI may have also been exposed to other STIs by their partner and should be tested and treated according to CDC guidelines.

 If one sexually transmitted infection is identified, investigate for others, especially chlamydia, gonorrhea, herpes, HIV, and syphilis.

If an STI that was treated early in pregnancy recurs, take the following steps:
- Reevaluate the treatment that was administered.
- Reassess whether all sexual partners were identified.
- Treat or re-treat partners as necessary. Know the legal status of *expedited partner treatment* in your state.
- Re-treat the woman with the same or different medication, depending on your findings, and then
  — Retest to see if the therapy has been effective.
  — Evaluate the woman for occurrence of nonconsensual sex.

Although failure of treatment does occur (for some infections more often than others), *recurrence of most STIs results most often from reinfection from exposure to an inadequately treated partner.*

The exceptions are

- Herpes simplex virus (HSV) or human papillomavirus (HPV) infections, which are likely to recur locally because even optimal treatment does not eliminate these viruses from the body.

and

- HIV, which will persist systemically because treatment may slow progression of the disease but does not eliminate the virus.

  1. Chlamydia
- *Disease in women: Chlamydia trachomatis* is the most common reportable STI in the United States. Infected women are often asymptomatic but may have urethritis or mucopurulent cervical infection. Untreated or recurrent *Chlamydia* infection may lead to premature rupture of membranes, which significantly increases the risk for preterm birth. Chlamydia may cause pelvic inflammatory disease (PID) in nonpregnant women, with inflammation and scarring of the fallopian tubes, which may later

Table 3.2. Sexually Transmitted Infections That May Affect a Fetus

STI and Screening Recommendation in Pregnancy	Method of Transmission	Is Isolation of the Woman or Newborn Indicated?	Notes
Chlamydia trachomatis			
All women < 25 years Women over 25 years with risk factors (new partner, >1 partner, partner with an STI)	Woman: sexual Newborn: direct exposure during labor/vaginal birth	No	Risk of preterm birth increased Retest an at-risk woman in the third trimester Specific treatment needed to prevent chlamydia conjunctivitis in the newborn
Neisseria gonorrhoeae			
All women < 25 years Women over 25 years with risk factors (new partner, >1 partner, partner with an STI)	Woman: sexual Newborn: direct exposure during labor/vaginal birth	No	Risk of preterm birth increased Retest an at-risk woman in the third trimester Ophthalmic prophylaxis for all newborns Single-dose ceftriaxone for the newborn of a woman with active infection
Herpes simplex virus			
Test for the virus in symptomatic women General screening is not recommended	Woman: sexual Newborn: direct exposure during labor/vaginal birth. Postpartum mother-to-child transmission is possible from oral lesions (or from genital lesions if hand hygiene is inadequate).	If a baby is suspected of having this infection, isolate the baby from other babies and pregnant women. Perform a culture 24–48 hours after birth. Breastfeeding is OK if there are no breast lesions. Having a private room and rooming-in with the mother is OK.	Risk of preterm birth is increased with primary maternal infection. Neonatal morbidity and mortality are high. Vaginal delivery is OK if no lesions are present. Cesarean delivery is recommended when lesions are present.
HIV			
Screen all women at entry to prenatal care. Rescreen in the third trimester if a woman is at increased risk.	Woman: sexual, injection drug use Newborn: transplacental or via exposure to blood and vaginal fluid during labor in women who have increased viral load	No	Recommendations are updated regularly. Consult infectious disease specialists. www.cdc.gov www.aidsinfo.nih.gov
HPV			
Screen women according to established cervical cancer screening guidelines.	Woman: sexual Newborn: exposure to cervical and vaginal secretions	No	Neonatal genital warts and laryngeal papillomas are very rare.
Syphilis (*Treponema pallidum*)			
Screen all women at entry to prenatal care Rescreen in the third trimester if at increased risk	Woman: sexual Newborn: transplacental or via exposure during labor or vaginal birth if an active genital lesion is present	Body fluids of mother and baby may remain infectious for 24 hours after penicillin is started. Visitors, parents, and health professionals should wear gloves to handle the baby.	Penicillin is the only antibiotic that reliably treats syphilis. If the mother is allergic to penicillin, desensitize her to it. Maternal serologic status should be known before every baby's discharge.

Abbreviations: HPV, human papillomavirus; STI, sexually transmitted infection.

result in infertility and an increased risk for ectopic pregnancy. PID is uncommon in pregnancy.
- *Risks for the fetus and newborn: C trachomatis* is not known to cross the placenta. About one-half of the babies born vaginally to infected women will acquire *Chlamydia* organisms during passage through the birth canal. Ascending infection can occur, and some babies born via cesarean delivery with intact membranes will also be infected. Neonatal infection most often takes the form of conjunctivitis, developing at a few days to several weeks of age, but can also manifest as pneumonia, developing at several weeks or months of age.

a. Prenatal considerations
   - The CDC recommends screening the following groups of pregnant women for chlamydia infections at the initial visit and again in the third trimester:
     — Women younger than 25 years
     — Women with a new partner
     — Women with more than one partner or whose partner has more than one partner
     — Women whose partner has an STI
   - If a woman's chlamydia screening result is positive, treat with
     — Azithromycin, 1 g, given orally, in a single dose
     or
     — Erythromycin base, 500 mg, given orally, every 6 hours for 7 days (or, to reduce gastrointestinal side effects, 250 mg, given orally, every 6 hours for 14 days)
     Note: Erythromycin estolate is contraindicated during pregnancy.
   - Test and treat the woman's partner(s). Investigate for other STIs.
   - Retest 3 to 4 weeks after the completion of antibiotic therapy and again 3 months after treatment to screen for reinfection.

b. Intrapartum considerations
   If antibiotic treatment was started earlier but is not yet complete, continue treatment.

c. Postpartum considerations
   Maternal
   - Reassess maternal treatment and be sure it is adequate prior to discharge.
   - Women with inadequately treated infection have an increased risk for postpartum endometritis. Onset may be soon after delivery or as late as 1 to 2 weeks after birth.
   - Investigate the need to treat the woman's partner(s).

   Neonatal (See also Book 3: Neonatal Care, Unit 8, Infections.)
   - Babies born to women with untreated or incompletely treated chlamydia infection should be monitored for development of conjunctivitis or pneumonia. Prophylactic antibiotics are *not* recommended. Cesarean delivery is performed only for usual obstetric indications.
   - Topical treatment of chlamydial conjunctivitis is ineffective. If chlamydial conjunctivitis or pneumonia develops, systemic antibiotics are needed. Administer to the baby oral erythromycin, 50 mg/kg/day, in 4 divided doses for 14 days.
   - Erythromycin is only about 80% effective, so a second course of antibiotics may be needed. Follow-up with the baby is recommended.

Routine prophylactic eye treatment with ophthalmic preparations of erythromycin, tetracycline, or silver nitrate used to prevent gonococcal eye infection will not reliably prevent chlamydial conjunctivitis.

2. Gonorrhea
   - *Disease in women:* Infection is passed by sexual contact and is highly contagious. The symptoms may be minor and include minimal vaginitis or urethritis, with or without discharge. Untreated maternal infection may lead to premature rupture of membranes, which significantly increases the risk for preterm birth. Progression to PID is unlikely during pregnancy. Although rare, systemic disease with arthritis, high fever, and abdominal pain from liver involvement can occur.
   - *Risks for the fetus and newborn: Neisseria gonorrhoeae* does not cross the placenta. Transmission to the baby usually occurs during passage through the vagina. Although rare, ascending infection can also occur through intact or ruptured membranes and cause chorioamnionitis. Neonatal infection is usually confined to the eye (if untreated, it can cause blindness) but can (rarely) become a life-threatening systemic disease, affecting multiple organs.
   a. Prenatal considerations
      - The CDC recommends screening the following groups of pregnant women for gonorrhea infections at the initial visit and again in the third trimester:
        — Women younger than 25 years
        — Women with a new partner
        — Women with more than one partner or whose partner has more than one partner
        — Women whose partner has an STI
        — Women with a prior personal history of STI
        — Women who exchange sex for money or drugs
      - An extended-spectrum (third-generation) cephalosporin is recommended as initial therapy for all patients.
        — Ceftriaxone, 500 mg, administered intramuscularly, in a single dose (preferred because of its effectiveness in treating all infection sites, including the pharynx)
          or
        — Spectinomycin, 2 g, administered intramuscularly, in a single dose (for those who cannot tolerate a cephalosporin)
          plus
        — Azithromycin, 1,000 mg, given orally, in a single dose, for concurrent coverage for *Chlamydia* infections and for coverage of resistant strains of *N gonorrhoeae*. (*Chlamydia* infection is common and may be presumed to be present without testing for it.)
      - A test of cure is not routinely done for uncomplicated urogenital gonorrhea, but it is recommended for pharyngeal gonorrhea.
      - Test and treat the woman's partner(s). Investigate for other STIs.
      - Retest 3 months after treatment to screen for reinfection.

b. Intrapartum considerations
   If the woman is inadequately treated at the time of labor, use internal fetal monitoring judiciously because a scalp abscess may develop at the site where the electrode is attached.
c. Postpartum considerations
   Maternal
   - The risk for endometritis is increased if active infection is present at the time of delivery. Administer a single dose of ceftriaxone, intramuscularly, soon after delivery.
   - Reassess maternal treatment and be sure it is adequate prior to discharge.
   - Investigate the need to treat the woman's partner(s). Presumptive treatment of all previously untreated partners is recommended.

   Neonatal (see also Book 3: Neonatal Care, Unit 8, Infections)
   - Provide routine prophylactic eye treatment to *all* newborns with ophthalmic preparation of 1% tetracycline, 0.5% erythromycin, or 1% silver nitrate *to prevent* gonococcal ophthalmia neonatorum. Infection can cause blindness.

    Do not irrigate the baby's eyes after instillation. After 1 minute, excess medication may be wiped away with sterile cotton.

   - If maternal gonococcal infection is active at the time of delivery, give the baby a single dose of ceftriaxone, 25 to 50 mg/kg (not to exceed 125 mg), intravenously or intramuscularly.
   - If infection develops, topical antibiotic therapy will *not treat* it adequately. Systemic antibiotics are needed for treatment. The baby should be hospitalized for complete evaluation and treatment.

3. Herpes simplex virus (HSV-1 or HSV-2)
   - *Disease in women:* HSV infection is extremely common. The CDC estimates that 16% of adults in the United States are infected, with most unaware of their infection. The virus, once acquired, remains for the person's lifetime. It may be latent and asymptomatic for long periods, broken by episodes of recurrence of symptoms. Primary infection usually causes painful genital vesicles but may also be relatively asymptomatic. Recurrent infection is usually less symptomatic. Asymptomatic viral shedding is common in men and women, with most herpes infections transmitted by sexual contact during asymptomatic periods.
   - *Risks for the fetus and newborn:* Transplacental transmission is rare but can occur at any time during pregnancy. Transmission to the baby usually occurs via direct contact with lesions or virus shed from the cervix or lower genital tract during passage through the birth canal. Ascending infection, though uncommon, also can occur, even with intact membranes. Risk of transmission to the newborn during vaginal delivery is much lower for recurrent (1%–2%) than for primary (33%–50%) infections. Neonatal herpes infection carries a high risk of mortality and severe damage in the survivors, even when antiviral therapy is provided. Presentation is split about equally among
     — Disseminated disease involving multiple organs, particularly the lungs and liver
     — Disease localized to the central nervous system
     — Disease localized to the skin, eyes, and mouth

a. Prenatal considerations
- If lesions occur during pregnancy, obtain culture specimens from the lesions.
- Clinical evaluation, laboratory testing of fluid from the lesion, and type-specific (HSV-1 or HSV-2) serology are important for disease classification and, therefore, patient management. Clinical evaluation alone is frequently unable to indicate infection.
- Oral acyclovir or valacyclovir is used to treat initial or recurrent infection. Treatment may be episodic or suppressive therapy. Consultation should be considered.
- Prophylactic treatment with acyclovir in late pregnancy reduces the number of recurrences at term and reduces the need for cesarean delivery.
- Intravenous (IV) acyclovir is used for patients with complicated or severe infection.
- Treatment with topical acyclovir ointment is ineffective.

Optimal prenatal, intrapartum, and neonatal care depends on identification of maternal infection as primary, non-primary first episode, or recurrent episode. Consultation with regional perinatal center experts is recommended.

b. Intrapartum considerations
- Women with active genital herpes at the onset of labor (any visible herpes lesion in the lower genital tract) should be counseled to undergo cesarean delivery. Women with a prior history of genital herpes but no active lesions at the time of labor may deliver vaginally. If membranes rupture at or near term in a woman with active genital HSV infection, *prompt* cesarean delivery is recommended.
- There is no evidence that a particular duration of rupture of membranes exists beyond which the fetus does not benefit from cesarean delivery. Even if a woman presents with prolonged rupture of membranes, cesarean delivery is recommended if active lesions are present.
- Appropriate management with preterm premature rupture of membranes, fetal lung immaturity, and active maternal HSV infection is unclear. Some experts recommend IV acyclovir in this situation, especially when the fetus is extremely preterm and may benefit from corticosteroids for fetal lung maturation and delayed delivery. Consult with regional perinatal center specialists.
- Avoid internal fetal monitoring whenever possible in women suspected of having active genital herpes.
- If active lesions, genital or non-genital, are present, contact precautions (in addition to standard precautions) should be used during labor, delivery, and postpartum care.

c. Postpartum considerations
Maternal
- If maternal lesions are present, the baby may room-in with the mother. *Good handwashing* techniques should be used, and maternal lesions should be covered with an occlusive barrier. Educate parents and caregivers about the importance of good handwashing at home.
- If there are no breast lesions, the mother may breastfeed.
- If oral cold sores are present, the mother should use caution to avoid transmission

of the virus to her baby until the lesions have crusted and dried. Such cautions may include not kissing the baby and careful hand hygiene, especially at the time of diaper changing.

Neonatal (See also Book 3: Neonatal Care, Unit 8, Infections.)
- Isolate any newborn suspected of having HSV infection from all other babies and pregnant women. This may occur in a single-patient room with mother and baby rooming-in continuously. Use standard precautions, as well as contact precautions if lesions are present.
- The risk of neonatal HSV infection ranges from less than 5% in the setting of recurrent maternal infection to more than 50% when the woman has a primary outbreak.
- Symptoms of systemic or central nervous system infection may be present shortly after birth or not appear until as late as 4 to 6 weeks of age. Infected babies do not always develop skin lesions during the neonatal period.
- Refer to Book 3, Neonatal Care, Unit 8, Infections, and other resources for specific guidance regarding testing and treatment for possible HSV infection in a newborn.
- Consider delaying circumcision for a month in boys born vaginally to women with active genital lesions, because herpes infection is more likely to occur at a site of skin trauma.
- Teach parents about signs of late-onset neonatal herpes infection, including rash or skin lesions, respiratory distress, seizures, or general signs of illness, and counsel them to seek *immediate* care if any signs develop.

Most babies who develop herpes infection are born to women with asymptomatic or unrecognized herpes simplex virus (HSV) infection.

Consultation with regional perinatal center experts on neonatal management of a baby with potential or suspected HSV infection is recommended.

Self-test A

Now answer these questions to test yourself on the information in the last section.

A1. In the following list, match each condition or situation on the left with the best choice on the right.

_____	Mother with chlamydia	a. Ceftriaxone for mother and baby
_____	Mother with active genital herpes	b. Cesarean delivery
_____	Mother with active gonorrhea	c. Asymptomatic maternal infection

A2. True False The risk of premature rupture of membranes and preterm birth is increased when a pregnant woman has gonorrhea.

A3. True False Neonatal herpes infection is life-threatening.

A4. True False When a pregnant woman has an infection, any organism in her bloodstream will cross the placenta and infect the fetus.

A5. True False Internal fetal heart rate monitoring should be avoided with maternal gonorrhea.

A6. True False Ascending infection can occur only after rupture of membranes.

A7. True False Silver nitrate or certain ophthalmic antibiotic ointments are used to treat gonococcal ophthalmia neonatorum.

A8. True False Women with untreated chlamydia infection have an increased risk for developing endometritis after birth.

A9. True False Routine prophylactic eye medications given to prevent gonorrheal ophthalmia will also prevent neonatal chlamydial conjunctivitis.

A10. True False A newborn suspected of being infected with herpes simplex virus should be isolated from other newborns.

A11. True False Infection by the same organism at different gestational ages may have different effects on the fetus.

A12. True False The degree of maternal illness corresponds directly with how seriously an infection will affect a fetus.

A13. If maternal gonorrhea infection is present, you should investigate for the presence of

Yes	No	
_____	_____	Toxoplasmosis
_____	_____	Syphilis
_____	_____	Chlamydia
_____	_____	Parvovirus
_____	_____	Herpes
_____	_____	HIV

Check your answers with the list that follows the Recommended Routines. Correct any incorrect answers and review the appropriate section in the unit.

4. HIV
   - *Disease in women:* Women with a history of any STI (syphilis, genital herpes, gonorrhea, or chlamydia) are at increased risk for HIV infection for 2 reasons.
     — The occurrence of one STI indicates the woman or her partner(s) has had an additional partner(s), thus increasing the risk of exposure to HIV.
     — Local inflammation of genital tissue may create a relatively easy portal of entry for the HIV virus.

   Pregnancy itself demonstrates a history of unprotected sexual intercourse. Unprotected intercourse is a common route of HIV transmission to women.

   Sharing of needles by injected drug users is also a common route of HIV transmission. It accounts for about half of all infections in women.

   Because of the extremely complex and rapidly changing management needed for maternal/fetal and neonatal HIV disease, consultation with regional perinatal center experts is strongly recommended.

   In addition, refer to recommendations from the Centers for Disease Control and Prevention (www.cdc.gov) and the National Institutes of Health (www.aidsinfo.nih.gov).

   - *Risks for the fetus and newborn:* HIV infection in pregnancy is associated with an increased risk of fetal growth restriction and preterm birth. In addition, HIV-positive women are more likely to have other infections or risk factors that may jeopardize maternal health or fetal development. The precise timing of mother-to-child transmission of HIV is unknown, but evidence suggests (in the absence of breastfeeding) that 30% of transmissions occur before birth but late in pregnancy and 70% of transmissions occur around the time of delivery. The risk of transmission is significantly correlated with higher maternal viral load.

   Both the virus and maternal antibodies can cross the placenta. All babies (100%) born to HIV-positive women will test positive for HIV antibodies of maternal origin at birth. Without appropriate treatment of women with HIV during pregnancy, 15% to 25% of babies will become infected with HIV.

   The risk of mother-to-child transmission of HIV is lowest ($\leq 1\%$) when maternal combination antiretroviral therapy (cART) is taken consistently throughout pregnancy and the maternal viral load near term is less than 1,000 copies/mL. In these women, labor and vaginal birth may be planned. Women with a viral load of at least 1,000 copies/mL should undergo a planned cesarean delivery prior to the onset of labor, preceded by a 3-hour period of IV zidovudine (ZDV) administration to minimize the risk of mother-to-child transmission.

   IV ZDV may be considered during labor for women with a viral load between 50 and 999 copies/mL. It is not thought to be necessary to administer IV ZDV during labor to women with a viral load less than 50 copies/mL, who are adherent to their cART regimen.

Antiretroviral therapy for HIV-positive women dramatically reduces the risk of neonatal infection.

a. Prenatal considerations
- Women with no known risk factors may be infected with HIV. They may not feel ill and may not be aware they are infected until neonatal HIV is diagnosed.

The American Academy of Pediatrics and the American College of Obstetricians and Gynecologists recommend routine HIV testing for all pregnant women (American Academy of Pediatrics, American College of Obstetricians and Gynecologists. Guidelines for Perinatal Care. *Kilpatrick SJ, Papile L, Macones GA, Watterberg KL, eds. 8th ed. American Academy of Pediatrics; 2017; American Academy of Pediatrics.* Red Book: 2021 Report of the Committee on Infectious Diseases. *Kimberlin DW, Brady MT, Jackson MA, Long SS, eds. 32nd ed. American Academy of Pediatrics; 2021).*

Extensive pretest counseling and informed consent may be a barrier to universal prenatal HIV testing. The CDC and the American College of Obstetricians and Gynecologists (ACOG) recommend HIV screening for all pregnant women as part of the routine panel of prenatal blood tests, after notifying them that they will be tested, unless they decline the test (ie, opt-out screening). The American Academy of Pediatrics (AAP) also endorses the recommendation of the National Academy of Medicine for universal (routine) testing, with notification. Know your state's laws, because this recommendation may conflict, in some states, with laws governing consent for testing. Women who are at increased risk for HIV infection but who test negative at the initiation of prenatal care should be retested in the third trimester.
- Women at increased risk for HIV infection include
  — Injection drug users (IV, intramuscular, intradermal) or those who exchange sex for money or drugs
  — Women exposed to contaminated blood. Blood or blood products transfused after 1983 are extremely unlikely to carry HIV. The current risk of HIV acquisition from blood transfusion is estimated to be 1 in 250,000 or lower.
  — Women with a history of any other STIs
  — Women who have had a new sex partner or more than one sex partner during this pregnancy
  — Partners of men who engage in high-risk behaviors (eg, drug use, multiple partners, same-sex partners)
  — Partners of men who are HIV positive
- If HIV is found, test for syphilis and other STIs and for tuberculosis. An HIV-positive individual is at increased risk for other infections, which should be treated immediately and, in some cases, should be treated prophylactically.
- Establish the gestational age as early and as accurately as possible by using ultrasonography (US) and clinical findings.

- Obtain a baseline plasma viral RNA load (number of viral RNA copies per milliliter of plasma) and again every 3 months during pregnancy.
- cART used routinely for nonpregnant adults is highly effective in suppressing HIV viral RNA load and is generally recommended during pregnancy. Refer to www.aidsinfo.nih.gov for the most up-to-date recommendations for antiretroviral therapy regimens, as the recommendations change regularly.

Performing cesarean delivery before the onset of labor and rupture of membranes may significantly reduce the risk of HIV transmission to the fetus or newborn in women with viral loads >1,000 copies/mL (ACOG Committee Opinion No. 751: Labor and delivery management of women with human immunodeficiency virus infection. Obstet Gynecol 2018;132[3]:e131–e137).

- Appropriate antiretroviral therapy may reduce the risk of HIV transmission to the fetus to as low as 1%. No combination of therapies can guarantee that a newborn will not become infected.
- As early in pregnancy as possible, to allow time for adequate consideration, provide information on the risks and benefits of vaginal or scheduled cesarean delivery to all HIV-positive women.
  — Cesarean delivery is associated with a higher risk of complications than vaginal delivery. Preoperative maternal health affects the degree of maternal risk associated with surgery.
  — Decision-making about delivery route needs to include the woman and to weigh the benefits to the newborn versus maternal health status and risks (Table 3.3).
  — HIV-positive women with a viral load of at least 1,000 copies/mL are at highest risk for transmission of the virus to their fetuses and newborns; therefore, their babies stand to benefit most from a planned cesarean delivery before the onset of labor. It has not been shown that babies of women with plasma viral load less than 1,000 copies/mL benefit from scheduled cesarean birth; thus, cesarean delivery should not be routinely planned solely for prevention of HIV transmission. Women with a viral load of less than 1000 copies/mL may have other indications for cesarean delivery or may request an elective cesarean delivery.
  — The reduction in mother-to-child transmission from cesarean delivery undertaken after the onset of labor is not known.
b. Intrapartum considerations
  - If labor begins spontaneously and is allowed to continue, or if vaginal delivery is the woman's chosen delivery route
    — Do not use internal fetal monitoring.
    — Limit the use of operative vaginal delivery to only those cases with a clear clinical indication.
  - Continue all scheduled antiretroviral therapy during labor, whether ZDV is indicated or not.
  - IV ZDV is not indicated if the viral load is less than 50 copies/mL. If the viral load is between 50 and 999 copies/mL, ZDV may be considered, as there may be some

Table 3.3. Recommendations for Medication Management at Delivery and Route of Delivery for Women with HIV Infection

Maternal HIV Viral Load	IV ZDV During Labor	Maternal Oral cART	Cesarean Delivery
<50 copies/mL	Not recommended	Continue during labor	Recommended for obstetric indications only
50–999 copies/mL	May be considered	Continue during labor	Recommended for obstetric indications only
≥1,000 copies/mL	Recommended: 2 mg/kg IV loading dose over 1 hour 1 mg/kg IV continuous infusion	Continue during labor	Scheduled at 38 weeks of gestation Complete ≥3 hours of ZDV infusion before delivery

Abbreviations: cART, combination antiretroviral therapy; IV, intravenous; ZDV, zidovudine.

benefit in the reduction of transmission. ZDV should be given during labor in women with a viral load of at least 1,000 copies/mL who have declined a cesarean delivery.
- Intrapartum and pre-cesarean dosage of ZDV
  — Provide a 1-hour loading dose of 2 mg/kg intravenously.
  — Follow with a continuous IV infusion of 1 mg/kg per hour until delivery.
- When planning a scheduled cesarean delivery for an HIV-positive woman, ACOG recommends that it be performed at 38 0/7 weeks to reduce the likelihood of the onset of labor or rupture of membranes before delivery.
  — Provide IV ZDV prophylaxis, starting 3 hours before surgery, to achieve adequate drug levels.
  — Provide prophylactic, presurgical antibiotic therapy according to usual practice to reduce the risk of postpartum maternal infection.

c. Postpartum considerations

Maternal
- HIV can be transmitted in breast milk. In the United States, breastfeeding is contraindicated in HIV-positive women. In low- and middle-income countries, the risk of mother-to-child HIV transmission via breast milk must be weighed against the risks of malnutrition and enteric infections from preparing infant formula with an unsafe water supply. Rooming-in is recommended, as it is for all well newborns.
- Inform neonatal care practitioners of a mother's HIV status. Know the laws in your state, however, because some states require a mother's written consent before this information can be given to anyone not a part of her own health care team—including neonatal care practitioners.

Neonatal (see also Book 3, Neonatal Care, Unit 8, Infections)
- For babies born to mothers with unknown HIV status, rapid HIV antibody testing of the mother is recommended as soon as possible after birth, with the initiation of newborn antiretroviral prophylaxis immediately if the rapid test result is positive.
- Intramuscular injections (immunizations, vitamin K) should be delayed until after the baby is thoroughly bathed to remove any maternal blood and body fluids.
- Begin ZDV treatment of the baby within 8 to 12 hours of birth and continue treatment for the first 6 weeks after birth.

Even without maternal zidovudine therapy or scheduled cesarean delivery, zidovudine treatment of the baby can significantly reduce the incidence of neonatal HIV infection.

- Test babies born to HIV-positive women with HIV RNA or DNA polymerase chain reaction assay during the first 48 hours after birth to try to identify in utero HIV transmission. Test again at 1 to 2 months, although testing at 14 days may aid in decision-making about antiretroviral therapy. Early antiviral therapy is indicated for most HIV-infected babies. Consult www.aidsinfo.nih.gov for treatment recommendations and for further information about testing and requirements for confirmation of HIV-positive or HIV-negative status in perinatally exposed babies.
- Arrange for comprehensive follow-up care for HIV-positive babies, their mothers, and their families.
- Information changes rapidly. Consult with regional perinatal center experts and refer to www.cdc.gov and www.aidsinfo.nih.gov.
- The effects of antiviral medications on the fetus and newborn are unknown. Long-term follow-up of babies born to women treated during pregnancy with antiretroviral drugs is recommended, as is reporting of these women and their newborns to the Antiretroviral Pregnancy Registry (800-258-4263 or www.apregistry.com). Follow-up of children with antiretroviral exposure should continue into adulthood.

5. Human papillomavirus
   - *Disease in women:* There are numerous papillomaviruses, several of which cause warts on the skin and mucous membranes. Genital warts are called *condylomata acuminata*. Genital HPV transmission occurs primarily by sexual contact. Infection with HPV is common (up to 40% of sexually active women). It may persist for life or be transient and clear spontaneously. About 90% of cervical cancers and a considerable proportion of vulvar, anal, and penile cancers are associated with HPV, as well as some head and neck cancers. A Papanicolaou test can be used to detect the cervical dysplasia typical of HPV infection. Other tests can be used to more specifically detect several high-risk types of HPV DNA in cervical cell samples. Cervical cancer screening strategies acknowledge the role of HPV in the etiology of cervical cancer. HPV vaccines have been approved for primary prevention of genital HPV infections and are recommended for all girls and boys between the ages of 9 and 26 years, ideally between the ages of 9 and 14 years and adults up to 45 years of age. HPV vaccination is not recommended during pregnancy. If a woman becomes pregnant during the vaccination schedule, it is recommended that she delay completion until after delivery.

     Warty lesions on the perineum may grow rapidly during pregnancy, but they rarely grow large enough to interfere with vaginal delivery. Extensive condylomata may also severely limit the distensibility of the vagina and vulva, increasing the risk of vulvovaginal lacerations, with subsequent intrapartum and postpartum bleeding.
   - *Risks for the fetus and newborn:* HPV does not cross the placenta. The fetus is unaffected by maternal infection. There is a small risk that, over months or years, a baby exposed to HPV during vaginal delivery may develop laryngeal papillomas due to aspirating vaginal secretions that contain viral particles.

a. Prenatal considerations
- Treatment focuses on elimination of the lesions that result from HPV infection, rather than elimination of the virus. Chemical or physical treatment methods are used, but lesions often recur.
- During pregnancy, genital warts may proliferate because of relative immune suppression. Treatment may be delayed until after birth to evaluate the degree of spontaneous resolution.

b. Intrapartum considerations
- Because the risk of laryngeal papillomas is low, cesarean delivery is not indicated to protect the baby from infection. Cesarean delivery may be necessary, however, if the size or location of condylomas obstructs vaginal delivery or threatens hemorrhage from lacerations.
- Notify pediatric staff of maternal infection so that follow-up of the baby for possible laryngeal papillomas can be arranged, if necessary.

c. Postpartum considerations
Maternal
Provide follow-up for cervical dysplasia. A routine cervical cytologic study (Papanicolaou test) is performed, with reflexive HPV testing for atypical results.
Neonatal (See also Book 3: Neonatal Care, Unit 8, Infections.)
Neonates born to women with HPV do not need to be managed with special precautions in the nursery.

6. Syphilis
- *Disease in women:* In the United States, the incidence of primary and secondary syphilis has been increasing steadily since 2013. Its incidence varies geographically and is more common among adults with HIV infection.
  — *Primary stage:* A chancre (painless ulcer) develops at the site of infection within *weeks* of exposure. While the chancre is present, the disease is highly contagious to sexual partners or anyone who comes in direct contact with the lesion. Chancres last 4 to 10 weeks, and then they heal spontaneously. Depending on the location of a lesion, an infected person may not be aware of its presence.
  — *Secondary stage:* Systemic disease with a widespread rash (including the palms of the hands and soles of the feet), fever, general malaise, lymphadenopathy, and splenomegaly develop 1 to 2 months after the initial infection and may last for months. The infected person may have several episodes of illness before the disease becomes latent. A flat-appearing condyloma (*condyloma lata*) may develop on the vulvar-perineal area as a sign of secondary syphilis. Syphilis can be passed to sexual partners at any time, whether the disease is active or latent. Secondary syphilis is particularly infectious, especially with direct contact with the cutaneous rash or condyloma lata.
  — *Latent stage:* Syphilis may enter a latent period of variable duration (years to decades) after untreated primary and secondary syphilis.
  — *Tertiary stage:* Involvement of the central nervous system, skin, bones, and visceral organs becomes apparent years or decades after untreated primary infection and follows secondary-stage syphilis and a subsequent asymptomatic latent period of variable duration. Sexual partners can be infected, but the rate of transmission is lower than during the primary stage.

Transplacental passage of the spirochete *Treponema pallidum* can cause spontaneous abortion, fetal death, or congenital syphilis. During the primary stage, transmission to the fetus occurs in approximately one-half of infected pregnant women and results in a high rate of fetal loss. Transplacental transmission during the secondary stage is 60% to 100%. Transplacental infection of the fetus declines as the duration of infection lengthens and, during the tertiary stage, occurs in only about 10% of infected pregnant women.

Transmission to the fetus can occur at any stage of maternal syphilis infection.

- *Risks for the fetus and newborn:* Fetal infection may involve multiple organs and may cause fetal growth restriction, nonimmune hydrops, or stillbirth. Congenital syphilis can cause varying degrees of damage to the fetal heart, spleen, liver, lung, bone, cartilage, skin, and brain tissue. Some consequences of congenital syphilis, such as eighth cranial nerve deafness, may take years to become apparent. The infection may manifest at birth as rhinitis or more severe respiratory distress, with skin rash, hepatosplenomegaly, anemia, and fever. Some babies will display the characteristic facial appearance (broad, flat face and nose), physical features, and radiographic findings of congenital syphilis. Many infected babies, however, have normal appearance and no symptoms.

  Congenital syphilis in an infected but untreated baby may not become apparent for 2 years or longer. During this time, however, serious, irreversible damage may be done to the central nervous system, bones, teeth, eyes, and other organs.
  a. Prenatal considerations
     - Screen *all* pregnant women for syphilis with a nontreponemal serologic test at the first prenatal visit and, among those at high risk for infection or reinfection, again at 28 to 36 weeks of gestation. Test and treat the women's partner(s).
     - Use Venereal Disease Research Laboratories, rapid plasma reagin, or automated reagin testing for screening tests. Some centers have adopted treponemal antibody tests for initial screening, but if this result is positive, a quantitative nontreponemal test is also needed to monitor the response to treatment. Confirm positive results with a test specific for *Treponema pallidum* (ie, fluorescent treponemal antibody absorption or microhemagglutination test for *T pallidum*).
     - All women who have syphilis should be tested for HIV infection and other STIs.
     - Treat with penicillin. (See footnote in Table 3.4.) Treatment with erythromycin is *not* recommended because it does not adequately treat the fetus.
     - Treatment in the second half of pregnancy may trigger the Jarisch-Herxheimer reaction (fever, headache, and myalgias) in the first 24 hours after treatment, which may lead to preterm birth.
     - Wear gloves if lesions are present, until 24 hours of treatment have been completed.

Only penicillin reliably treats syphilis in the mother and fetus.

UNIT 3: INFECTIOUS DISEASES IN PREGNANCY

Table 3.4. Penicillin Treatment of Syphilis During Pregnancy[a]	
Disease Stage	**Treatment**
Primary or secondary syphilis Latent syphilis < 1-yr duration	Benzathine penicillin G 2.4 million units, IM, 1 dose
Latent syphilis ≥ 1-yr duration Latent syphilis of unknown duration	Benzathine penicillin G 2.4 million units, IM, 1 dose per week for 3 weeks
Neurosyphilis (tertiary stage)	Aqueous crystalline penicillin G 3–4 million units, IV every 4 h for 10–14 d **then give** Benzathine penicillin G 2.4 million units, IM, 1 dose per week for 3 weeks

Abbreviations: IM, intramuscularly; IV, intravenously.

[a] If a woman is allergic to penicillin, she should be desensitized to it, and then treated with it. Desensitization is complicated, time-consuming, and potentially hazardous. Consult with infectious disease specialists. About 1% of women are allergic to penicillin and are at risk for a fatal reaction if they are not identified with the usual hypersensitivity testing. Use penicillin cautiously whenever penicillin-allergy status is unknown.

    b. Intrapartum considerations
- If genital lesions (chancre or condyloma lata) are present, the baby may become infected through direct contact during delivery.
- If a woman was not tested prenatally or is at risk for reinfection, test and begin treatment if results are positive.
- If a woman has a positive test result for syphilis, inform the pediatrician who is caring for the newborn so evaluation and treatment can begin promptly.

    c. Postpartum considerations
Maternal
- Reassess maternal treatment and be sure it is adequate prior to discharge.
- Investigate the need to treat the woman's partner(s).
- The mother may breastfeed if her infection was adequately treated or if she is currently undergoing adequate antibiotic therapy.
- Arrange for clinical and serologic follow-up of the woman 6 and 12 months after treatment for primary and secondary syphilis and also 24 months after treatment for latent syphilis. Consider retreatment if treatment failure is suspected.
- Teach the parent(s) that careful serial evaluation of the baby will be needed according to CDC recommendations, and treatment will be determined on the basis of these evaluations.

No newborn should be discharged from a hospital without determination of the mother's serologic status for syphilis (American Academy of Pediatrics, American College of Obstetricians and Gynecologists. Guidelines for Perinatal Care. *Kilpatrick SJ, Papile L, Macones GA, Watterberg KL, eds. 8th ed. American Academy of Pediatrics; 2017:393).*

Neonatal (See also Book 3: Neonatal Care, Unit 8, Infections.)
- Testing of cord blood or newborn sera is *not* adequate for syphilis screening because these tests can be nonreactive when the mother has syphilis.
- False-positive and false-negative test results can occur. Maternal and neonatal test results need to be interpreted jointly. Review Figure 8.3 in Book 3: Neonatal Care, Unit 8, Infections, for comprehensive interpretation guidelines.
- Infected newborns can be severely ill or completely asymptomatic at birth. Even if asymptomatic, consider body fluids infectious until 24 hours after drug therapy has started. Parents, visitors, and health professionals should wear gloves to handle the baby for any reason during that time.
- Treat an infected baby with penicillin according to guidelines given in Table 8.4 in Book 3: Neonatal Care, Unit 8, Infections.
- Arrange for follow-up examinations and testing.

Self-test B

Now answer these questions to test yourself on the information in the last section.

B1. All babies born to HIV-positive women will

Yes	No	
____	____	Test positive for HIV antibodies.
____	____	Be infected with the virus.

B2. For each of the following organisms, indicate whether the fetus may become infected during pregnancy or at the time of delivery.

Pregnancy	Delivery	
____	____	Syphilis
____	____	Herpes simplex virus
____	____	Human papillomavirus

B3. **True** **False** In the United States, it is appropriate for a woman with HIV infection to breastfeed her baby.

B4. **True** **False** Sharing of needles by injected drug users is a common route of HIV transmission to women.

B5. **True** **False** Syphilis infection can pass to the fetus only during the primary stage of maternal infection.

B6. **True** **False** Women with one sexually transmitted infection are at increased risk for having other sexually transmitted infections.

B7. **True** **False** Babies with untreated congenital syphilis may not develop signs and symptoms of the illness until 2 years or longer after birth.

B8. **True** **False** Treatment of HIV-positive women with zidovudine during pregnancy and labor or neonatal treatment after delivery significantly reduces the number of babies infected with HIV.

B9. **True** **False** Blood and body fluid precautions need to be used only for HIV-positive patients.

B10. **True** **False** When maternal human papillomavirus infection is known, neonatal treatment should begin soon after birth.

B11. Indicate whether screening of all pregnant women is recommended for these infections.

Yes	No	
____	____	HIV
____	____	Human papillomavirus
____	____	Syphilis
____	____	Gonorrhea
____	____	Herpes simplex virus

Check your answers with the list that follows the Recommended Routines. Correct any incorrect answers and review the appropriate section in the unit.

B. Other maternal infections that may affect a fetus (Table 3.5)
   1. Cytomegalovirus
      - *Disease in women:* The infection may be asymptomatic or accompanied by nonspecific, mild, flu-like symptoms, making it difficult to identify primary cytomegalovirus (CMV) infection in pregnant women. Diagnosis of primary infection is most commonly established by a change in serologic titers. After recovery from the primary infection, the virus may remain latent for years between episodes of recurrent infection. During primary or recurrent infection, the virus is shed in body fluids and may continue to be shed long after all symptoms of the illness have disappeared.

        CMV is widespread, with transmission occurring by sexual contact or contact with body fluids such as urine (changing diapers) or saliva. Most babies and children are asymptomatic, but most young children excrete the virus, thus exposing child care workers and household members to CMV. CMV-negative women should be counseled about the potential hazards of CMV infection and the particular importance of good handwashing. Routine screening of pregnant women is not recommended because of the relatively high prevalence of maternal antibodies, the potential for infection via reactivation of latent virus in antibody-positive women, and the lack of specific treatment to prevent congenital infection. Serial testing of pregnant women suspected of having been exposed to CMV, to establish seroconversion and thus identify a primary infection, may be appropriate. Maternal seroconversion and fetal infection are most commonly diagnosed after US shows features consistent with possible CMV infection.

Table 3.5. Other Maternal Infections That May Affect a Fetus				
Infection	**Transmission**		**Isolation**	**Notes**
Recommended Screening	**Woman**	**Fetus/Newborn**	**Standard Precautions (all patients, at all times)**	**(See Book 3: Neonatal Care, Unit 8, Infections, for more details of neonatal care)**
Cytomegalovirus General screening is not recommended.	• Sexual contact • Casual contact with infected fluids, including urine and saliva • Transfusion of contaminated blood (rare)	*Transplacental:* yes *Ascending:* no *Delivery:* yes; direct contact with organisms in the birth canal *Postpartum:* CMV can be transmitted in human (breast) milk (preterm babies are at higher risk).	Isolation is not needed for mother or baby. CMV is passed in breast milk but does not cause neonatal disease in term babies, probably due to passage of maternal antibodies.	Approximately 1% of all newborns are infected and excrete CMV at birth. Most babies are asymptomatic. Consult experts on breastfeeding of preterm babies by CMV-positive mothers and antiviral therapy for neonatal CMV.

(continued)

UNIT 3: INFECTIOUS DISEASES IN PREGNANCY

Table 3.5. Other Maternal Infections That May Affect a Fetus (*continued*)				
Infection	**Transmission**		**Isolation**	**Notes**
Recommended Screening	**Woman**	**Fetus/Newborn**	**Standard Precautions (all patients, at all times)**	**(See Book 3: Neonatal Care, Unit 8, Infections, for more details of neonatal care)**
Hepatitis B virus Screen all women at first prenatal visit	• Intimate contact, usually sexual (most common) • Sharing needles with users of injected drugs • Transfusion of contaminated blood (rare)	*Transplacental:* rare *Ascending:* no *Delivery:* yes; through direct contact with mother's blood *Postpartum:* yes; close personal contact with an HBsAg-positive adult or child, unless the baby is immunized	Isolation is not needed for mother or baby. Breastfeeding is not contraindicated, but breastfed babies should receive HBIG and HBV vaccine.	HBV vaccine may be given to HBsAg-negative women during pregnancy or lactation. The delivery route does not alter the transmission rate. All newborns should receive HBV vaccine, with the first dose given within 12 hours of birth. Babies born to HBsAg-positive women should also receive HBIG.
Listeriosis (*Listeria monocytogenes*)	Eating contaminated food Significantly increases risk of abortion, fetal death, preterm birth, and amnionitis	*Transplacental:* yes *Ascending:* yes *Delivery:* yes; through direct contact with mother's blood *Postpartum:* Yes; nosocomial outbreaks have occurred.	Isolation is not needed for mother or baby. Transmission in breast milk is not known to occur.	Provide prenatal instruction about foods to avoid and proper heating of prepared foods. This organism is common, but recognized infection is rare. Pregnant women, however, are at high risk for serious illness after contracting listeriosis. Maternal and neonatal mortality is high.
Parvovirus B19 (fifth disease or erythema infectiosum)	Contact with respiratory secretions or blood	*Transplacental:* yes *Ascending:* no *Delivery:* no	Isolation is not needed for mother or baby	Most babies are born healthy, but a few may have fetal anemia and heart failure from nonimmune hydrops. Affected fetuses may benefit from fetal transfusion.

(*continued*)

Table 3.5. Other Maternal Infections That May Affect a Fetus (*continued*)			
Infection	**Transmission**		**Isolation**	**Notes**
Recommended Screening	**Woman**	**Fetus/Newborn**	Standard Precautions (all patients, at all times)	(See Book 3: Neonatal Care, Unit 8, Infections, for more details of neonatal care)
Rubella (German measles)	• Droplets • Direct contact with nasopharyngeal secretions	*Transplacental:* yes *Ascending:* no *Delivery:* no	Babies with congenital rubella may shed virus for 1 year or longer. Isolate infected newborns from all babies and nonimmune adults.	Measure rubella antibodies at the first visit for every woman without documented immunity. If nonimmune, vaccinate after birth. Breastfeeding does not contraindicate maternal immunization.
Group B streptococcus Screen all women, every pregnancy, at 36 0/7–37 6/7 weeks of gestation	Sexual or direct contact Systemic maternal infection is rare. Colonization is common and increases the risk of bacteriuria, intra-amniotic infection, endometritis, preterm labor, and neonatal infection.	*Transplacental:* no *Ascending:* yes *Delivery:* yes; direct contact with organisms in the birth canal	Isolation is not needed for mother or baby	Treat all bacteriuria, whether symptomatic or not. Appropriate intrapartum maternal antibiotic therapy can dramatically reduce the risks of the following: 1. The baby becoming infected with GBS (neonatal infection is life-threatening) 2. The woman developing GBS endometritis *See Figure 3.1.*
Toxoplasmosis (*Toxoplasma gondii*) Screen all HIV-positive women	• Cats or cat feces (most common) • Raw or undercooked meat (rare) • Contaminated blood products or infected donor organs (rare)	*Transplacental:* yes *Ascending:* no *Delivery:* no	Isolation is not needed for mother or baby. No information is available about breast milk.	If infection is suspected during pregnancy, consult specialists, because treatment may reduce transmission to the fetus. Consult specialists about neonatal diagnosis, treatment, and long-term follow-up evaluation.

(*continued*)

UNIT 3: INFECTIOUS DISEASES IN PREGNANCY

Table 3.5. Other Maternal Infections That May Affect a Fetus (*continued*)				
Infection	**Transmission**		**Isolation**	**Notes**
Recommended Screening	**Woman**	**Fetus/Newborn**	**Standard Precautions (all patients, at all times)**	**(See Book 3: Neonatal Care, Unit 8, Infections, for more details of neonatal care)**
Tuberculosis Screen all high-risk women	Droplets	*Transplacental:* rare *Ascending:* no *Delivery:* aspiration or ingestion of infected maternal fluids (rare) *Postpartum:* droplets	Isolate (with respiratory precautions) women known to have or suspected of having TB. In certain situations, mother and baby may need to be separated temporarily. Delay breastfeeding (pump and discard the milk) until the mother is noncontagious (2 weeks or longer, depending on therapy). Isolate the baby (with respiratory precautions) until fully evaluated.	Treat the baby if the mother is considered to be contagious at the time of delivery. • Test mother and baby for HIV. • Consider BCG vaccine for the baby. • Consult with infectious disease specialists because prenatal and neonatal therapy is complicated. • Arrange for long-term follow-up because treatment may take 18 months for mother and baby.
Varicella-zoster virus (chickenpox)	Direct contact with respiratory droplets or skin lesions of an infected person (most common)	*Transplacental:* yes *Ascending:* no *Delivery:* yes, if the mother was infected at the time of delivery *Postpartum:* yes, if the mother develops a rash between 5 days before and 2 days after delivery	Isolate (contact, airborne, standard) women with active disease. Isolate women who receive VariZIG for 28 days. If hospitalized, isolate the baby from birth until 21 days of age, unless VariZIG was administered, in which case isolate the baby for 28 days.	Consider giving VariZIG to nonimmune pregnant women within 96 hours of exposure. If a woman develops a rash within 5 days before and 2 days after delivery, administer VariZIG to the baby as soon as possible. A term baby more than 2 days old does not need VariZIG when exposed to varicella because the risk of complications from infection is no greater than for older children.

Abbreviations: BCG, bacille Calmette-Guérin; CMV, cytomegalovirus; GBS, group B streptococcus; HBIG, hepatitis B immunoglobulin; HBsAg, hepatitis B surface antigen; HBV, hepatitis B virus; TB, tuberculosis; VariZIG, varicella-zoster immunoglobulin.

- *Risks for the fetus and newborn:* CMV transmission can occur by 3 routes.
  — *In utero,* with primary maternal infection having a significantly higher rate of transmission (approximately 40%) than recurrent illness (<1%)
  — *At birth,* through contact with vaginal fluids containing the virus
  — *After delivery,* through ingestion of CMV-positive breast milk or from transfusion of blood from a CMV-positive donor (rare)

Approximately 1% of all babies are infected in utero and excrete CMV at birth. Transplacental infection, particularly primary maternal infection during the first trimester, can cause varying degrees of damage to the fetus. Babies most severely affected (about 10% of infected fetuses) may show growth restriction, jaundice, and systemic disease, including thrombocytopenia, hepatosplenomegaly, microcephaly, intracerebral calcifications, chorioretinitis, and deafness.

Some babies with asymptomatic congenital infection or those infected at birth or soon after (clinical illness is rarely apparent) may be found later in childhood to have hearing loss, learning disability, or intellectual disability. Preterm babies are at higher risk for subsequent damage than are term babies.

a. Prenatal considerations
   - Consult with regional perinatal center specialists for assistance with diagnosis if maternal illness is suspected. Amniotic fluid or fetal blood sampling and US examination may be used to establish a prenatal diagnosis of congenital CMV infection. There is no established treatment that has been documented to prevent fetal damage or symptomatic illness in the newborn, and current antiviral drugs have limitations, side effects, and limited safety data in pregnancy.
   - If CMV infection occurs early in pregnancy, particularly if it is a woman's first infection, she may wish to consider termination of the pregnancy, based on the risks of fetal harm from infection.

b. Intrapartum considerations
   None specific to CMV infection

c. Postpartum considerations
   Maternal
   - Notify pediatric staff if maternal infection is suspected, so the baby can be evaluated.
   - Women who are CMV-positive may breastfeed their babies. Preterm newborns (<30 weeks' gestation or <1,500 g [<3 lb 5 oz]) have a higher risk for late-onset sepsis, and in these babies, the benefits of breastfeeding must be weighed against this risk. Consultation with regional perinatal center specialists about a CMV-positive mother breastfeeding her preterm neonate is recommended. Freezing and pasteurization of the milk may reduce transmission of the virus.

   Neonatal (See also Book 3: Neonatal Care, Unit 8, Infections.)
   - Determination of infection timing requires a positive viral culture result obtained within 3 weeks of birth, unless clinical signs of CMV infection are present, to be certain it is a congenital infection and not acquired during or after birth.

- Consult with regional perinatal center specialists on neonatal diagnosis, treatment, and long-term follow-up evaluation. Antiviral drugs may be appropriate.
- Evaluate the baby for congenital malformations.

2. Hepatitis A virus

    Hepatitis A virus causes a self-limited illness in the mother. It is not known to cause adverse effects for the fetus or newborn.

3. Hepatitis B virus
    - *Disease in women:* Infected persons carry the virus in all body fluids, with transmission primarily by intimate (usually sexual) contact and sharing of needles by drug users. Within households, nonsexual transmission occurs adult to child and child to child, although the exact mechanism is unknown. The virus can survive on inanimate objects for a week or longer but is killed by bleach and commonly used disinfectants. While there is no specific therapy for hepatitis B virus (HBV), most adult acute infections are self-limited, with complete recovery. Some infected persons develop chronic active hepatitis, and others become asymptomatic carriers of the virus and are therefore at risk for developing serious liver disease later in life. HBV may be transmitted during acute or chronic infection.

    Since standard precautions and vaccinations were introduced, the number of work-acquired hepatitis infections and the number of deaths from hepatitis have declined dramatically in health professionals.

    - *Risks for the fetus and newborn:* If untreated, up to one-half of the babies born to women with HBV infection will become infected, and up to 25% of those babies will eventually develop HBV-related liver disease (cirrhosis or hepatocellular carcinoma). Transplacental transmission occurs but is rare. The risk of transmission during amniocentesis is low, and this procedure is not contraindicated. Transmission seems to be mainly through direct contact with the mother's blood at the time of delivery. The rate of transmission is not affected by whether the mother is a chronic carrier or has an acute infection at the time of delivery. There is no evidence to suggest that cesarean delivery reduces the risk of transmission. Immunization of the baby and administration of hepatitis B immunoglobulin (HBIG) in the early newborn period markedly reduces the risk of infection from delivery exposures.
      a. Prenatal considerations
         - It is recommended that all pregnant women be screened with every pregnancy for HBV infection (American Academy of Pediatrics, American College of Obstetricians and Gynecologists. *Guidelines for Perinatal Care*. Kilpatrick SJ, Papile L, Macones GA, Watterberg KL, eds. 8th ed. American Academy of Pediatrics; 2017:486). More than one-third of infected adults have *no* identifiable risk factor.

    Test all pregnant women for hepatitis B surface antigen at the first prenatal visit.

- HBV vaccine should be offered to all women of reproductive age. It may be safely given to hepatitis B surface antigen (HBsAg)-negative women during pregnancy and lactation. Three doses are needed, with the second dose given 1 month and the third dose given 6 months after the first dose. Administer via intramuscular injection into the deltoid muscle, as injection into the gluteus muscle may be less effective.
- Screen other children, household contacts, and sexual partner(s) of HBsAg-positive persons. HBsAg–negative household members and partners should receive a single dose of HBIG and begin the HBV vaccine series.
- In late pregnancy, consider repeat testing of women at high risk for HBV infection.
  — Users of injected drugs and their partners
  — History of any other STI during pregnancy
  — Women with multiple sexual partners
- In women who have high HBV loads, treatment with antiviral agents in the third trimester may reduce mother-to-child transmission. Consult with specialists in liver or infectious disease, as well as maternal-fetal medicine specialists, for recommendations for managing active hepatitis B in pregnancy.

b. Intrapartum considerations
  - When women are admitted for delivery, test them if they were not screened earlier.
  - Route of delivery does not affect the rate of transmission from mother to baby.
  - Although it is not clear if internal fetal heart rate monitoring increases the rate of transmission from mother to baby, avoid internal monitoring because it is presumed to increase the risk.
  - Before delivery, notify postpartum and nursery personnel of HBsAg-positive women.

c. Postpartum considerations
  Maternal
  - Babies of HBsAg-positive mothers should receive HBV vaccine and HBIG.
  - Immunization of the baby nearly eliminates the risk of HBV infection by any route of transmission.

  Neonatal (See also Book 3: Neonatal Care, Unit 8, Infections.)
  - Wash maternal blood off the baby promptly and prior to administering injections.

All newborns should receive hepatitis B vaccine (American Academy of Pediatrics, American College of Obstetricians and Gynecologists. Guidelines for Perinatal Care. *Kilpatrick SJ, Papile L, Macones GA, Watterberg KL, eds. 8th ed. American Academy of Pediatrics; 2017:380). Babies born to hepatitis B surface antigen–positive women should also receive hepatitis B immunoglobulin.*

- HBV infection can be prevented for approximately 95% of babies born to HBsAg-positive women by administering HBIG and the HBV vaccine series.
- The first dose of hepatitis B vaccine *and* HBIG should be administered within 12 hours of birth for term and preterm babies born to HBsAg-positive women. The HBV vaccine dosage depends on the specific preparation used.
- HBV vaccine and HBIG can be administered at the same time but in different sites. Intramuscular injection into the anterolateral thigh or the deltoid muscles are the only recommended sites.
- Babies born to women whose HBsAg status is unknown should be given an HBV vaccine within 12 hours of birth. If maternal testing shows that she is HBsAg-positive, HBIG should be administered to the baby as soon as possible, within 24 hours after birth. The HBV vaccine series should be completed according to the usual schedule.
- Give the first dose of HBV vaccine series to *all* babies, according to the protocol given in Book 3: Neonatal Care, Unit 8, Infections.

4. Hepatitis C virus

In some patient populations, hepatitis C is as common as or more common than HBV. The U.S. Preventive Services Task Force and the CDC recommend universal screening for all adults and screening of women during each pregnancy for hepatitis C antibodies. Hepatitis C is usually asymptomatic in the early stages. A positive antibody test should be followed by determination of hepatitis C viral load and liver enzyme concentrations. Consultation with regional obstetric and infectious disease experts is recommended.

a. Prenatal considerations

Consult with regional perinatal center specialists, liver disease specialists, or infectious disease specialists if active maternal hepatitis C is suspected. Antiviral treatment for hepatitis C has not been established to be safe for administration during pregnancy.

b. Intrapartum considerations
- Although it is not clear if internal fetal heart rate monitoring increases the rate of transmission from mother to baby, avoid internal monitoring because of the presumed increased risk it poses.
- Currently available evidence suggests that cesarean delivery should be performed in hepatitis C virus–infected women only for standard obstetric indications.

c. Postpartum considerations

Maternal
- Women with hepatitis C may breastfeed their babies. Consult with a lactation consultant and/or reference resources for current information regarding the compatibility of maternal antiviral treatment with continued breastfeeding.
- Refer to a liver or infectious disease specialist for definitive maternal treatment.

Neonatal

Arrange follow-up testing to assess the newborn for hepatitis C congenital infection. This testing should be performed after the maternal antibodies would be expected to have cleared from the newborn's blood, which may be as long as 8 to 12 weeks after birth.

5. Listeriosis
   - *Disease in women: Listeria monocytogenes* is widespread in the environment, but infection in adults is rare and is often asymptomatic (about 2,500 reported cases of illness per year in the United States). Pregnant women, however, are much more susceptible to infection and clinical illness from *L monocytogenes*. Adult mortality for listeriosis is highly variable and depends on the patient's underlying immune status and comorbid conditions. Infection is associated with flu-like symptoms, including fever, malaise, headache, backache, abdominal pain or diarrhea, and, occasionally, more serious findings of endocarditis or encephalitis. Women can have asymptomatic vaginal and fecal reservoirs of the organism. The risk of early pregnancy loss, fetal death, preterm delivery, and chorioamnionitis is markedly increased with maternal infection.

     Most infections result from eating contaminated food. Pregnant women should avoid foods most likely to harbor *L monocytogenes*, including soft cheeses; raw or unpasteurized cow or goat milk or milk products, including blue-veined or Mexican-style cheeses; unwashed raw vegetables; undercooked poultry; leftover food; and refrigerated smoked fish. Pregnant women should not eat luncheon meats, bologna, or other delicatessen meats, or prepared meats, such as hot dogs, unless they are heated until steaming. The use of a microwave oven for cooking should be avoided, as uneven heating may occur. Because *L monocytogenes* can grow at refrigerator temperatures of 4°C (39.2°F) or colder, all precooked or ready-to-eat foods should be eaten as soon as possible.

     Canned smoked fish and meat; cottage cheese; cream cheese; hard, semisoft, or pasteurized cheeses; and food heated or reheated to steaming hot are safe to eat.
   - *Risks for the fetus and newborn:* Transplacental, ascending, and direct contact during delivery are all possible routes of transmission to the baby. Nosocomial outbreaks within nurseries have been documented. Pneumonia and septicemia are typical of early-onset neonatal disease. Late-onset (after the first postnatal week) illness probably occurs as a result of transmission during delivery but may result from environmental sources. Meningitis is typical with late-onset illness. Neonatal mortality for listeriosis is high (about 40%–50%).
     a. Prenatal considerations
        - Diagnosis can only be confirmed by positive culture results of blood or amniotic, cerebrospinal, or other body fluid. At microscopic examination, *L monocytogenes* can be mistaken for other organisms with a similar appearance, so laboratory notification that listeriosis is being considered is important.
        - IV antibiotic therapy with ampicillin for 10 to 14 days for maternal infection during pregnancy may prevent infection of the baby. Treatment of severe infection may benefit from the addition of an aminoglycoside—usually gentamicin—and a longer course (14–21 days) of therapy. *L monocytogenes* is not responsive to cephalosporins.
     b. Intrapartum considerations
        Fetal infection is often accompanied by passage of meconium before or during labor.
     c. Postpartum considerations
        Maternal
        - Abscesses may be evident within the placenta after delivery.
        - Transmission of *L monocytogenes* in breast milk is not known to occur.

Neonatal
- Symptoms are variable and vague and not unlike early and late group B streptococcus (GBS) onset. Granulomatosis infantisepticum (a red rash with scattered, small, pale microabscesses) can occur in severe neonatal infection.
- Ampicillin is highly effective against *L monocytogenes*, but gentamicin (or another aminoglycoside) is usually added.

6. Parvovirus B19 (fifth disease or erythema infectiosum)
   - *Disease in women:* Parvovirus B19 is widespread, and infection is mainly a disease of school-aged children. While there is no treatment for parvovirus B19, reinfection probably does not occur, and immunity is common. Primary infection may be asymptomatic, but findings are typically mild and include fever, myalgias, arthralgias, headache, and malaise, followed in 7 to 10 days by a rash. The rash is intensely red, with a slapped-cheek appearance on the face, but lacelike first on the trunk, and then spreading to the arms, buttocks, and thighs. The rash may come and go for weeks or months and is often less prominent in adults. Arthralgia and arthritis occur frequently in adults, especially women.

     Transmission is thought to occur via exposure to respiratory secretions and blood. Exposure to infected individuals is difficult to avoid because the infected person has viremia and is actively shedding virus prior to the onset of the rash and any other clinical symptoms. Once the rash appears, the infected person is no longer shedding the virus. Good handwashing and proper disposal of used facial tissues, especially by teachers and child care workers, may lessen the rate of transmission. Diagnosis is established with clinical evaluation and documentation of seroconversion from negative to positive antibody status.
   - *Risks for the fetus and newborn:* The virus readily crosses the placenta, but transplacental transmission is not known to cause congenital defects, even during early pregnancy infections. Early pregnancy infection may occasionally result in pregnancy loss, usually 4 to 6 weeks after maternal infection. Infection later in pregnancy may destroy immature red blood cells in the fetus, causing severe fetal anemia, which may lead to nonimmune fetal hydrops and fetal death. The degree of fetal illness is unpredictable. Most women with prenatal parvovirus B19 infection deliver healthy babies.
     a. Prenatal considerations
        - Serial US examinations should be performed to evaluate the fetus for signs of anemia, which may allow for intervention before the onset of fetal hydrops. Assessment of middle cerebral artery Doppler velocimetry is a reliable fetal anemia screening tool. Referral to a maternal-fetal medicine specialist is indicated for middle cerebral artery Doppler examination.
        - If there is suspicion for fetal anemia based on middle cerebral artery Doppler values or the presence of hydrops, referral to maternal-fetal medicine specialists for intrauterine transfusion is strongly recommended. Intrauterine transfusion(s) may be lifesaving for the fetus.
     b. Intrapartum considerations
        None specific to parvovirus

c. Postpartum considerations
Maternal
None specific to parvovirus
Neonatal
Check hematocrit values soon after birth.
7. Rubella (German measles)
- *Disease in women:* Before the widespread use of rubella vaccine, rubella was a common, mild illness, especially in children, displaying a typical pattern of rash, fever, and lymphadenopathy. Transmission occurs by exposure to respiratory droplets or direct contact with nasopharyngeal secretions. There is no treatment, but infection or immunization confers prolonged, probably lifelong, immunity. Since the introduction of rubella vaccine, the incidence of infection in the United States has declined by 99%. Outbreaks today generally occur only among college students, young adults in military or work settings, and certain underserved groups, such as migrant workers. Approximately 10% of young American adults are currently susceptible to rubella because of lack of vaccination, rather than declining immunity in those who were vaccinated. Maternal diagnosis is established with clinical condition and serologic testing.
- *Risks for the fetus and newborn:* The likelihood of transplacental transmission of the virus is high during the first trimester and somewhat lower later in pregnancy. Maternal infection, especially early during the first trimester, carries a high risk of miscarriage, fetal death, and congenital rubella syndrome, which typically includes serious visual, hearing, cardiac, and neurological disorders. Fetal growth restriction, hepatosplenomegaly, thrombocytopenia, and purpuric skin lesions may also occur. Second-trimester infection may be less damaging, but growth restriction, intellectual disability, or deafness is possible. Third-trimester infection is associated with less risk for fetal damage. Some infected babies will display little or no clinical evidence of their infection at birth but may show hearing defects, abnormal neuromuscular development, learning deficits, or behavioral disturbances later in childhood.
  a. Prenatal considerations
   - Determine immunity at the first prenatal visit for every woman who does not have documented rubella immunity.
   - Women should not be immunized during pregnancy. However, after accidental maternal vaccination, less than 2% of babies had asymptomatic infection, and none had evidence of congenital rubella syndrome.
   - If a nonimmune pregnant woman is exposed to rubella, test the woman serially to see if seroconversion occurs, indicating that infection occurred.
   - Routine use of immunoglobulin for nonimmune pregnant women exposed to rubella early in pregnancy is not recommended. Immunoglobulin may significantly reduce clinically apparent maternal infection but does not ensure prevention of fetal infection.
   - If maternal rubella infection occurs early in pregnancy, the woman may wish to consider termination of the pregnancy, based on the risks of fetal harm from infection. Accidental immunization of a pregnant woman is not an indication to recommend pregnancy termination.

b. Intrapartum considerations
Babies with congenital rubella may continue to shed the virus for a year or longer and can infect others. If congenital infection is suspected, nursery personnel should be notified, so that appropriate isolation of the baby can be instituted.

c. Postpartum considerations

Maternal
- Women who are not immune to rubella should receive rubella or measles-mumps-rubella vaccine early during the immediate postpartum period, before discharge from the hospital. Isolation of the newly immunized mother from the newborn is not indicated.
- Breastfeeding may continue in women who are receiving immunization.

Neonatal (See also Book 3: Neonatal Care, Unit 8, Infections.)
- Isolate newborns with congenital rubella from all other babies and from non-immune pregnant women and health professionals. *Contact precautions should be used for at least 1 year, unless nasopharyngeal and urine culture results are repeatedly negative.*
- Evaluate the baby for congenital malformations, particularly congenital heart defects.
- Conduct serology tests to establish the diagnosis of congenital infection (consult with regional perinatal center experts about appropriate tests and timing of testing) so that long-term follow-up and care can be planned. Most infants with congenital rubella infection are asymptomatic at birth, but over time they may develop hearing loss, vision problems, central nervous system abnormalities, or cardiac problems.

Self-test C

Now answer these questions to test yourself on the information in the last section.

C1. For which of the following maternal infections is the fetus at risk for transplacental infection?

Yes	No	
___	___	Gonorrhea
___	___	Primary parvovirus infection
___	___	Rubella (German measles)
___	___	Cytomegalovirus
___	___	Chlamydia
___	___	Listeriosis

C2. **True** **False** Maternal infection with parvovirus may cause severe fetal anemia.

C3. **True** **False** Listeriosis occurs most commonly after exposure to contaminated food.

C4. **True** **False** Hepatitis B virus vaccine is recommended for all newborns.

C5. **True** **False** Cesarean delivery decreases the rate of transmission of hepatitis B from hepatitis B surface antigen–positive women to their babies.

C6. **True** **False** Primary infection with cytomegalovirus during the first trimester can cause severe, permanent neurological damage in the fetus.

C7. **True** **False** Breastfeeding by women who are positive for hepatitis B surface antigen should be discouraged because hepatitis B is easily transmitted in breast milk.

C8. **True** **False** Cytomegalovirus rarely crosses the placenta, even during early pregnancy.

C9. **True** **False** When a mother tests positive for hepatitis B, treatment of the baby should begin within hours of birth.

C10. **True** **False** When a pregnant woman receives a diagnosis of parvovirus, treatment with acyclovir is indicated.

C11. **True** **False** A baby suspected of having or proven to have congenital rubella should be isolated from other babies.

C12. **True** **False** Hepatitis B virus screening is recommended for all pregnant women.

C13. **True** **False** Cytomegalovirus can be transmitted through sexual contact.

C14. **True** **False** Pregnant women are at much higher risk for listeriosis than are nonpregnant healthy adults.

C15. **True** **False** Maternal postpartum rubella vaccination is a contraindication to breastfeeding.

Check your answers with the list that follows the Recommended Routines. Correct any incorrect answers and review the appropriate section in the unit.

8. Group B streptococcus (See Figures 3.1–3.3 on pages 126–128.)
   (Recommendations for testing and management of GBS are based on ACOG Committee Opinion 797: Prevention of Group B Streptococcal Early Onset Disease in Newborns, February 2020)
   - *Colonization in women:* Streptococcus agalactiae, more commonly known as *group B streptococcus* or *GBS*, is a β-hemolytic gram-positive organism that asymptomatically colonizes the lower gastrointestinal tract and the genitourinary tract in 10% to 30% of women. Colonization may be brief, chronic, or intermittent, coming and going with no apparent cause.

     GBS vaginal or rectal colonization increases the risk of urinary tract infection (UTI), intra-amniotic infection, and endometritis. Urinary tract GBS infections complicate 2% to 4% of pregnancies. Systemic infection is possible, although rare, in healthy adults.
   - *Risks for the fetus and newborn:* Ascending infection from the lower genital tract to the uterus occurs most commonly during labor after the rupture of membranes, but it can also occur through intact membranes. Fetal exposure to GBS in the reproductive tract and especially to infected amniotic fluid can lead to neonatal sepsis, neonatal pneumonia, or death. Babies born to women with GBS colonization may acquire the organisms during vaginal delivery and become colonized themselves, although they usually remain asymptomatic. Less than 1% of newborns will develop symptomatic GBS infection, with preterm neonates much more susceptible than term neonates. Neonatal GBS infection (sepsis or pneumonia and, less often, meningitis, osteomyelitis, or septic arthritis) can be life-threatening for both term and preterm babies. Mortality and morbidity from GBS infection are high. Active screening and prophylaxis strategies markedly reduce the likelihood of neonatal infection.
   - *Illness and prevention in babies:* GBS disease occurs in babies in 2 forms: early onset (within first week after birth) and late onset (most infections are evident within 3 months after birth). The incidence of early-onset disease (most infections) began declining after ACOG and AAP first issued statements on prevention in the early 1990s. A decline in reported cases continued after the CDC consensus statement was published in 1996 and continued to decline until 1999, at which time a plateau in prevention efforts occurred. The current recommendations are based on research that has been conducted since these first guidelines were issued and are designed to promote further reduction in neonatal GBS disease. The incidence of late-onset GBS disease is much lower than that of early-onset illness and has not changed significantly over the past 20 years.
   a. Prenatal considerations
      - Maternal colonization early in pregnancy is not predictive of neonatal disease. Culture screening in late pregnancy can indicate women most likely to be colonized with GBS at the time of delivery and, therefore, to be at higher risk of transmitting GBS to the fetus.

        Treatment of colonization prior to the onset of labor does not eradicate GBS or prevent vertical transmission during labor.

Samples for group B streptococcus (GBS) culture should be obtained from the lower vagina and rectum at $36^{0/7}$ to $37^{6/7}$ weeks of gestation for every pregnant woman. Screen each pregnancy, regardless of a woman's GBS status in any previous pregnancy.

- Specimens may be collected by the pregnant woman or by a health professional by swabbing the lower vagina (a speculum is not needed) first and then through the anal sphincter into the rectum.
  — Women with a prior child who had early-onset neonatal GBS sepsis and women who had GBS bacteriuria any time in the current pregnancy do not require a rectovaginal culture. Either circumstance is an indication for intrapartum antibiotic prophylaxis.
  — Place the swab(s) into a nonnutritive transport medium. If separate vaginal and rectal swabs were used, both may be put in the same container because isolation of the colonization site is not important to clinical management and doing so minimizes laboratory costs.
  — Nucleic acid amplification tests are used in some centers. They offer similar sensitivity for GBS, but antibiotic sensitivity testing cannot be performed.
  — For women who are allergic to penicillin, specify that clindamycin susceptibility testing is needed if GBS is identified.
  — Follow laboratory guidelines to increase the likelihood that GBS, if present, will be identified and to determine the sensitivity to clindamycin for women who are allergic to penicillin.
- Except for asymptomatic GBS bacteriuria, antibiotics should not be used before the intrapartum period to treat asymptomatic GBS colonization.
- Treat all GBS bacteriuria with a colony count of at least 10^5 CFUs/mL.

Group B streptococcal urinary tract infections, with or without symptoms, should be treated whenever identified during pregnancy.

b. Intrapartum considerations
   IV antibiotics should be started when labor begins or when the membranes rupture for women in the following risk groups:
   - *Women with positive vaginal or rectal GBS culture results, obtained during the current pregnancy.*
   - *Women with either of the following risk factors* should also receive intrapartum antibiotics. Rectal and vaginal cultures do *not* need to be obtained for these women. Antibiotics are recommended in both situations, regardless of culture results, thus making cultures unnecessary.
     — Birth of a previous newborn with early-onset GBS infection
     — Group B streptococcal bacteriuria of any concentration during this pregnancy
   - *Women with the following risk factors and whose culture results are unknown:*
     — Rupture of membranes for 18 hours or longer
     — Temperature of 38°C (100.4°F) or higher
     — Preterm labor (<37 weeks of gestation)

   Note: Women with any of these 3 risk factors but whose *culture results are known to have been negative within 5 weeks of delivery* do *not* require intrapartum GBS antibiotic therapy. Women with intrapartum fever should be assessed for possible intra-amniotic infection and treated with an appropriate antibiotic regimen.

c. Cesarean delivery considerations
   - Maternal colonization with GBS is not an indication for cesarean delivery.
   - GBS–colonized women with a planned cesarean delivery and who have not entered labor or had rupture of membranes have a low risk for delivering a neonate with early-onset GBS disease and should *not* routinely receive GBS prophylaxis during cesarean delivery. These women should receive standard preoperative antibiotic prophylaxis to reduce surgical site infections. Perform vaginal and rectal cultures at $36^{0/7}$ to $37^{6/7}$ weeks of gestation because onset of labor and rupture of membranes may occur before the planned cesarean delivery date.
d. Antibiotic choice and administration
   - *IV antibiotics, when appropriate, should be administered throughout labor until delivery.*
   - *IV administration* is preferred, regardless of the antibiotic used, because higher intra-amniotic concentrations are achieved with IV administration than with intramuscular administration.
     — *The preferred antibiotic is penicillin G.* The initial dose of 5 million units intravenously over 2 hours is followed by 2.5 (or 3.0) million units intravenously every 4 hours until delivery.
     — *The alternative antibiotic is ampicillin,* with 2-g first dose given intravenously, and then 1-g dose administered intravenously every 4 hours until delivery. Ampicillin is used when penicillin is unavailable or when a patient's labor is advanced at her arrival to the hospital, because the initial dose can be administered over 30 minutes.
     — *For women who are allergic to penicillin,* assess the history of the allergy and the severity of the reaction(s) early in prenatal care. Consider referral for penicillin allergy testing, especially if the history of allergic reaction is not well documented or appears mild.
       - *For women not at high risk for anaphylaxis,* cefazolin is the drug of choice—2 g given in an initial dose, intravenously, and then 1 g given intravenously every 8 hours until delivery.
       - *For women at high risk for anaphylaxis,* use a prenatal screening culture specimen to test GBS susceptibility to clindamycin. If sensitive, administer clindamycin 900 mg intravenously, every 8 hours until delivery.
       - *When GBS is resistant to clindamycin or susceptibility is unknown,* use vancomycin 20 mg/kg, given intravenously every 12 hours until delivery.
   - Broad-spectrum antibiotics, including a drug effective against GBS disease, may be needed to treat intra-amniotic infection.

 Appropriate intrapartum maternal antibiotic therapy can significantly reduce the risk that
   - *The baby will become infected with GBS disease.*
   - *The woman will develop endometritis.*

e. Onset of preterm labor (at 37 weeks of gestation or earlier)
   - *If GBS culture status is unknown*
     — Conduct vaginal and rectal cultures.

- After cultures have been performed, begin IV penicillin (or an alternative for women who are allergic to penicillin).
- If there is no growth in cultures after 48 hours, stop the penicillin (the penicillin should be administered until preterm labor is deemed to have stopped progressing).
- If preterm labor recurs more than 5 weeks after a negative GBS culture result, or if the woman reaches $36^{0/7}$ weeks of gestation, repeat the culture.
- If the GBS culture result is positive, manage as for GBS-positive women.

- *For GBS-positive women*
  - Administer penicillin for 48 hours until labor has stopped progressing or until delivery if labor progresses.
  - If preterm labor stops progressing but recurs at a later time, restart antibiotic prophylaxis.

- *For GBS-negative women*

  There is no indication for intrapartum antibiotic therapy *unless* the woman had a previous neonate with early-onset GBS disease (see part b, Intrapartum considerations).

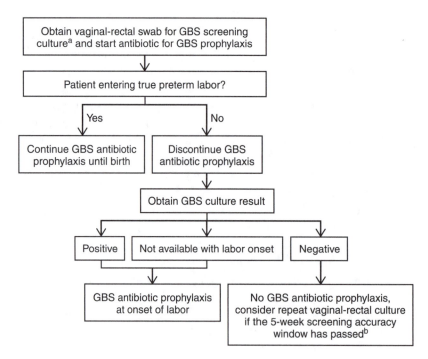

Figure 3.1. Algorithm for Screening for Group B Streptococcal (GBS) Colonization and Use of Intrapartum Prophylaxis for Women With Preterm Labor

[a] If a patient has undergone vaginal-rectal GBS screening culture within the preceding 5 weeks, the results of that culture should guide management. Women colonized with GBS should receive intrapartum antibiotic prophylaxis. Although a negative GBS culture result is considered valid for 5 weeks, the number of weeks is based on early-term screening, and data in preterm gestations are lacking. [b] A negative GBS culture result is considered valid for 5 weeks. However, the number of weeks is based on early-term screening, and data in preterm gestations are lacking. If a patient with preterm labor is entering true labor and had a negative GBS culture result more than 5 weeks previously, she should be rescreened and treated according to this algorithm at that time.

From American College of Obstetricians and Gynecologists. Prevention of group B streptococcal early-onset disease in newborns. Committee Opinion Number 797, February 2020.

UNIT 3: INFECTIOUS DISEASES IN PREGNANCY

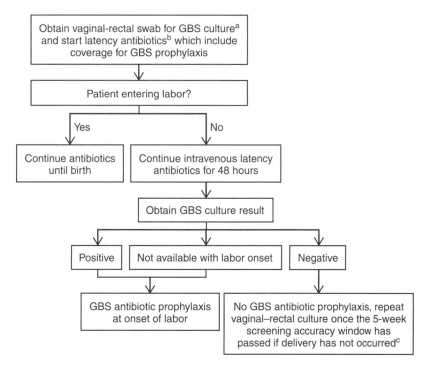

Figure 3.2. Algorithm for Screening for Group B Streptococcal (GBS) Colonization and Use of Intrapartum Prophylaxis for Women With Preterm Rupture of Membranes

[a] If a patient has undergone vaginal-rectal GBS culture within the preceding 5 weeks, the results of that culture should guide management. Women colonized with GBS should receive intrapartum antibiotic prophylaxis. Although a negative GBS culture result is considered valid for 5 weeks, the number of weeks is based on early-term screening, and data in preterm gestations are lacking. [b] Latency antibiotics that include ampicillin given in the setting of preterm prelabor rupture of membranes are adequate for GBS prophylaxis. The optimal latency antibiotic regimen is unclear, but one of the published protocols should be used (see ACOG Practice Bulletin No. 188, Prelabor Rupture of Membranes [*Obstet Gynecol* 2018; 131:e1-e14]). If other regimens are used that do not provide appropriate GBS coverage, CBS prophylaxis should be initiated in addition. [c] A negative CBS culture result is considered valid for 5 weeks. However, the number of weeks is based on early-term screening, and data in preterm gestations are lacking. If a patient with preterm prelabor rupture of membranes is entering labor and had a negative GBS culture result more than 5 weeks previously, she should be rescreened and managed according to this algorithm at that time.

From American College of Obstetricians and Gynecologists, Prevention of Group B Streptococcal Early-Onset Disease in Newborns. Committee Opinion Number 797, February 2020.

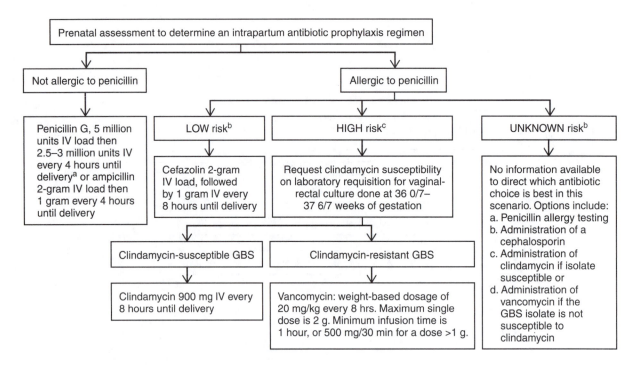

Figure 3.3. Intrapartum Antibiotic Prophylaxis Regimen for Women Colonized with Group B Streptococcus (GBS). Abbreviation: IV, intravenous

[a] Doses ranging from 2.5 to 3.0 million units are acceptable for the doses administered ever 4 hours after the initial dose. The choice of dose within that range should be guided by which formulations of penicillin G are readily available to reduce the need for pharmacies to specially prepare doses. [b] Individuals with a history of any of the following: nonspecific symptoms unlikely to be allergic (gastrointestinal distress, headaches, yeast vaginitis), nonurticarial maculopapular (morbilliform) rash without systemic symptoms, pruritis without rash, family history of penicillin allergy but no personal history, or patient reports history but has no recollection of symptoms or treatment. [c] Individuals with a history of any of the following after administration of a penicillin: a history suggestive of an immunoglobulin E-mediated event: pruritic rash, urticaria (hives), immediate flushing, hypotension, angioedema, respiratory distress or anaphylaxis; recurrent reactions, reactions to multiple beta-lactam antibiotics, or positive penicillin allergy test result; or severe rare delayed-onset cutaneous or systemic reactions, such as eosinophilia and systemic symptoms/drug-induced hypersensitivity syndrome, Stevens-Johnson syndrome, or toxic epidermal necrolysis.

From American College of Obstetricians and Gynecologists, Prevention of Group B Streptococcal Early-Onset Disease in Newborns. Committee Opinion Number 797, February 2020.

9. Toxoplasmosis
   - *Disease in women:* Toxoplasmosis is a common infection caused by the protozoan parasite *Toxoplasma gondii.* As many as one-third of women in the United States have evidence of being infected at some point in their lifetime. Diagnosis of primary or acute infection is established with documentation of maternal seroconversion. Initial infection almost always confers lifelong immunity. Because toxoplasmosis infection in adults is most often either asymptomatic or a mild and self-limited illness, serologic testing is rarely performed, and most active infections go undetected. In a pregnant woman with symptoms indicative of mononucleosis but with a negative heterophile antibody test result, toxoplasma antibody titers should be considered as part of the diagnostic evaluation. Routine screening of pregnant women is not recommended, except for HIV-positive women. A reference laboratory, such as the Palo Alto Medical Foundation Research Institute Toxoplasma Serology Laboratory, should be used to confirm acute infection (www.pamf.org).

     T gondii is common in house cats and many other mammals. Transmission of the infection to humans occurs by exposure to cat feces that contain infectious oocysts or by eating raw or undercooked meat that contains tissue cysts of the parasite. Except for rare cases of infected donor organs and contaminated blood products, the only person-to-person transmission is by transplacental transfer from a pregnant woman to her fetus.
   - *Risks for the fetus and newborn:* *T gondii* can cross the placenta. Fetal infection early in pregnancy can cause miscarriage or may lead to growth restriction and fetal systemic disease, resulting in permanent, severe damage. Typically, hydrocephalus, microcephaly, cerebral calcifications, seizures, deafness, or chorioretinitis is present, along with lymphadenopathy, hepatosplenomegaly, jaundice, or thrombocytopenia. Most infected fetuses will be asymptomatic at birth, but many of those will go on to demonstrate intellectual disabilities, learning disabilities, impaired vision, or blindness months or years later.
     a. Prenatal considerations
        - Screening pregnant women for toxoplasma antibody status is not currently recommended in the United States.
        - Women with negative or unknown *Toxoplasma* serology results should avoid
          — Cleaning cat litter boxes or gardening in areas that cats frequent
          — Cats, especially those with access to wild rodents
          — Eating raw or undercooked meat, especially red meat
        - Consider obtaining *preconception* toxoplasmosis titer for women at high risk for contracting the infection. This titer would provide a baseline level in the event an infection is suspected during pregnancy, as well as indicate preexisting immunity if the result is positive.

- Consult with regional center specialists if an acute maternal infection is identified. Medication therapy may reduce *T gondii* transmission to the fetus and improve neonatal outcome, but appropriate drugs vary by trimester, and some need special authorization.
- Congenital infection is confirmed by *T gondii* found in fetal blood or amniotic fluid.
- When congenital *T gondii* infection is suspected, serial US examinations are recommended to detect ventricular enlargement in the brain or any other signs of fetal infection.
- Discuss pregnancy termination if infection occurs early in pregnancy.
- Coexisting HIV infection complicates maternal and neonatal evaluation and treatment. Consult with specialists.

b. Intrapartum considerations
 None specific to toxoplasmosis

c. Postpartum considerations
 Maternal
- Notify pediatric staff if maternal infection is suspected.
- Breastfeeding is recommended for women who have contracted toxoplasmosis during pregnancy. There are no reports of documented breast milk transmission of toxoplasma in humans (for additional information, see www.cdc.gov/parasites/toxoplasmosis/gen_info/pregnant.html).

 Neonatal (See also Book 3: Neonatal Care, Unit 8, Infections.)
- If neonatal diagnosis of *T gondii* is suspected at birth or if there is evidence of primary *T gondii* maternal infection during pregnancy, *Toxoplasma*-specific tests should be performed. (For specific recommendations, see American Academy of Pediatrics. *Toxoplasma gondii* infections. In: Kimberlin DW, Brady MT, Jackson MA, Long SS, eds. *Red Book: 2021 Report of the Committee on Infectious Diseases*. 32nd ed. American Academy of Pediatrics; 2021.) It may also be possible to isolate the organism from the placenta, umbilical cord, or baby's blood.
- Treatment with pyrimethamine and sulfadiazine (plus folinic acid) is usually recommended. Treatment is prolonged, often continuing for 1 year or longer. Consult with infectious disease specialists.
- Evaluate the baby for congenital malformations and obtain consultations as indicated for care of the baby and family.

10. Tuberculosis
- *Disease in women:* Tuberculosis is an infection with *Mycobacterium tuberculosis* that has progressed over weeks or years to the point that radiographic findings, clinical signs, symptoms, or positive culture results are present. Infection may be present in a latent form, before radiographic and clinical findings develop. The incidence of tuberculosis has increased dramatically in the United States, including infections with drug-resistant organisms.

Treatment recommendations vary according to latent and active phases and primary infection site. Most commonly, the infection is pulmonary, but extrapulmonary infection is possible and can involve many organ systems.

- *Risks for the fetus and newborn:* Extrapulmonary tuberculosis is associated with an increased likelihood of antenatal hospitalization, low Apgar scores, and low birth weight. Transmission in utero through infected amniotic fluid or at the time of delivery through aspiration or ingestion of infected maternal fluids is thought to be rare. When congenital tuberculosis is suspected, the newborn and mother need prompt evaluation.

In most cases, transmission occurs by person-to-person exposure to droplets from the respiratory tract. Respiratory droplet exposure represents the most common way a mother or household contact with active tuberculosis passes the infection to a newborn.

  a. Prenatal considerations
   - All pregnant women at risk for tuberculosis should be screened with a skin test early in their prenatal care. High-risk factors include
     — Close contact with an individual(s) known to have tuberculosis
     — Poverty
     — Community settings, such as urban environments; residents or employees of correctional or mental institutions, nursing homes, and long-term care facilities
     — Birth in a tuberculosis endemic area
     — Medically underserved group, such as migrant workers
     — Persons with any other systemic disease, such as diabetes mellitus
     — Malnutrition
     — HIV infection, or other immunocompromised medical condition, such as transplant recipient, or chronic immunosuppressant medications, such as glucocorticoids or tumor necrosis factor α inhibitors
     — Substance abuse, including alcohol or injection drug use (tobacco use also increases the risk of tuberculosis infection)
   - If a positive skin test result is found for the first time during pregnancy, obtain a chest radiograph and conduct sputum cultures.
   - If active disease is found, treat promptly and aggressively with multidrug therapy, in consultation with infectious disease specialists. Management is complex, especially during pregnancy, and must be individualized. Drug resistance can further complicate therapy.
   - If infection is latent, with normal chest radiographic findings and no clinical signs, prompt treatment may be advisable for recent (<2 years) infection or immunosuppression. For all other pregnant women with latent tuberculosis, treatment may be delayed until after delivery.
   - Arrange for testing and treatment of home contacts. Public health departments have protocols for identifying and screening contacts and monitoring adherence with therapy. Individuals with tuberculosis should also be tested for HIV because people who are HIV positive have an increased risk of contracting tuberculosis.

b. Intrapartum considerations
Isolate (with respiratory precautions) women with suspected or known active disease from other pregnant women and all newborns.

c. Postpartum considerations
Maternal
- Maintain isolation (respiratory precautions) of the mother.
- In certain situations, the mother and baby need to be separated until the mother (or sometimes the mother and the newborn) is receiving appropriate therapy and considered noncontagious (American Academy of Pediatrics, American College of Obstetricians and Gynecologists. *Guidelines for Perinatal Care*. Kilpatrick SJ, Papile L, Macones GA, Watterberg KL, eds. 8th ed. American Academy of Pediatrics; 2017:538).
- Delay breastfeeding in women with active tuberculosis until the mother is noncontagious (usually 2 weeks after medication is started). If the mother wishes to breastfeed, she may pump her breasts to establish and maintain a milk supply, but the milk should be discarded until the mother becomes noncontagious.
- Breastfeeding is not contraindicated for noninfectious women being treated with first-line antituberculosis drugs. The drug concentration in breast milk is low and is not known to cause toxicity in the nursing newborn. For the same reason, drugs in breast milk are not an effective treatment for tuberculosis disease or latent tuberculosis infection in a nursing baby. Breastfeeding women who are taking isoniazid should also take pyridoxine (vitamin B_6) supplementation. Consult with medication safety databases or infectious disease experts.
- Arrange for follow-up of mother and baby. Treatment with antituberculosis drugs can require 18 months of therapy, and compliance with the drug regimen can be difficult. Adherence to the treatment regimen is essential for providing effective therapy and for limiting the development of drug-resistant strains of *M tuberculosis*.

Neonatal (See also Book 3: Neonatal Care, Unit 8, Infections.)
- Treat the baby if the mother was incompletely treated or is considered to be contagious at the time of delivery. Consult with infectious disease specialists; maternal and neonatal therapy should be coordinated.
- Consider giving the baby a bacille Calmette-Guérin (BCG) vaccine. BCG vaccine does not prevent infection but rather prevents disseminated and life-threatening complications of *M tuberculosis* infection. In the United States, its use is generally confined to non-infected babies who cannot be given long-term preventive therapy but who are likely to have prolonged exposure to persistently infectious individuals.
- Reassess testing and treatment of home contacts. Test the baby for HIV.
- Isolate the baby (with respiratory precautions) from other newborns and pregnant women until a full evaluation of the baby has been conducted.

11. Varicella-zoster virus (chickenpox)
    - *Disease in women:* Varicella-zoster virus (VZV) infection is characterized by a typical rash, fever, and mild systemic symptoms, although adolescents and adults are likely to be much sicker than children with chickenpox. While rare in children, pneumonia is the most common complication in adults and can be life-threatening. Pregnant women are more likely than non-pregnant women to become seriously ill. After recovery from the primary infection, the virus remains in latent form. Transmission is usually by direct contact with an infected person, although droplet spread also occurs. Reactivation results in herpes zoster infection (shingles).
    - *Risks for the fetus and newborn:* The likelihood of transplacental transmission of the virus is high if maternal infection occurs during the first 20 weeks of pregnancy. First-trimester infection carries an increased risk of spontaneous abortion. In a small number of infected fetuses, congenital varicella syndrome will result, which is characterized by limb atrophy and scarring of the skin; neurological and ophthalmic damage and microcephaly may also occur.

    If a woman delivers during active varicella illness, the baby may become infected at delivery and become seriously ill. Neonatal illness may develop between 1 and 16 days after birth, although the usual time from onset of maternal rash to onset of neonatal illness is 9 to 15 days.

    Shingles is a painful vesicular rash that usually occurs in the distribution of a dermatome. It is caused by reactivation of latent VZV in an individual who previously had chickenpox. Shingles in a pregnant woman is not known to cause adverse effects on the fetus or newborn. If a pregnant woman who is not immune to varicella is exposed to someone with shingles, the risk of her getting chickenpox is low. Caution is recommended, including avoiding contact between the pregnant woman and the person with shingles until the rash has crusted. People with shingles should also avoid contact with preterm babies.

    Varicella in the newborn carries a mortality rate as high as 30%.
    a. Prenatal considerations
        - Most women with negative or uncertain history of VZV infection are, in fact, immune. Serologic testing can be used to document immunity. VZV vaccine has been available since 1995 and is widely used to immunize children, including newborns, and susceptible adults.
        - Women should not receive varicella immunization during pregnancy because the possible effects of the vaccine on the fetus are not completely known. The Pregnancy Registry for Varicella Zoster Virus-Containing Vaccines (now closed) received more than 900 reports of women receiving varicella-zoster vaccine in pregnancy over the course of 18 years without any documented cases of congenital varicella syndrome. Nonimmune women should be immunized at least 1 month before conception, or anytime after delivery.
        - Nonimmune pregnant women who are exposed to varicella infection should receive varicella zoster immunoglobulin (VariZIG) (a VZV-specific immunoglobulin), ideally within 96 hours of exposure but as long as 10 days after exposure. The dose to be administered is 125 IU/10 kg to a maximum dose of 625 IU, given intramuscularly or intravenously. It is intended to prevent or reduce the severity of maternal disease but is not thought to have effectiveness

after the disease has become established. It is not known to reduce the risk of fetal varicella infection.
- Acyclovir antiviral therapy for VZV infections during pregnancy may be appropriate for some women. Consult with infectious disease specialists.
- Discuss the risks of fetal infection and the option of pregnancy termination if infection occurs early in pregnancy.

b. Intrapartum considerations
- Administer VariZIG to nonimmune pregnant women if they are exposed to varicella within 96 hours of delivery.
- Women with active varicella should be isolated from other pregnant women and all newborns. Those who receive VariZIG should be observed carefully until 28 days after exposure to varicella, as treatment with VariZIG may prolong the latency period to active infection.
- Notify pediatrics personnel if the mother was recently exposed to chickenpox or develops a rash between 5 days before and 2 days after delivery. Initiate IV acyclovir for women who present with active varicella infections while in labor.

c. Postpartum considerations

Maternal
- Review intrapartum guidelines. Institute isolation precautions, as appropriate.
- Breastfeeding mothers who are not immune to varicella should be immunized and do not require isolation from their baby or others. The first dose of VZV vaccine should be administered before hospital discharge, with the second dose given 4 to 8 weeks later.

Neonatal (See also Book 3: Neonatal Care, Unit 8, Infections.)
- If a woman develops a rash within 5 days before and 2 days after delivery, administer VariZIG to the baby as soon as possible. Prevention or reduction in severity is important because neonatal varicella infection carries a high mortality rate.
- A term baby who is more than 2 days old when first exposed to varicella (including one whose mother developed a rash >48 hours after delivery) may not require VariZIG treatment, because of a lower risk for severe infection. A preterm baby may need to receive VariZIG regardless of maternal history, due to the higher risk of death among these babies; consult with infectious disease specialists.
- Newborns with VZV infection should be isolated with standard, airborne, and contact precautions for the duration of their illness. A baby born to a mother who was exposed to varicella close to delivery should be isolated from birth until 21 days of age, unless VariZIG was administered, in which case the baby should be isolated for 28 days. Babies born with congenital VZV infection contracted earlier in gestation do not need isolation.
- Consult with regional perinatal center specialists about treatment of individual babies.
- Having a pregnant woman in a family or household is not a contraindication to immunizing children within the family or household. Children who are susceptible to VZV infection should be immunized just as they would be if not in contact with a pregnant woman.

12. Coronavirus disease 2019 (COVID-19)

    Coronavirus disease 2019 (COVID-19) is the clinical illness caused by infection with SARS-CoV-2 (severe acute respiratory syndrome coronavirus 2), a novel coronavirus that caused a global pandemic beginning in late 2019. Nearly every country in the world has been affected; millions of individuals have been diagnosed with COVID-19, and millions of deaths have been caused by infection with this virus. SARS-CoV-2 is spread via respiratory droplets and potentially via aerosol. Although the knowledge base regarding this virus and the clinical illness it causes has grown rapidly, many details of its behavior and clinical course are not yet fully understood. For example, it is not yet clear if transplacental passage of the virus may occur from mother to fetus, although this method of transmission is suspected to be possible. Current information about COVID-19 from the CDC can be found at https://www.cdc.gov/coronavirus/2019-nCoV/hcp/index.html.

    COVID-19 is a respiratory infection with a spectrum of clinical illness that includes severe viral pneumonia, respiratory failure, and death. Pregnant women are more susceptible to severe cases of COVID-19, which is similar to the clinical experience with other forms of viral pneumonia during pregnancy, including influenza, varicella-zoster, and infection with other coronaviruses (severe acute respiratory syndrome [SARS] and Middle Eastern respiratory syndrome [MERS]). Pregnant women should be encouraged to follow appropriate precautions to minimize their risk of exposure to SARS-CoV-2. These precautions include frequent handwashing with soap and water (substituting an alcohol-based hand sanitizer if soap and water are not readily available), maintaining social distancing of at least 6 feet, and wearing a cloth face covering or mask while around individuals other than immediate household members. Some pregnant women with COVID-19 will have a mild clinical course and do not require hospital admission or special care. Others may be critically ill and require treatment in an intensive care unit. The medical decision-making surrounding a critically ill pregnant patient is complex and will often require transfer to a regional referral center.

Self-test D

Now answer these questions to test yourself on the information in the last section.

D1.	True	False	Maternal vaginal colonization with group B streptococcus can lead to neonatal sepsis.
D2.	True	False	A woman with varicella-zoster virus infection at the time of delivery should be isolated from all pregnant women and newborns.
D3.	True	False	It is safe for a woman with active tuberculosis to breastfeed her baby as soon as her treatment is started.
D4.	True	False	A woman with diagnosed or suspected active tuberculosis at the time of delivery should be isolated from all pregnant women and newborns.
D5.	True	False	When a woman has active tuberculosis at the time of delivery, 18 months of therapy with antituberculosis drugs may be needed for adequate treatment of the mother and the baby.
D6.	True	False	When a woman develops a rash from varicella-zoster virus infection within 5 days before delivery, administration of varicella zoster immunoglobulin (VariZIG) to the newborn is indicated.
D7.	True	False	Neonatal varicella-zoster (chickenpox) infection at 2 days of age or younger is usually much less severe than in older children.

D8. For each of the following organisms, indicate how the fetus may become infected:
- a. Transplacental _____ Gonorrhea
- b. Ascending _____ Toxoplasmosis
- c. At delivery _____ Varicella-zoster virus (chickenpox)

D9. A woman's group B streptococcus culture results are unknown. Which of the following complications are indications for antibiotics during labor for the prevention of neonatal group B streptococcal infection?

Yes	No	
_____	_____	Maternal temperature of 38°C (100.4°F)
_____	_____	Rupture of membranes for 20 hours
_____	_____	Post-term labor
_____	_____	Maternal thrombocytopenia
_____	_____	Previous baby with group B streptococcal infection
_____	_____	Group B streptococcal bacteriuria early in pregnancy

D10. Which of the following pathways is the most common way for a newborn to acquire group B streptococcal infection?
- A. Direct contact with organisms during passage through the birth canal
- B. Transplacental passage from organisms in the mother's blood to the fetus, near term
- C. Direct contact with organisms on the skin of caregivers, soon after birth
- D. Through breastfeeding, from organisms on the mother's skin and in the breast milk

Check your answers with the list that follows the Recommended Routines. Correct any incorrect answers and review the appropriate section in the unit.

C. Sites of maternal infection with a variety of causative organisms
  1. Bacterial vaginosis
     - *Condition in women:* This is not an infection in the usual sense but, rather, an abnormal distribution of organisms that normally inhabit the vagina. Hormonal changes (including pregnancy) or antibiotic administration are thought to cause an imbalance in the normal vaginal flora, with the usual lactobacilli largely replaced by other organisms. *Gardnerella vaginalis* is the organism most often associated with bacterial vaginosis. A woman with bacterial vaginosis may be asymptomatic or have a foul-smelling white or yellowish vaginal discharge. The odor is often described as "fishy" and may be accentuated after sexual intercourse (due to the pH level of semen). Bacterial vaginosis may increase the risk of intra-amniotic infection, preterm delivery, and postpartum endometritis.
     - *Risks for the fetus and newborn:* The risks to the fetus and newborn are those associated with preterm birth, premature rupture of membranes, or intra-amniotic infection, if any of those conditions develop.
        a. Prenatal considerations
           - Pregnant women with symptoms of bacterial vaginosis should be evaluated and treated on the basis of the evaluation results.
           - Treatment recommendations include
             — Metronidazole, 500 mg, given orally, twice daily for 7 days
             or
             — Metronidazole 0.75% vaginal gel, 5 g, used daily for 5 days
             or
             — Clindamycin 2% vaginal cream, 5 g, used daily for 7 days
           - Sexual transmission does not seem to play a role in this condition because treating sexual partners does not reduce recurrence.
           - Screening for bacterial vaginosis is not recommended as a strategy to reduce the incidence of preterm birth.
        b. Intrapartum considerations
           None specific to bacterial vaginosis
        c. Postpartum considerations
           Maternal
           The risk of endometritis is increased, particularly with cesarean delivery.
           Neonatal
           None specific to bacterial vaginosis
  2. Urinary tract infection and acute pyelonephritis
     - *Disease in women:* Asymptomatic bacteriuria and symptomatic UTI are more common during pregnancy because of the anatomical and physiological changes that lead to urinary stasis. Bacteriuria and UTI may progress to pyelonephritis during pregnancy. Pyelonephritis can cause serious maternal illness (systemic infection or kidney damage).
     - *Risks for the fetus and newborn:* Maternal UTI is associated with increased risk of preterm labor and premature rupture of membranes.
        a. Prenatal considerations
           Bacteriuria (symptomatic or asymptomatic)
           - Conduct a urine culture for asymptomatic bacteriuria routinely for *all* women at the first prenatal visit.

- A positive screening test result (eg, a point-of-care test) during pregnancy should be confirmed with a urine culture prior to treatment.
- Treat positive cultures, with or without UTI symptoms (burning, urinary frequency, urinary urgency), promptly with appropriate antibiotics. Recommended antibiotics, until sensitivities are known, include trimethoprim-sulfamethoxazole, nitrofurantoin, and cephalexin.
- *Escherichia coli* is most commonly the infecting organism and is often resistant to ampicillin. Treatment with ampicillin or amoxicillin is not recommended unless culture and antibiotic sensitivity results are known.
- It is commonly recommended to conduct a follow-up urine culture after completion of antibiotic therapy, although data to support this practice are limited.
- Women who are treated for bacteriuria should be periodically rescreened during pregnancy. If asymptomatic bacteriuria recurs, daily antibiotic suppressive therapy for the remainder of the pregnancy is generally recommended.

Screen all pregnant women for bacteriuria. If found, whether symptomatic or asymptomatic, treat bacteriuria promptly.

Acute pyelonephritis
- Women with a temperature of 38°C (100.4°F) or higher with flank pain (usually the right side) and urinary symptoms should be evaluated without delay. Treatment for pyelonephritis may be administered on an outpatient basis for stable pregnant women. Many women require hospitalization. Treatment includes
  — IV fluid infusion
  — IV antibiotics, followed by oral antibiotics after hospital discharge
  — Investigation for the presence of renal stones, especially in patients with recurrent urinary infections or a history of stones
- After treatment for pyelonephritis, daily antimicrobial suppressive therapy is recommended for the remainder of the pregnancy.

b. Intrapartum considerations

Continue antibiotic therapy if it was started earlier and the course is not yet completed.

c. Postpartum considerations

Maternal

Monitor the mother for symptoms of UTI after delivery. If cesarean delivery is performed, remove the Foley catheter early to reduce the risk of catheter-associated UTI.

Neonatal

If maternal infection is active at time of delivery
- Conduct blood cultures.
- Check the complete blood cell count with differential.
- Consider starting antibiotics.
- Observe the baby closely for evidence of respiratory distress or sepsis. If any signs of illness develop, treat promptly with antibiotics.

3. Intra-amniotic infection

   Intra-amniotic infection puts a woman at risk for sepsis and postpartum endometritis and puts a fetus at risk for preterm birth or neonatal sepsis. Management is presented in Unit 8, Prelabor Rupture of Membranes and Intra-amniotic Infection, in this book.

4. Puerperal endometritis
   - *Maternal illness:* Endometritis is an infection of the endometrium (the lining of the uterus) after delivery that was once a major cause of maternal mortality but is rarely fatal today. The likelihood of infection is increased after cesarean delivery. It can occur in any woman, but those with prelabor rupture of membranes, prolonged labor, or GBS colonization are at highest risk.

     Infection of the endometrium may include the myometrium, adnexae, and pelvic peritoneum. In some women with endometritis, *septic pelvic thrombophlebitis* (multiple small thrombi in the pelvic veins with bacterial seeding) may develop. Septic pelvic thrombophlebitis may be life-threatening if untreated because of the possibility of pulmonary embolism and overwhelming sepsis. Treatment involves heparin infusion and IV antibiotic therapy.
   - *Risks for the newborn:* The reason the mother developed endometritis may also pose a serious risk for neonatal infection.

     a. Signs and symptoms
        - Temperature of 38°C (100.4°F) or higher more than 24 hours after delivery
        - Abdominal cramping pain
        - Foul-smelling lochia
        - Leukocytosis (increased white blood cell count)

     b. Diagnosis
        - Uterine tenderness (diagnosed with abdominal and/or bimanual examination of the uterus and adnexa)
        - Foul-smelling lochia
        - No indication of other infections, including
          — Mastitis
          — Pneumonia (consider obtaining a chest radiograph)
          — Pyelonephritis (check urinalysis and culture)

     c. Treatment

        Initial
        - Begin IV antibiotic therapy. Recommended treatment is gentamicin, 1.5 mg/kg, plus clindamycin, 900 mg, administered intravenously every 8 hours. Some regimens call for once-daily gentamicin, 5 mg/kg.
        - Continue treatment until the woman has been afebrile and symptom free for 24 to 48 hours.

        If fever persists more than 48 hours after antibiotics are started
        - Suspect *Bacteroides* or *Enterococcus* infection or drug-resistant organisms.
        - Repeat pelvic examination to evaluate the mother for pelvic abscess.
        - Consider pelvic imaging (computed tomography or US) to assess the mother for retained placental tissue or abscess.
        - Review the antibiotic regimen: Consider adding ampicillin for coverage of *Enterococcus*. Consider substituting metronidazole for clindamycin. If an abscess is suspected, aztreonam may be more effective than gentamicin.

- Metronidazole may be detected in breast milk and reach the newborn, and it may lead to loose stools and growth of *Candida* in the newborn. Some authorities recommend discontinuing breastfeeding during metronidazole therapy and for 12 to 24 hours after the end of therapy to allow maternal excretion of the drug. During this time, the mother may pump her breasts to establish and maintain her milk supply, but the milk should be discarded.

If the fever persists further
- Repeat the pelvic examination and consider pelvic imaging, if not conducted earlier. If imaging has already been performed, it may need to be repeated. If an abscess is identified, surgical or imaging-directed drainage may be indicated. Consider nonpelvic sources of infection, such as appendicitis or pyelonephritis. Drug fever is also a possibility.
- Consider heparin therapy for septic pelvic thrombophlebitis.
- Consult with regional perinatal center specialists; consider transfer of the patient.

5. Group A streptococcus

Group A streptococcus (*Streptococcus pyogenes*) is a particularly important cause of serious postpartum infections (puerperal sepsis) due to its rapid clinical course and high case fatality rate. As many as 30% of adults are colonized with group A streptococcus, and most do not experience clinical illness. The patient may demonstrate symptoms during the delivery hospitalization or may return after discharge with symptoms of infection. The clinical symptoms that should lead to the suspicion for a group A streptococcal infection include
- Fever (>38.0°C)
- Tender, non-involuted uterus
- Chills, malaise
- Lower abdominal pain
- Foul-smelling, purulent lochia

If a postpartum group A streptococcal infection is suspected, the management must be rapid and coordinated to protect the patient against permanent disability or death. The antibiotic regimen chosen to treat the postpartum infection must include penicillin G, which is the most effective antibiotic against this organism. Fluid resuscitation should be initiated, with vasopressor support as indicated by maternal vital signs. Obtain cultures and pursue source control (debridement of infected tissue, which may include perineal debridement and debridement of the abdominal wound for patients who underwent cesarean delivery and/or hysterectomy). More information about the management of sepsis can be found at the website of the Surviving Sepsis Campaign, https://www.sccm.org/SurvivingSepsisCampaign/Home.

6. Mastitis
    - *Maternal illness:* Postpartum infection and inflammation of the breasts rarely develop while the woman is still hospitalized but can become a significant problem after she has been discharged. Proper breastfeeding technique that encourages milk drainage from all areas of the breast decreases the likelihood of mastitis developing.
    - *Risks for the newborn:* Infectious mastitis does not pose a threat to a healthy newborn unless an abscess has formed. If an abscess is present, breastfeeding with the affected breast will need to be interrupted temporarily.
    a. Signs and symptoms
        - Systemic signs: Fever (temperature $\geq$ 38.5°C [$\geq$101.3°F]), myalgias, chills
        - Breast (usually only one is affected) is swollen, reddened, tender, and hot
        - Red streaks (infected lymph vessels) may lead away from the tender area
    b. Treatment
        - Begin dicloxacillin, a penicillinase-resistant penicillin, as first-line treatment. A first-generation cephalosporin (eg, cephalexin) may also be used, but it has a broader spectrum and may promote antibiotic resistance or reduce counts of beneficial bacteria in the mother. Clindamycin is used if the woman is allergic to penicillin.
        - A culture of the mother's milk may be conducted if she does not respond well to treatment. This may be done by the woman expressing a sample of milk, after careful cleansing of her breast.
        - Breastfeeding should continue and is encouraged at frequent intervals to ensure emptying of the affected breast. Mastitis usually resolves with antibiotic therapy and continued lactation. Pain medication may be needed for several days to allow breastfeeding.
        - Breast abscess is rare. If one occurs
            — Drain the abscess as soon as it becomes fluctuant.
            — Rupture of an abscess into the ductal network of the breast can release large numbers of organisms into the breast milk. For this reason, nursing with the affected breast is not recommended when an abscess is present (nursing on the unaffected side may continue). A breast pump, with the milk discarded, may be used on the affected side to empty the breast and facilitate lactation.
            — Nursing with the affected breast may resume after the abscess has been surgically drained and antibiotic therapy instituted.

Self-test E

Now answer these questions to test yourself on the information in the last section.

E1.	True	False	All pregnant women should be screened for asymptomatic bacteriuria.
E2.	True	False	Bacterial vaginosis may increase the risk for maternal complications and preterm delivery.
E3.	True	False	Women with asymptomatic urinary tract infection should be treated with antibiotics.
E4.	True	False	Septic pelvic thrombophlebitis may develop in women with endometritis.
E5.	True	False	Bacterial vaginosis is spread through sexual contact.
E6.	True	False	When mastitis is present, breastfeeding must stop completely to avoid infection of the baby.
E7.	True	False	Acute pyelonephritis in a pregnant woman requires hospitalization, intravenous antibiotics, and fluid infusion.
E8.	True	False	Physiological changes during pregnancy increase the risk of urinary tract infection, even for women who have never had a urinary tract infection.
E9.	True	False	Urinary tract infection, whether it is symptomatic or asymptomatic, increases the risk of premature rupture of membranes and preterm labor.
E10.	True	False	Antibiotic treatment for puerperal mastitis is penicillinase-resistant penicillin.
E11.	True	False	Initial treatment of puerperal endometritis includes intravenous administration of antibiotics.
E12.	True	False	Bacterial vaginosis is often associated with a "fishy" odor.

E13. List at least 3 signs of postpartum endometritis.
_____
_____
_____

Check your answers with the list that follows the Recommended Routines. Correct any incorrect answers and review the appropriate section in the unit.

UNIT 3: INFECTIOUS DISEASES IN PREGNANCY

INFECTIOUS DISEASES IN PREGNANCY

Recommended Routines

All the routines listed below are based on the principles of perinatal care presented in the unit you have just finished. They are recommended as part of routine perinatal care.

Read each routine carefully and decide whether it is standard operating procedure in your hospital. Check the appropriate blank next to each routine.

Procedure Standard in My Hospital	Needs Discussion by Our Staff	Recommended Routines
_____	_____	1. Establish a system to ensure the use of standard precautions by all staff members.
_____	_____	2. Establish a written protocol to conduct lower vaginal and rectal cultures for group B streptococcus (GBS) from all women at $36^{0/7}$ to $37^{6/7}$ weeks of gestation (unless a woman had an earlier baby with early-onset GBS infection or had GBS bacteriuria in the current pregnancy).
_____	_____	3. Establish a written protocol for prenatal and intrapartum management for the prevention of neonatal GBS infection.
_____	_____	4. Establish a policy to screen *all* women early in pregnancy for • Bacteriuria • Gonorrhea and chlamydia • Hepatitis B virus • Hepatitis C virus • HIV • Syphilis
_____	_____	5. Establish a protocol for treatment of bacteriuria, whether symptomatic or asymptomatic.
_____	_____	6. Establish a system for timely transfer of information about possible or proven maternal infections to neonatal practitioners.
_____	_____	7. Establish written guidelines for isolation of • Women with active genital herpes and their babies • Babies with congenital rubella • Women with active tuberculosis and their babies • Women with varicella-zoster infection, or recent exposure, and their babies
_____	_____	8. Establish written guidelines or protocol orders for • Prophylactic eye care of all newborns • Newborns at risk for chlamydial conjunctivitis

PCEP BOOK 2: MATERNAL AND FETAL CARE

_____   _____   9. Establish a policy to ensure administration of
- Hepatitis B virus vaccine to *all* babies, with the first vaccine of a 3-dose series given soon after birth and prior to discharge (see Book 3: Neonatal Care, Unit 8, Infections).
- Hepatitis B virus vaccine (first dose) and hepatitis B immunoglobulin to preterm and term babies born to women positive for hepatitis B surface antigen, given within 12 hours of birth.

_____   _____   10. Establish a system to ensure that maternal serologic status for syphilis is known for *every* newborn before discharge.

Self-test Answers

These are the answers to the Self-test questions. Please check them with the answers you gave and review the information in the unit wherever necessary.

Self-test A

A1. Mother with chlamydia = c. Asymptomatic maternal infection
Mother with active genital herpes = b. Cesarean delivery
Mother with active gonorrhea = a. Ceftriaxone for mother and baby

A2. True

A3. True

A4. False *Reason:* Most organisms cannot cross the placenta and infect the fetus. The ones that can, however, are often capable of causing serious damage to the fetus.

A5. True

A6. False *Reason:* Ascending infection is more likely to occur after the membranes have ruptured but can occur through intact membranes.

A7. False *Reason:* Prophylactic eye treatment with silver nitrate or antibiotic ointment is used to prevent neonatal gonorrheal ophthalmia. If an infection develops, topical treatment is not adequate. Systemic antibiotics must be used to treat it.

A8. True

A9. False *Reason:* Routine prophylactic eye treatment with silver nitrate, erythromycin, or tetracycline will *not* reliably prevent neonatal chlamydial conjunctivitis. Some experts advise that all babies born to women with untreated chlamydia infection receive oral erythromycin for 14 days.

A10. True

A11. True

A12. False *Reason:* A woman may have a mild or asymptomatic viral illness that causes serious fetal illness or damage. Likewise, certain serious maternal illnesses may not affect the fetus at all.

A13.
Yes	No	
	X	Toxoplasmosis
X		Syphilis
X		Chlamydia
	X	Parvovirus
X		Herpes
X		HIV

Note: The presence of any one sexually transmitted infection should prompt investigation for other sexually transmitted infections.

Self-test B

B1.
Yes	No	
X		Test positive for HIV antibodies.
	X	Be infected with the virus.

B2.
Pregnancy	Delivery	
X	X	Syphilis
X	X	Herpes simplex virus
	X	Human papillomavirus

B3. False *Reason:* HIV can be passed from an infected woman to her newborn in her breast milk.

B4. True

B5. False *Reason:* Syphilis infection can pass to the fetus during any stage of maternal infection. Transplacental transfer rates are
- Primary stage, approximately 50%
- Secondary stage, approximately 100%
- Tertiary stage, approximately 10%

B6. True

B7. True

B8. True

B9. False *Reason:* Standard precautions need to be used for all patients at all times. Use of these precautions has dramatically lowered the incidence of work-acquired hepatitis infections in health professionals.

B10. False *Reason:* There is no treatment for neonatal human papillomavirus. Only a very small number of babies born to women with human papillomavirus become infected, but if infection occurs at the time of delivery, symptoms may not be evident for months or years.

B11.
Yes	No	
X		HIV
	X	Human papillomavirus
X		Syphilis
X		Gonorrhea
	X	Herpes simplex virus

Self-test C

C1.
Yes	No	
	X	Gonorrhea
X		Primary parvovirus infection
X		Rubella (German measles)
X		Cytomegalovirus
	X	Chlamydia
X		Listeriosis

C2. True

C3. True

C4. True

C5. False *Reason:* The route of delivery does not affect the rate of transmission of hepatitis B virus from women who test positive for hepatitis B surface antigen to their babies. Cesarean delivery should be used only for obstetric reasons.

C6. True

C7. False *Reason:* Breastfeeding by women who test positive for hepatitis B surface antigen does not increase the risk of infection for the baby. Vaccination of the baby eliminates nearly all risk. Administration of hepatitis B virus vaccine and hepatitis B immunoglobulin is recommended for breastfed babies of women who test positive for hepatitis B surface antigen.

C8. False *Reason:* Cytomegalovirus, particularly during a primary infection, easily crosses the placenta in early pregnancy. Because maternal illness is mild, such infections are rarely detected.

C9. True

C10. False *Reason:* Acyclovir is used in the treatment of herpes simplex virus infection. There is no treatment for parvovirus B19. If maternal parvovirus infection is identified during pregnancy, the fetus should be monitored for possible (although uncommon) serious complications.

C11. True

C12. True

C13. True

C14. True

C15. False *Reason:* Breastfeeding is not a contraindication to postpartum rubella vaccination of a nonimmune mother.

Self-test D

D1. True

D2. True

D3. False *Reason:* A woman with active tuberculosis needs to maintain respiratory precautions and delay breastfeeding until she is noncontagious. Depending on the specific therapy and strain of tuberculous bacilli, this will take 2 weeks or more after appropriate medications are started.

D4. True

D5. True

D6. True

D7. False *Reason:* The reverse is true. Neonatal varicella-zoster (chickenpox) infection at 2 days of age or younger is usually much more severe than in older children.

D8.
a. Transplacental   b, c   Gonorrhea
b. Ascending   a   Toxoplasmosis
c. At delivery   a, c   Varicella-zoster virus (chickenpox)

D9. | Yes | No | |
|---|---|---|
| X | ___ | Maternal temperature of 38°C (100.4°F) |
| X | ___ | Rupture of membranes for 20 hours |
| ___ | X | Post-term labor |
| ___ | X | Maternal thrombocytopenia |
| X | ___ | Previous baby with group B streptococcal infection |
| X | ___ | Group B streptococcal bacteriuria early in pregnancy |

D10. A. Direct contact with organisms during passage through the birth canal

Self-test E

E1. True

E2. True

E3. True *Reason:* Women with asymptomatic bacteriuria, as well as women with symptomatic urinary tract infection, should be treated with antibiotics. All women should be checked routinely at the first prenatal visit for asymptomatic bacteriuria. Positive culture results, with or without symptoms, should be treated promptly with appropriate antibiotics.

E4. True

E5. False *Reason:* Sexual transmission does not appear to play a role in bacterial vaginosis. Treating sexual partners does not reduce recurrence.

E6. False *Reason:* There is no reason to stop breastfeeding when mastitis is present, unless an abscess develops (which rarely happens). If an abscess develops, breastfeeding from the affected breast should be temporarily interrupted.

E7. True

E8. True

E9. True

E10. True

E11. True

E12. True

E13. Any 3 of the following signs:
- Maternal temperature of 38°C (100.4°F) or higher more than 24 hours after delivery
- Increased white blood cell count
- Abdominal cramping
- Foul-smelling lochia

Unit 3 Posttest

After completion of each unit there is a free online posttest available at www.cmevillage.com to test your understanding. Navigate to the PCEP pages on www.cmevillage.com and register to take the free posttests.

Once registered on the website and after completing all the unit posttests, pay the book exam fee ($15) and pass the test at 80% or greater to earn continuing education credits. Only start the PCEP book exam if you have time to complete it. If you take the book exam and are not connected to a printer, either print your certificate to a .pdf file and save it to print later or come back to www.cmevillage.com at any time and print a copy of your educational transcript.

Credits are only available by book, not by individual unit within the books. Available credits for completion of each book exam are as follows: Book 1: 14.5 credits; Book 2: 16 credits; Book 3: 17 credits; Book 4: 9 credits.

For more details, navigate to the PCEP webpages at www.cmevillage.com.

Unit 4: Other Medical Risk Factors in Pregnancy

Objectives 152

1. How do maternal medical problems affect pregnancy? 154
2. How does maternal cardiovascular disease affect pregnancy? 154
   - A. Classes I and II 155
   - B. Classes III and IV 157
3. How do maternal endocrine disorders affect pregnancy? 157
   - A. Hyperthyroidism 157
   - B. Hypothyroidism 158
   - C. Diabetes mellitus 159
4. How does maternal hematologic disease affect pregnancy? 162
   - A. Severe anemia 162
   - B. Hemoglobinopathy 162
   - C. Thrombocytopenia 164
   - D. Thromboembolic disease 165
5. How does maternal immunologic disease affect pregnancy? 166
   - A. Antiphospholipid antibody syndrome 166
   - B. Systemic lupus erythematosus 168
6. How does maternal renal disease affect pregnancy? 170
7. How does maternal neurological disease affect pregnancy? 172
   - A. Seizure disorders 172
8. How does maternal respiratory disease affect pregnancy? 173
   - A. Asthma 173

Table

Table 4.1. Clinical and Laboratory Criteria for the Diagnosis of Antiphospholipid Antibody Syndrome 167

PCEP BOOK 2: MATERNAL AND FETAL CARE

Objectives

In this unit you will learn

A. What medical conditions place a pregnant woman or her fetus at risk

B. How to evaluate and monitor medical risk factors during pregnancy, labor, and the postpartum period

C. What implications maternal medical conditions have for the baby after birth

D. How to evaluate and monitor the baby for possible complications from maternal medical conditions

Note: Not all management and treatment details are presented in this unit. Hypertension and gestational diabetes are covered in detail in other units in this book. The scope of this unit does not allow the inclusion of material on *all* maternal medical conditions and how they may affect pregnancy. The problems covered here are relatively common, serious, or both, and each section provides an overview of the risks associated with that condition and the basic evaluation needed. Many of these high-risk conditions necessitate consultation with or referral to maternal-fetal medicine specialists and medical specialists—for example, an endocrinologist or cardiologist. Several of these conditions may pose significant risk to the woman's health during pregnancy, and pregnancy may result in a permanent effect on the woman's health. These conditions may also pose significant risk to fetal health and well-being. A woman needs to have specific, detailed, and current information about the risks and management options to make informed decisions. If pregnancy continues, management is often complex.

Unit 4 Pretest

Before reading the unit, please answer the following questions. Select the *one best* answer to each question (unless otherwise instructed). Record your answers on the test and check them with the answers at the end of the book.

1. Which of the following medical conditions is associated with an increased risk of maternal death?
   A. Teen pregnancy
   B. Severe, but well-controlled, asthma
   C. Twin gestation
   D. Maternal cardiac disease

2. **True** **False** Maternal immune thrombocytopenic purpura may place the fetus and newborn at risk for intracranial hemorrhage.

3. **True** **False** Women with antiphospholipid antibody syndrome should use only oral contraceptives that contain estrogen.

4. **True** **False** The dosage of an anticonvulsant medication to a woman with a seizure disorder should not be adjusted during pregnancy.

5. **True** **False** A fetus may develop goiter if maternal hyperthyroidism was treated during pregnancy.

6. All of the following statements are accurate concerning severe maternal anemia, except:
   A. Anemia may be a consequence of chronic medical illnesses.
   B. If postpartum hemorrhage occurs in a woman with severe anemia, it is more likely to be fatal.
   C. A fetus generally adapts better to chronic maternal anemia than to acute blood loss.
   D. Non–iron deficiency anemia should be treated with vitamin B_{12}.

7. **True** **False** Heparin use is contraindicated in women with antiphospholipid antibody syndrome.

For each condition presented in this unit, sections are given for *prenatal considerations, intrapartum considerations,* and *postpartum considerations, maternal* and *neonatal*. Lists within each section identify the procedures or tests that comprise the minimum basic evaluation for all women, fetuses, and babies with that particular risk factor. Women and their babies may each have several risk factors that may be the same or may be different from each other. Tests or procedures beyond those listed may also be needed. In addition, the lists do not include routine evaluation and care measures.

1. How do maternal medical problems affect pregnancy?

A preexisting medical illness may adversely affect the outcome of pregnancy, or pregnancy may affect the underlying medical condition. These effects are often most prominent in late pregnancy. Care requires a balance between treatment of the medical condition and management of the pregnancy and between fetal and maternal considerations.

Preconception counseling is advised for all women, particularly those with chronic medical conditions. This should include a discussion of the following:

- Risks to the fetus from maternal disease, including the likelihood of the fetus acquiring the condition through heredity
- Short-term and long-term risks to the woman's health, caused by worsening of a medical condition during pregnancy
- Probable medical management during pregnancy
- Risks and benefits of medications that may be needed during pregnancy and medication changes that should occur before conception

Any medical condition can affect pregnancy or be affected by pregnancy. Some conditions are especially likely to place a pregnant woman or her fetus at risk. Hypertension and infectious diseases are each covered in separate units in this book.

2. How does maternal cardiovascular disease affect pregnancy?

Cardiovascular disease has become a more prevalent issue during pregnancy. Women with a congenital heart defect that has been repaired may reach reproductive age with impaired cardiac function but normal fertility. The increase in obesity, diabetes, and hypertension, as well as delayed childbearing, has resulted in more women with acquired heart disease (eg, coronary artery disease) becoming pregnant. As pregnancy progresses, oxygen consumption, blood volume, heart rate, and cardiac output all increase. Women with heart disease may have difficulty responding to the demands these changes place on heart function. As a result, preexisting cardiac disease represents a leading and growing cause of maternal death.

Evaluation and treatment of women with heart disease in pregnancy will vary, depending on the specific heart disease and its severity. Consultation with cardiac, maternal-fetal, and pediatric specialists is recommended for the care of the woman and her fetus, especially if there is any evidence of maternal cardiac decompensation. Symptoms of concern include shortness of breath, decreased tolerance of physical activity, inability to sleep lying flat (orthopnea), and palpitations. Concerning physical findings include peripheral edema, rales, and rhonchi with auscultation of the lungs, and distension of the jugular veins.

 The effect of pregnancy on a woman with heart disease is closely related to her prepregnancy clinical status.

New York Heart Association Functional Classification of heart disease: This system uses symptoms a person experiences during physical activity to classify the relative severity of heart disease. The categories are as follows:

Class I.   Patients with cardiac disease but without resulting limitation of physical activity. Ordinary physical activity does not cause undue fatigue, palpitation, dyspnea, or anginal pain.

Class II. Patients with cardiac disease resulting in slight limitation of physical activity. They are comfortable at rest. Ordinary physical activity causes fatigue, palpitation, dyspnea, or anginal pain.

Class III. Patients with cardiac disease resulting in marked limitation of physical activity. They are comfortable at rest. Less than ordinary activity causes fatigue, palpitation, dyspnea, or anginal pain.

Class IV. Patients with cardiac disease resulting in an inability to carry on any physical activity without discomfort. Symptoms of heart failure or the anginal syndrome may be present even at rest. If any physical activity is undertaken, discomfort increases.

A. Classes I and II

Although patients usually tolerate pregnancy well, this degree of heart disease poses a risk to a woman and her fetus. Limitation of physical activity may be needed, especially for women with class II heart disease. Medical management of cardiac decompensation may be required during the second and third trimesters, and invasive hemodynamic monitoring during labor and the postpartum period may be necessary. Maternal health status should be optimized before pregnancy, including medication adjustments and weight loss.

1. Prenatal considerations
   - Be aware of the possible influence of maternal medications on fetal condition.
     — Oral anticoagulants are associated with abnormal fetal development and fetal intracranial hemorrhage and should be replaced with low-molecular-weight heparin (if possible, before conception). Women with a mechanical heart valve are at high risk for valve thrombosis, and management is complex, sometimes including continuation of oral anticoagulants. Consult with specialists.
     — Diuretics may interfere with placental perfusion, although this is much less likely in women chronically treated with diuretics prior to conception.
     — Angiotensin-converting enzyme inhibitors and angiotensin receptor blockers are associated with fetal renal abnormalities and, potentially, with fetal heart defects and are not used in pregnancy.
   - If a woman has congenital heart disease, a fetal echocardiogram is recommended because there is an increased risk the baby will also have congenital heart disease. The fetus will not necessarily have the same type of congenital heart disease as the mother.
   - Counsel the woman to avoid excessive weight gain, as appropriate for her initial body mass index.
   - Encourage reduction in strenuous activities and work schedule, as dictated by maternal symptoms. In general, bed rest is not recommended in pregnancy, as it has not been shown to improve outcomes and is associated with an increased risk of deep venous thrombosis and pulmonary embolism.

- Schedule regular prenatal visits tailored to the woman's specific needs. Watch for evidence of congestive heart failure—question the woman specifically about changes in activity and work tolerance, dyspnea, and orthopnea; auscultate her chest thoroughly to evaluate the lungs; assess whether weight gain is normal (weight gain from retained fluid may indicate congestive heart failure); and consider chest radiography or pulmonary function tests if there is uncertainty about cardiopulmonary status. Cardiac symptoms and shortness of breath may be expected to worsen at 30 to 34 weeks of gestation as intravascular blood volume reaches its maximum level for the pregnancy, and then remain stable until delivery. Labor is another high-risk period because of fluid administration and increased cardiac work.

2. Intrapartum considerations
   - Perform cesarean delivery only for obstetric indications (for most patients with heart disease, anesthesia and surgery pose a greater risk than labor).
   - Consider starting antibiotics.
     — The American Heart Association does *not* recommend prophylactic antibiotic therapy against infective endocarditis for women with heart disease for vaginal or cesarean delivery *except* for women who are *febrile* at the time of delivery. Mitral valve prolapse syndrome is not typically considered an indication for prophylactic antibiotics.
     — For women with unrepaired congenital heart disease, nonbiological prosthetic material in situ, or a history of endocarditis, who show no signs of infection at the time of delivery, antibiotic prophylaxis is individualized. Consult with the woman's cardiologist or maternal-fetal medicine specialist.
     — If a woman with heart disease has a fever at the time of delivery, the recommended prophylactic antibiotic regimen is as follows:
       - Ampicillin, 2 g, administered intramuscularly or intravenously, plus gentamicin, 1.5 mg/kg (not to exceed 120 mg), within 30 minutes of delivery, followed 6 hours later by ampicillin, 1 g, administered intramuscularly or intravenously, or amoxicillin, 1 g, given orally.
       - If a woman is allergic to ampicillin, administer 1 g of vancomycin intravenously over 1 to 2 hours and completed within 30 minutes of delivery; no postpartum dose is needed.
   - Monitor the fluid balance and avoid fluid overload.
   - Minimize the cardiac workload.
     — Minimize pain (increased heart rate due to reaction to pain may lead to heart failure).
     — Use narcotic analgesia or regional anesthesia as needed for pain relief.
     — Consider starting epidural anesthesia, which is appropriate for most patients once normal labor has been achieved.
   - Watch for congestive heart failure during the second stage of labor and the first few days after delivery.

3. Postpartum considerations

   Maternal
   - If antibiotic prophylaxis was given, provide a follow-up dose after delivery, as appropriate, to complete the course of antibiotics. (See Intrapartum considerations.)
   - Continue to monitor for deterioration of cardiac function.

UNIT 4: OTHER MEDICAL RISK FACTORS IN PREGNANCY

Neonatal
- Recommended actions depend on the fetal response to labor and delivery.
- If the mother has congenital heart disease, evaluate the newborn for evidence of congenital heart disease.
- If the mother has been taking thiazide diuretics and the baby has petechiae or otherwise shows evidence of bleeding, check the neonate's platelet count because neonatal thrombocytopenia has been reported.

B. Classes III and IV

Because of considerable risk to maternal health from heart failure during pregnancy, labor, or delivery, prompt consultation with a cardiologist or a maternal-fetal medicine specialist is needed. These women should receive prenatal care and plan to deliver at a tertiary care center.

 Women with class III or IV heart disease have a significant risk of decompensation during pregnancy or after birth. Care by specialists at a regional perinatal center is strongly advised.

3. How do maternal endocrine disorders affect pregnancy?

A. Hyperthyroidism

Consultation with specialists who are trained and experienced in the treatment of hyperthyroidism during pregnancy is recommended. If a woman's thyroid status is not stable before pregnancy, management can be especially complex. Even if hyperthyroidism is well controlled, it may worsen during pregnancy.

A pregnant woman should plan her medication management with her health professional before conception. Methimazole is most commonly used to treat hyperthyroidism; however, it may be associated with an increased risk of fetal scalp anomalies when used in the first trimester. Propylthiouracil is usually substituted in the first trimester; however, it is not used long term because of reports of liver damage associated with its use. An initial diagnosis of hyperthyroidism during pregnancy can be difficult because serum levels of certain thyroid hormones normally change with pregnancy. The use of radioactive iodine for treatment of hyperthyroidism is contraindicated.

1. Prenatal considerations
   - Thyroid-stimulating hormone (TSH) and free thyroxine levels should be followed and medication adjusted accordingly. The total thyroxine level increases with pregnancy and is more difficult to interpret; therefore, it is generally not used.
   - Monitor the woman for hypertensive disorders of pregnancy because the risk is increased. If found, manage according to guidelines in Unit 1, Hypertension in Pregnancy, in this book.
   - Monitor fetal well-being and growth because there is an increased risk for growth restriction.
   - Women who have uncontrolled hyperthyroidism, especially with increased concentrations of thyroid-stimulating immunoglobulins, may develop fetal goiter, although this is uncommon. Large fetal goiters can cause hyperextension of the head, which may require cesarean delivery. Performing routine ultrasonographic (US) evaluation specifically for the presence of fetal goiter is not recommended.

- If signs of thyroid crisis (storm) develop (maternal heart rate above 130 beats per minute, sweating, fever, tremor, and shortness of breath), the woman will need intensive care. Treatment with propranolol, thyroid inhibitors, saturated solution of potassium iodide, and antipyretics will be necessary.

Thyroid crisis can be life-threatening. Consultation with endocrinologists and maternal-fetal medicine specialists is strongly recommended.

2. Intrapartum considerations
   - In stable patients, continue the same dosage of autonomic drugs (eg, propranolol) and antithyroid medication during the intrapartum period.
   - Although rare, sudden development of thyroid crisis can occur, particularly in pregnant women with uncontrolled hyperthyroidism.
3. Postpartum considerations

   Maternal
   - Hyperthyroidism may become unstable. Monitor the woman carefully for several weeks after birth for tachycardia, palpitations, increased sweating, or unexplained diarrhea.
   - The mother may breastfeed if she requires treatment with methimazole.

   Neonatal
   - Consultation with pediatric specialists is recommended.
   - Evaluate the baby for hypothyroidism, hyperthyroidism, or goiter, because any of these conditions may be present.
   - Initially, the baby may develop transient hypothyroidism from placentally transferred antithyroid medication.
   - After several weeks, the baby may develop hyperthyroidism from thyroid-stimulating immunoglobulins, which also cross the placenta.
   - Monitoring or treatment may be needed for weeks or months.

B. Hypothyroidism

   A woman may be stable while taking thyroid hormone replacement therapy, with her serum TSH level within the reference range throughout pregnancy. If her condition is unstable, consultation with specialists who are trained and experienced in the treatment of this disease during pregnancy is recommended.

   Note: Women with untreated hypothyroidism are more likely to be anovulatory or have recurrent first-trimester losses. Pregnancy can occur unexpectedly during early treatment of the disease.

   1. Prenatal considerations
      - Check the woman's TSH level at the first prenatal visit and at least each trimester. The TSH should be checked within 4 to 6 weeks of a change in the dose of L-thyroxine.
      - Continue thyroid hormone replacement therapy throughout pregnancy to maintain a TSH level within reference range. For most women, the drug dosage may need to be increased. Some authorities recommend an automatic 30% L-thyroxine dose increase upon diagnosis of pregnancy.

UNIT 4: OTHER MEDICAL RISK FACTORS IN PREGNANCY

- Monitor fetal well-being because there is an increased risk for adverse events, including hypertensive disorders of pregnancy, placental abruption, low birth weight (secondary to preterm delivery due to preeclampsia), perinatal mortality, and neuropsychological impairment.

2. Intrapartum considerations
   None specific to hypothyroidism
3. Postpartum considerations
   Maternal
   - Monitor TSH levels and readjust thyroid replacement dosage as necessary.
   - Maternal medication treatment for hypothyroidism is not a contraindication to breastfeeding.

   Neonatal
   - The baby is usually unaffected; however, evaluate the baby for hypothyroidism, owing to *(a)* antithyroid antibodies that may cross the placenta or *(b)* goiter.
   - Consultation with pediatric specialists is recommended.

C. Diabetes mellitus

Women with preexisting type 1 or type 2 diabetes mellitus have an increased risk for early pregnancy loss, fetal congenital malformations, large size for gestational age, intrauterine fetal death (stillbirth), hypertensive disorders of pregnancy, shoulder dystocia, maternal and fetal birth injury, and cesarean delivery. Neonatal risks include macrosomia, hypoglycemia, hyperbilirubinemia, hypocalcemia, polycythemia, and respiratory distress syndrome. The likelihood of early miscarriage and congenital anomalies is related to how well the maternal blood glucose level is controlled around the time of conception. The risk of late pregnancy and newborn complications is related to how well the maternal blood glucose is controlled throughout the pregnancy; the existence of maternal end-organ complications, such as renal function impairment; and comorbidity such as chronic hypertension.

The management of diabetes mellitus in pregnant women is complex. Individualized evaluation and ongoing management of maternal glycemic control and comorbidities, as well as fetal growth and development, are essential for optimal pregnancy outcome. Collaborate with maternal-fetal medicine and/or endocrinology specialists who have experience in managing preexisting diabetes. It may be recommended that prenatal care and delivery occur at a regional perinatal center.

1. Prenatal considerations
   - Assess baseline maternal health status, including hemoglobin A_{1C} level, serum electrolytes and creatinine level, and urine protein excretion (urine protein to creatinine ratio on a spot urine sample, or a 24-hour urine total protein). Conduct early US examination to confirm gestational age and fetal viability.
   - Confirm that the woman has undergone a recent assessment for diabetic retinopathy.
   - Recommend the initiation of low-dose aspirin (81 mg daily) beginning at 12 weeks of gestation to reduce the risk of hypertensive disorders of pregnancy.
   - Recommend assessments for congenital anomalies, including maternal serum α-fetoprotein level at 16 to 18 weeks of gestation for open neural tube defects, detailed US at 18 to 20 weeks for congenital anomalies, and fetal echocardiography at 18 to 22 weeks for fetal congenital heart defects.

- In the third trimester, monitor fetal growth with serial US and fetal well-being with antenatal testing. Monitor the woman for the development of hypertensive disorders of pregnancy.
2. Intrapartum considerations
    - Monitor maternal blood glucose levels frequently, and maintain blood glucose values within reference range to avoid both hypoglycemia and hyperglycemia. This may require the use of a continuous intravenous insulin infusion.
    - Assess estimated fetal weight at the onset of labor. Monitor progress of labor carefully.
3. Postpartum considerations

Maternal
- After delivery, monitor blood glucose levels closely. Many women with type 1 diabetes will have a period of low insulin requirements and may experience hypoglycemia. Consider reducing insulin doses immediately after delivery.
- Breastfeeding is encouraged for all women who have diabetes. Careful attention to blood glucose control is needed, especially for women with type 1 diabetes.

Neonatal
- In the early newborn period, monitor the baby for hypoglycemia. Initiate breastfeeding within the first hour after birth, or formula feeding if the mother has chosen not to or is unable to breastfeed.

UNIT 4: OTHER MEDICAL RISK FACTORS IN PREGNANCY

Self-test A

Now answer these questions to test yourself on the information in the last section.

A1. True False Oral anticoagulants, rather than heparin, should be used during pregnancy.

A2. True False Thyroid crisis (storm) can be life-threatening.

A3. True False A woman with congenital heart disease was treated for congestive heart failure and pulmonary edema early in pregnancy. Near term, she is stable, without symptoms, and has a clear chest radiograph. You can anticipate that her labor and delivery will be uncomplicated.

A4. True False Thyroid crisis may develop in a woman with hypothyroidism.

A5. True False Cesarean delivery is usually less of a risk for a woman with heart disease than labor would be.

A6. True False Antibiotics are recommended during labor and for 6 hours after birth for all women with heart disease.

A7. True False With maternal hyperthyroidism, postpartum monitoring and treatment of the woman and her baby may be needed for months.

A8. True False A woman with congenital heart disease is at increased risk for delivering a baby with congenital heart disease.

A9. Which of the following actions are appropriate care measures for a woman with class II heart disease?

Yes	No	
___	___	Plan for cesarean delivery.
___	___	Frequent evaluation for evidence of congestive heart failure.
___	___	Maintain careful intravenous fluid balance.

A10. Which of the following complications may be signs of thyroid crisis?

Yes	No	
___	___	Maternal heart rate of 60 beats per minute
___	___	Sweating
___	___	Shortness of breath
___	___	Fever
___	___	Dry skin
___	___	Deep, labored breathing
___	___	Maternal heart rate of 150 beats per minute

A11. True False A woman with preexisting diabetes is at increased risk of delivering a baby with a congenital heart defect.

A12. Which of the following actions are recommended for the prenatal care of a woman with type 2 diabetes mellitus?

Yes	No	
___	___	Check maternal hemoglobin A_{1C} levels in early pregnancy
___	___	Confirm gestational age with early ultrasonography
___	___	Assess the fetus for congenital anomalies in the second trimester
___	___	Counsel the mother that the newborn will also have diabetes
___	___	Maintain control of the woman's blood glucose level throughout pregnancy

Check your answers with the list that follows the chapter. Correct any incorrect answers and review the appropriate section in the unit.

4. How does maternal hematologic disease affect pregnancy?

A. Severe anemia
   1. Prenatal considerations
      - Generally, a fetus can adapt better to chronic maternal anemia than to sudden maternal blood loss.
      - Investigate the cause of the woman's anemia.

       Accurate identification of the cause of severe anemia is the most important aspect of care.

      — Rule out chronic gastrointestinal blood loss with a stool guaiac test. If a stool guaiac test result is positive, investigate likely causes (eg, ulcers, hemorrhoids) and treat the underlying condition.
      — If the cause is iron deficiency, prescribe iron, folic acid, and vitamin supplements. Provide nutritional counseling.
      — Non–iron deficiency anemia may be caused by chronic medical conditions, particularly renal failure. Check urinalysis and renal function tests.
      — Non–iron deficiency anemia may also originate from a maternal hemoglobinopathy or other primary hematologic (non–pregnancy-related) cause.
   2. Intrapartum considerations
      If obstetric hemorrhage occurs, it is more likely to be fatal for a woman with preexisting severe anemia. A hemoglobin level below 7 g/dL represents a greatly diminished number of red blood cells and, therefore, a greatly reduced oxygen-carrying capacity. In the face of severe anemia, bleeding does not need to be massive for a critical volume of red blood cells to be lost, resulting in a lack of oxygen delivery to all body tissues. The normal function of the coagulation system may be impaired in the setting of severe chronic anemia. Steps that may be taken to minimize and quantify blood loss at delivery are described in Unit 2, Obstetric Hemorrhage, in this book.
   3. Postpartum considerations
      Maternal
      - Check hematocrit and hemoglobin levels.
      - Reassess or begin treatment, accordingly, per the cause.
      - Monitor carefully for postpartum hemorrhage.

      Neonatal
      Evaluate the baby for neonatal anemia.

B. Hemoglobinopathy
   Hemoglobinopathy is the condition of having abnormal hemoglobin molecules in the red blood cells. A genetic mutation in the β-globin gene leads to substitution of an amino acid in the β-globin protein, which reduces oxygen-carrying capacity of these molecules. Normal hemoglobin is designated *hemoglobin A;* known genetic variants include hemoglobin S (or sickle hemoglobin), hemoglobin A_2 (or β-thalassemia), and hemoglobin C. It is necessary to inherit 2 abnormal β-globin genes (one from each parent) to have clinically significant illness. Variants also exist in the α-globin gene, leading to 4 forms of α-thalassemia that range in severity from clinically silent to fatal. People of African, Mediterranean, and Asian descent, among others, are at increased risk for abnormal hemoglobin.

An individual with one hemoglobin A gene and one abnormal β-globin gene is a carrier for the abnormal gene and is referred to as having a hemoglobinopathy *trait*—for example, *sickle cell trait (hemoglobin AS)*. Carriers may be asymptomatic, have mild symptoms intermittently, or be symptomatic only in specific circumstances (eg, at high altitude).

Individuals with 2 abnormal β-globin genes have a hemoglobinopathy, as they have no normal hemoglobin molecules. *Sickle cell disease* is the prototype condition, which is present when an individual has 2 copies of the sickle hemoglobin gene (hemoglobin SS) and no copies of hemoglobin A. Other less common variant conditions exist, such as hemoglobin SC and hemoglobin SA_2, with variable clinical severity. Sickle cell disease is a serious, painful, and debilitating condition that results from reduced oxygen-carrying capacity of sickle hemoglobin and deformation of the red blood cells in small vessels, leading to occlusion of the vessels and inadequate tissue oxygen delivery.

A woman with hemoglobinopathy can experience frequent painful crises during pregnancy, which seriously jeopardize her health and the pregnancy. Consultation with or referral to maternal-fetal medicine specialists and hematologists at a regional perinatal medical center is strongly recommended.

1. Prenatal considerations
   - Pregnant women should be tested with a hemoglobin electrophoresis, unless they are already known to have a hemoglobinopathy. If a pregnant woman has an abnormal hemoglobin electrophoresis, her partner should also be tested. If both parents have an abnormal β-globin gene, the fetus is at risk for hemoglobinopathy, and prenatal diagnosis is possible through amniocentesis or chorionic villus sampling. Consult with maternal-fetal medicine staff on recommended procedures and laboratory tests as needed.
   - Maternal hemoglobinopathy significantly increases the risk for fetal growth restriction, fetal death, preterm prelabor rupture of membranes, and preterm labor. Fetal well-being and growth need extremely close monitoring.
   - Maternal sickle crises may occur more frequently during pregnancy and may be life-threatening because of thromboembolism, infection, or heart failure. Nursing considerations during a crisis include the provision of pain medication, ensuring adequate intravenous hydration, administration of supplemental oxygen, and blood transfusion.
   - Urinary tract infections are more common in women with sickle hemoglobin. Treat all infections promptly with antibiotics. Screen women at least once per trimester for asymptomatic bacteriuria.
2. Intrapartum considerations
   - Women with a sickle cell trait generally require no special treatment during labor. If they are anemic, giving oxygen by mask may be helpful. Consider pulse oximetry to monitor maternal oxygenation.
   - Intrapartum management of women with sickle cell disease can be complex. Labor and delivery at a regional perinatal medical center are strongly recommended.
3. Postpartum considerations
   Maternal
   The risk of thromboembolism is increased, especially after cesarean delivery or with prolonged immobilization.

Neonatal
- Many states include testing for hemoglobinopathies as part of routine newborn screening. Know the requirements of your state.
- An affected baby will not show signs of illness for several months, when concentrations of fetal hemoglobin begin to decrease.
- Provide counseling for the parent or parents about future pregnancies and treatment for the baby, as appropriate, early in infancy.

C. Thrombocytopenia

Thrombocytopenia, defined as a maternal platelet count less than 150,000/mm^3, is a relatively common finding in pregnancy, with many possible causes. Gestational thrombocytopenia and immune thrombocytopenic purpura (ITP) are among the most common causes of thrombocytopenia. Thrombocytopenia may also occur in the setting of hypertensive disorders of pregnancy; refer to Unit 1, Hypertension in Pregnancy, in this book for more information.

1. Gestational thrombocytopenia

   This is a benign condition that occurs only during pregnancy. It occurs in 7% to 8% of pregnancies, but it has no maternal symptoms and does not result in fetal or neonatal thrombocytopenia.

   Gestational thrombocytopenia is characterized by
   - No history of easy bruising or bleeding
   - Platelet count within reference range or slightly decreased in early pregnancy
   - Low platelet count, generally between 70,000/mm^3 and 150,000/mm^3, in late pregnancy
   - Platelet count in reference range between pregnancies

2. Immune thrombocytopenic purpura

   ITP is not caused by pregnancy and is usually diagnosed when a non-pregnant woman is found to have easy bruising and abnormal bleeding. If thrombocytopenia is found for the first time when a woman is pregnant, it is necessary to distinguish gestational thrombocytopenia from ITP, which is characterized by
   - History of easy bruising and bleeding
   - Medical records that show a previously low platelet count (non-pregnant state)
   - Low platelet count, below 150,000/mm^3, in early pregnancy
   - Low platelet count, generally less than 70,000/mm^3, in late pregnancy

   If previous (non-pregnant) platelet counts are not available, it may not be possible to make the distinction between gestational thrombocytopenia and ITP. Platelet counts below 70,000/mm^3 are usually, but not always, associated with ITP rather than gestational thrombocytopenia.

   With ITP, maternal platelet counts may be extremely low. Treatment for symptomatic ITP is complex. Consultation with maternal-fetal medicine and hematology specialists is recommended.

   In addition, some women with ITP have antiplatelet antibodies that cross the placenta. These maternal antibodies attach to proteins on the surface of the fetus's platelets, destroying the fetal platelets. Currently available tests cannot differentiate between antibodies in the pregnant woman's blood that will affect fetal platelets and antibodies that will not. Estimates of the risk of neonatal thrombocytopenia vary widely; a summary of case series suggests a 10% chance of platelet count less than

50,000/mm³ and a 5% chance of platelet count less than 20,000/mm³. Platelet counts of babies born to women with ITP may decrease sharply in the days immediately after birth because of an increase in neonatal splenic function.

3. Prenatal considerations
   - It is especially important to instruct the woman with low platelet counts (from ITP or gestational thrombocytopenia) not to use aspirin or aspirin-containing medications, which inhibit the ability of platelets to aggregate and control bleeding.
   - Delivery should be planned to occur at a center where the newborn can be evaluated for thrombocytopenia. The route of delivery is determined by usual obstetric considerations and is not based solely on the maternal history of ITP. Percutaneous umbilical blood sampling to determine fetal platelet count was formerly recommended to determine fetal platelet counts, but this practice has been discontinued, as the risk of complications of the procedure exceed the risk to the neonate of vaginal birth. Delivery should occur at term with a stable maternal platelet count.

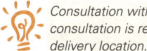
Consultation with or referral to maternal-fetal medicine specialists for consultation is recommended. Maternal status may influence preferred delivery location.

4. Intrapartum considerations

   Current recommendations are to manage labor and delivery in the usual fashion and to reserve cesarean delivery for the usual obstetric indications. Operative vaginal delivery is not contraindicated in a woman with ITP but should be undertaken with caution. For women with ITP and a platelet count below 70,000/mm³, epidural and spinal anesthesia are usually contraindicated because of the risk of epidural hematoma.

5. Postpartum considerations

   Maternal

   Monitor for excessive bleeding.

   Neonatal
   - Check the platelet count; the level may decrease, so monitor the count daily for several days.
   - Consider cranial US or computed tomography to check for intracranial hemorrhage if the neonatal platelet count is low.
   - Delay newborn circumcision until neonatal thrombocytopenia has been ruled out.

D. Thromboembolic disease

Pregnancy is a period of high risk for deep venous thrombosis and pulmonary embolism, due to the physiological changes associated with pregnancy. Women with a prior history of thromboembolism are at risk for a recurrent venous thromboembolism (VTE), and women with no prior history of VTE may experience the new onset of deep venous thrombosis or pulmonary embolism.

The management of pregnant women with a prior history of VTE is complex. Individualized evaluation and ongoing management of maternal anticoagulation is essential for optimal pregnancy outcome. Collaborate with maternal-fetal medicine and/or hematology specialists who have experience in managing thromboembolism and anticoagulation in pregnancy.

1. Prenatal considerations
   - Obtain a thorough medical history from the woman, detailing her prior history of thromboembolism, including the circumstances and treatments.
   - Refer the woman to a hematologist or maternal-fetal medicine specialist for anticoagulation treatment, based on her degree of risk.
   - Warfarin is contraindicated during pregnancy, and there are limited data regarding the use of oral agents such as apixaban and rivaroxaban during pregnancy. If a woman conceives while taking one of these agents, facilitate a medication change to either low-molecular-weight heparin (enoxaparin, dalteparin) or to unfractionated heparin.
   - Obtain a thorough medical history and family history from all pregnant women; in addition to a prior personal history of VTE, in some cases anticoagulation therapy is recommended during pregnancy on the basis of family history of thromboembolism.
2. Intrapartum considerations
   - Women receiving any form of anticoagulation therapy during pregnancy require careful coordination of care around the time of delivery. Low-dose (prophylactic) anticoagulation therapy will not affect the risk of bleeding at either vaginal or cesarean delivery, but full-dose (therapeutic) anticoagulation therapy may.
   - The timing of the last dose of anticoagulation therapy and the safe administration of neuraxial (epidural or spinal) anesthesia must be carefully coordinated.
3. Postpartum considerations

   Maternal
   - The postpartum period is a period of high risk for VTE. Women with a prior history of VTE should continue anticoagulation therapy for at least 6 weeks.
   - After delivery, assess all women for risk of VTE. Some women with no prior history of VTE will be at risk and should receive prophylactic anticoagulation therapy.
   - Breastfeeding is encouraged for all women with a history of VTE. Anticoagulant medications are compatible with breastfeeding.

   Neonatal
   None specific to a history of thromboembolism

5. How does maternal immunologic disease affect pregnancy?

A. Antiphospholipid antibody syndrome

This is an autoimmune disease characterized by clinical findings, including recurrent early pregnancy loss, unexplained fetal death, and venous or arterial thrombosis, as well as the presence of clinically significant titers of antiphospholipid antibodies (APAs) (Table 4.1). The diagnostic criteria are based on the detection of anticardiolipin immunoglobulin M (IgM) and/or immunoglobulin G (IgG) antibodies, anti-β_2 glycoprotein I IgM and/or IgG antibodies, and lupus anticoagulant. The use of a specialty reference lab will result in the most reliable results. Although some panels include other APAs (eg, antiphosphatidylserine, antiphosphatidylinositol) and other antibody classes, such as immunoglobulin A, these are not included in the diagnostic criteria.

Table 4.1. Clinical and Laboratory Criteria for the Diagnosis of Antiphospholipid Antibody Syndrome

Clinical Criteria	Laboratory Criteria

One or both of the following clinical events:
1. Vascular thrombosis (one or more episodes, whether arterial, vascular, or small vessel)
2. Obstetric morbidity
  a. One or more deaths of a morphologically normal fetus after 10 weeks of gestation; or
  b. One or more preterm births of a morphologically normal fetus before 34 weeks of gestation due to eclampsia, preeclampsia, or features consistent with placental insufficiency; or
  c. Three or more consecutive unexplained spontaneous pregnancy losses before 10 weeks of gestation, after hormonal, anatomic, and genetic causes have been excluded.
	Any one of the following results, on 2 assays performed at least 12 weeks apart:
	1. Positive for lupus anticoagulant (while the patient is not being treated with anticoagulants), or
	2. Positive for anti-cardiolipin IgG or IgM antibodies in medium or high titers (>40 GPL or MPL, or greater than the 99th percentile), or
	3. Positive for anti-β_2 glycoprotein 1 IgG or IgM antibodies (greater than the 99th percentile)

Abbreviations: GPL, IgG phospholipid units; IgG, immunoglobulin G; IgM, immunoglobulin M; MPL, IgM phospholipid units.

Derived from Miyakis S, Lockshin MD, Atsumi T, et al. International consensus statement on an update of the classification criteria for definite antiphospholipid syndrome (APS). *J Thromb Hemost.* 2005;4:295–306.

The most significant maternal complication associated with antiphospholipid antibody syndrome (APS) is thrombosis. Most thrombotic events are venous—most commonly a blood clot in a lower extremity or a pulmonary embolism. Arterial thrombosis is also possible, with stroke being the most common clinical picture. Venous and arterial thrombosis due to APS can appear in uncommon locations, and a clot found in such a site should prompt investigation for APS. Pregnancy and the use of estrogen-containing oral contraceptives are associated with thrombosis in women with APS.

While women with systemic lupus erythematosus (SLE) may also have APAs, most women with APS do not have SLE. Women with APAs but without SLE may be asymptomatic. Women with APS or APA-related disorders are often first identified as having APAs when evaluated for repeated pregnancy losses.

Treatment of women with antiphospholipid antibody syndrome during pregnancy requires careful management. Consultation with or referral to maternal-fetal medicine specialists at a regional perinatal center is recommended.

1. Prenatal considerations
   - Certain APAs cause a false-positive reaction in maternal and newborn nontreponemal tests for syphilis. Use treponemal tests for women with APAs.
   - Women with APS or APA-related disorders are at increased risk for
     — Early pregnancy loss
     — Fetal growth restriction
     — Second and third trimester fetal death

— Abnormal fetal heart rate patterns (often preceding second or third trimester fetal death)
— Early-onset preeclampsia (often before 34 weeks of gestation)
— Medically indicated preterm birth, due to pregnancy complications such as preeclampsia

Several theories exist as to the mechanism of fetal loss and growth restriction, but none fully explain the clinical findings.

- Low-molecular-weight heparin and low-dose aspirin is the recommended therapy for women with APS. The dosage and timing of initiation of therapy should be determined in consultation with specialists.
- Appropriate treatment for women with a history of pregnancy morbidity but non-diagnostic levels of APAs is not clearly defined.
- Antenatal surveillance of fetal status should start in the third trimester and should include US assessments of fetal growth and biophysical profiles or nonstress tests (NSTs).

2. Intrapartum considerations
Careful monitoring of maternal and fetal status

3. Postpartum considerations

Maternal

- Rarely, the course of APS becomes life-threatening. A small number of women with APS develop fever, multiple thromboses, and renal and cardiopulmonary failure postpartum.
- Oral contraceptives that contain estrogen should *not* be used, because estrogen increases the likelihood of VTE.
- Women with a previous thrombotic event may be advised to take lifelong anticoagulation. Warfarin is usually the anticoagulant medication used, except during pregnancy. During pregnancy, low-molecular-weight heparin should be used for women with a history of thrombosis. It is not clear whether women with APS but without a history of thrombosis should undergo long-term anticoagulation therapy.

Neonatal

- Anticipate the possible need for neonatal resuscitation.
- A baby may be preterm and small for gestational age. Screen for corresponding risk factors. Provide care appropriate for size and gestational age. (See Book 1: Maternal and Fetal Evaluation and Immediate Newborn Care, Unit 6, Gestational Age and Size and Associated Risk Factors.)

B. Systemic lupus erythematosus

SLE is an autoimmune condition that most often affects women of childbearing age. It is a multisystem, progressive disease characterized by periods of exacerbation and remission. Women with clinically significant SLE activity are more likely to experience complications during pregnancy.

Women with SLE produce a variety of autoantibodies that can affect nearly every organ system, causing an inflammatory immune response. Signs and symptoms may include joint or muscle pain, nephritis, hypertension, low white blood cell or platelet counts, anemia, rash over the nose and cheeks, pneumonitis, pleurisy, intermittent low-grade fever, pericarditis, myocarditis, or central nervous system involvement with seizures, irritability, headaches, or psychosis.

Current consensus criteria for the diagnosis of SLE include the detection of antinuclear antibodies (ANAs) as an obligatory finding, with additional clinical and immunologic criteria assessed and assigned a score. The criteria are regularly reviewed and updated jointly by the European League Against Rheumatism and the American College of Rheumatology.

Medication therapy for a woman with SLE should be coordinated with maternal-fetal medicine and rheumatology specialists.

1. Prenatal considerations
   - *Effects of pregnancy on SLE:* Pregnancy probably does not affect the long-term prognosis for SLE, but "flares" or periods of exacerbation seem to occur more often during pregnancy. Women with SLE should carefully plan their pregnancies for times when they have low disease activity and are taking stable doses of medication. Symptoms of an SLE flare may resemble preeclampsia, eclampsia, or HELLP (*h*emolysis, *e*levated *l*iver enzyme levels, and *l*ow *p*latelet count occurring in association with preeclampsia) syndrome. Worsening proteinuria, hypertension, or thrombocytopenia, or the onset of seizures, can be presumed to represent superimposed preeclampsia or eclampsia and should be treated accordingly.
   - *Effects of SLE on pregnancy*
     — *Miscarriage and fetal death during early pregnancy:* Risk is increased significantly, particularly if the woman also has APS or has active SLE disease activity around the time of conception.
     — *Fetal growth restriction, abnormal fetal heart rate testing, or fetal death during late pregnancy:* Risk is increased significantly if maternal hypertension, renal compromise, or placental insufficiency are present.
     — *Fetal heart block:* Maternal antibodies against SS-A and SS-B (formerly called *Ro* and *La*) proteins may cross the placenta during pregnancy and damage the conduction system of the fetal heart, causing fetal heart block. In some cases, this may lead to the onset of fetal hydrops and fetal death.
     — *Preterm delivery:* Risk of preterm birth is increased with SLE and may be owing to spontaneous onset of labor or to maternal or fetal indications for preterm delivery.
   - Consider delivery at a regional perinatal center, even for stable women, because SLE can worsen suddenly during labor or immediately after birth.
   - In addition to obstetric and medical care, physical therapy, exercise and dietary planning, psychiatric care, pain management, or the assistance of social services may be needed for the pregnant or postpartum woman.
   - Frequent antenatal testing of fetal growth and well-being should start at approximately 28 weeks of gestation and may include serial US examinations, NSTs, biophysical profile, and amniotic fluid assessment. Doppler assessment of umbilical blood flow is also performed if fetal growth restriction is present.

Surveillance and care of maternal and fetal health during pregnancy in a woman with systemic lupus erythematosus is often extremely complex. Consultation with or referral to maternal-fetal medicine specialists is strongly recommended.

2. Intrapartum considerations
   - Care should be individualized, based on the presence of complicating conditions such as fetal growth restriction, hypertensive disorders of pregnancy, lupus flare, or other complications.
   - Continuous electronic fetal monitoring is recommended during labor.
   - If the woman was receiving chronic steroid treatment during the pregnancy, stress-dose steroids are recommended at the time of labor or cesarean delivery.
   - Epidural or spinal anesthesia may be contraindicated if thrombocytopenia is present.

For women with systemic lupus erythematosus, delivery at a facility equipped and staffed to provide maternal, fetal, and neonatal intensive care is recommended.

3. Postpartum considerations
   Maternal
   - If maternal medications include steroids, the risk for infection (eg, endometritis, surgical wound, urinary tract) may be increased. Monitor closely and treat aggressively.
   - SLE exacerbation can occur after birth.
   - Although rare, severe renal or cardiopulmonary complications can develop, especially for women with SLE who also have APS.

   Neonatal
   - Anticipate a possible need for neonatal resuscitation.
   - Occasionally, babies born to women with SLE will have "transient neonatal SLE," a benign and self-limited condition characterized by a rash, briefly increased ANA levels, and—less often—by transient hematologic abnormalities, hepatosplenomegaly, and pericarditis.
   - Evaluate cardiac status. Monitor the baby for arrhythmias, particularly heart block. The prognosis for babies with congenital heart block depends on several factors, including the degree of heart block. A pacemaker may be needed.
   - The baby may be preterm and small for gestational age. Screen for corresponding risk factors. Provide care appropriate for the baby's size and gestational age (see Book 1: Maternal and Fetal Evaluation and Immediate Newborn Care, Unit 6, Gestational Age and Size and Associated Risk Factors).

6. How does maternal renal disease affect pregnancy?

Women with renal disease are at increased risk for preterm birth, fetal growth restriction, in utero death, and preeclampsia. The risk for these complications is directly related to the severity of the maternal renal dysfunction. If the renal disease is mild and uncomplicated by any other medical illness, the risk for development of these complications is relatively low.

Women with renal disease complicated by chronic hypertension or poor renal function are at much higher risk for development of complications. Severe renal disease may be permanently worsened by pregnancy.

Early detection of hypertension or deteriorating renal function is essential for the optimal care of women with renal disease.

A. Prenatal considerations
   - Preconception consultation is recommended to determine the best treatment during pregnancy.
   - Evaluate renal function early in pregnancy and periodically as the pregnancy progresses.
   - If renal function deteriorates, investigate other causes, such as urinary tract infection, dehydration, nephrotoxic drugs, and preeclampsia.
   - Monitor the woman for the development of preeclampsia. If renal function remains normal, follow the management guidelines presented in Unit 1, Hypertension in Pregnancy, in this book.
   - In the third trimester, begin closer maternal-fetal surveillance.
     — More frequent prenatal visits
     — Daily fetal activity determinations
     — Weekly to twice-weekly antenatal testing of fetal well-being, starting at 28 to 34 weeks of gestation, depending on the severity
     — Serial US evaluation of fetal growth

   Note: *Renal transplant patients* usually tolerate pregnancy well if they enter pregnancy with normal renal function and are taking stable doses of immunosuppressive medications. If renal function begins to deteriorate, it is necessary to differentiate between hypertensive disorders of pregnancy and transplant rejection. Intrapartum management has no special requirements. Medication management after delivery should be coordinated with the transplant specialist and include considerations of lactation status.

    Consultation with maternal-fetal medicine specialists is strongly recommended for the care of pregnant women with renal disease, especially if hypertension or declining renal function develops.

B. Intrapartum considerations
   Abnormal fetal heart rate patterns are more likely if fetal growth restriction or hypertensive disorders of pregnancy are present.

C. Postpartum considerations
   Maternal
   Monitor renal function and blood pressure.

   Neonatal
   - Anticipate the need for possible neonatal resuscitation.
   - Feed the baby early and screen for hypoglycemia. (See Book 1: Maternal and Fetal Evaluation and Immediate Newborn Care, Unit 8, Hypoglycemia.)
   - If resuscitation is needed, monitor for post-resuscitation complications.

7. How does maternal neurological disease affect pregnancy?

A. Seizure disorders
Consultation with a maternal-fetal medicine physician and a neurologist is recommended.
1. Prenatal considerations
   - Folate supplementation is recommended, beginning *before conception* or as early in pregnancy as possible. The neural tube, which develops into the brain and spinal cord, is formed during the first month of gestation. Many anticonvulsants interfere with folic acid metabolism, and folic acid deficiency has been associated with neural tube defects. Many authorities recommend higher daily folic acid dosage (4 mg/d) to decrease the risk of spina bifida, although the evidence to support higher doses for women taking antiepileptic drugs is limited.
   - Women with seizure disorders are at increased risk for delivering a baby with congenital anomalies. This is thought to be primarily due to exposure to medications, although some risk may be attributed to the seizure disorder and genetic susceptibility.
   - Seizure control is important to the woman's general health and day-to-day ability to function and engage in work and other activities. The regimen that best controls the woman's seizure activity should be continued throughout the pregnancy. Some anticonvulsant medications (eg, phenytoin, phenobarbital, carbamazepine) are associated with an increased risk for congenital anomalies, while others (lamotrigine, levetiracetam) are not. Anticonvulsant therapy with valproic acid should be avoided during pregnancy, as this medication is associated with a high risk for structural anomalies and developmental delays.
   - Serum anticonvulsant concentrations tend to decrease during pregnancy, owing to the increased volume of distribution and altered protein binding. Obtain serum levels at least each trimester and after dose adjustments, and adjust the dosage as needed.
   - Monitor the woman closely for the development of hypertensive disorders of pregnancy. If preeclampsia develops and seizures occur, eclampsia should be considered, rather than simply attributing the convulsion to her seizure disorder. Women with seizure disorders are at no higher risk for hypertensive disorders of pregnancy than other pregnant women. (See Unit 1, Hypertension in Pregnancy, in this book.)
2. Intrapartum considerations
   - If a woman's seizure disorder is under good control, with no recent symptoms, continue usual medication therapy during labor.
   - If a woman has had recent seizures, check the level of anticonvulsant medication in her blood. Adjust the medication dosage as needed.
   - If seizures are accompanied by hypertension and proteinuria, consider that they may be caused by eclampsia, and treat according to the guidelines in Unit 1, Hypertension in Pregnancy, in this book.
   - If uncontrollable seizures occur, which is rare, administer oxygen and anticonvulsant medication.
     — Phenytoin (Dilantin), 10 to 15 mg/kg, administered intravenously
       - Deliver slowly so as not to exceed the 50-mg/min infusion rate.
       - Initiate continuous cardiac monitoring during phenytoin infusion.
     or
     — Diazepam (Valium), 10 mg, administered intravenously

- Consult with a maternal-fetal medicine specialist, a neurologist, and an anesthesiologist (for airway management as necessary).
3. Postpartum considerations
Maternal
- Reevaluate the anticonvulsant medication dosage and adjust as necessary.
- All anticonvulsant medications enter breast milk in small amounts. If the mother takes anticonvulsants and wishes to breastfeed, consult a reference database for up-to-date information related to the potential risks of exposure to the newborn. A lactation consult may also be useful and would ideally be performed prior to delivery so that the infant nutrition plan will be established. Resources include *Hale's Medications and Mothers' Milk*; Briggs' *Drugs in Pregnancy and Lactation*; the National Institutes of Health LactMed database (https://toxnet.nlm.nih.gov/newtoxnet/lactmed.htm); and the Reprotox database (www.reprotox.org).

Neonatal
- Evaluate the baby for congenital malformations, depending on the anticonvulsant medication used to treat the mother.
- Check clotting studies; consider giving the baby additional vitamin K if the mother was taking phenytoin.

8. How does maternal respiratory disease affect pregnancy?

A. Asthma
1. Prenatal considerations
   - Encourage the woman to maintain her usual asthma treatment regimen. No fetal concerns have been attributed to maternal asthma treatments, and prevention of a severe exacerbation is preferred.
   - Treat acute asthma exacerbations medically. While medications used to treat asthma do not pose any risk to the fetus, a severe or prolonged asthma exacerbation poses a significant threat to the mother.
   - Target fetal surveillance, such as US for growth and fetal monitoring, to the severity of the maternal asthma and any associated conditions.
   - If maternal asthma is severe and persistent, monitor the fetus for growth restriction.
2. Intrapartum considerations
   - Plan to deliver vaginally. Perform cesarean delivery only for the usual obstetric indications and not exclusively because the woman has asthma. Be sure anesthesia staff are aware of the patient's asthma so bronchospasm-inducing agents can be avoided.
   - Avoid bronchospasm during labor. Treat with steroids or bronchodilators.
3. Postpartum considerations

Maternal
Be aware that asthma exacerbations can occur at any time.

Avoid the use of carboprost tromethamine for uterine atony, as this agent is associated with bronchoconstriction.

Neonatal
None specific

Self-test B

Now answer these questions to test yourself on the information in the last section.

B1.	True	False	Because of the risk of causing congenital anomalies, women with seizure disorders should not take phenytoin (Dilantin) during pregnancy.
B2.	True	False	Carboprost tromethamine given for postpartum hemorrhage may cause an asthma exacerbation.
B3.	True	False	Limited placental function in a woman with renal disease may result in growth-restriction.
B4.	True	False	In some cases of maternal immune thrombocytopenic purpura, fetal platelets can be destroyed, putting the fetus and newborn at risk for intracranial bleeding.
B5.	True	False	If hemorrhage occurs in a woman with severe anemia, it is more likely to be life-threatening than it would be in a non-anemic woman.
B6.	True	False	A woman with systemic lupus erythematosus may be stable or become seriously ill during pregnancy.
B7.	True	False	Sickle cell disease may be life-threatening to a woman and her fetus during pregnancy.
B8.	True	False	A severe asthma exacerbation that necessitates hospitalization of the pregnant woman increases the risk to the fetus.
B9.	True	False	Women with seizure disorders treated with phenytoin (Dilantin) maintain stable serum levels throughout pregnancy, making periodic readjustment of the drug dosage unnecessary.
B10.	True	False	Women with a sickle cell trait may benefit from receiving oxygen by mask throughout labor.
B11.	True	False	Women with renal disease are at increased risk for developing preeclampsia.
B12.	True	False	Cardiac arrhythmias may occur in babies born to women with systemic lupus erythematosus.
B13.	True	False	The risk of venous thromboembolism is increased during pregnancy for women with antiphospholipid antibody syndrome.
B14.	True	False	The risk of recurrent miscarriage is increased for women with antiphospholipid antibody syndrome and for women with systemic lupus erythematosus.
B15.	True	False	Regardless of maternal medical illness, worsening hypertension increases the risk of complications for a woman and her fetus.

Check your answers with the list that follows. Correct any incorrect answers and review the appropriate section in the unit.

Self-test Answers

These are the answers to the Self-test questions. Please check them with the answers you gave and review the information in the unit wherever necessary.

Self-test A

A1. False *Reason:* The reverse is accurate. Oral anticoagulants are harmful to the fetus and should be replaced with heparin therapy during pregnancy.

A2. True

A3. False *Reason:* A woman with that degree of heart disease is likely to develop complications, especially congestive heart failure, during labor or after birth.

A4. False *Reason:* Thyroid crisis (storm) is a possible complication of hyperthyroidism.

A5. False *Reason:* For most women with heart disease, anesthesia and surgery pose a greater risk than labor.

A6. False *Reason:* Antibiotics are recommended only for women who have a fever.

A7. True

A8. True

A9.
Yes	No	
	X	Plan for cesarean delivery.
X		Frequent evaluation for evidence of congestive heart failure.
X		Maintain careful intravenous fluid balance.

A10.
Yes	No	
	X	Maternal heart rate of 60 beats per minute
X		Sweating
X		Shortness of breath
X		Fever
	X	Dry skin
	X	Deep, labored breathing
X		Maternal heart rate of 150 beats per minute

A11. True

A12.
Yes	No	
X		Check maternal hemoglobin A_{1C} levels in early pregnancy
X		Confirm gestational age with early ultrasonography
X		Assess the fetus for congenital anomalies in the second trimester
	X	Counsel the mother that the newborn will also have diabetes
X		Maintain control of the woman's blood glucose level throughout pregnancy

Self-test B

B1. False *Reason:* While phenytoin therapy during pregnancy carries increased risk for congenital anomalies, the risk of serious injury to the woman is greater if anticonvulsant medication is stopped and seizures occur.

B2. True

B3. True

B4. True

B5. True

B6. True

B7. True

B8. True

B9. False *Reason:* Anticonvulsant levels tend to decrease during pregnancy and should be checked every 2 to 4 weeks, with the dosage readjusted as necessary to maintain therapeutic levels in the woman.

B10. False

B11. True

B12. True

B13. True

B14. True

B15. True

Unit 4 Posttest

After completion of each unit there is a free online posttest available at www.cmevillage.com to test your understanding. Navigate to the PCEP pages on www.cmevillage.com and register to take the free posttests.

Once registered on the website and after completing all the unit posttests, pay the book exam fee ($15) and pass the test at 80% or greater to earn continuing education credits. Only start the PCEP book exam if you have time to complete it. If you take the book exam and are not connected to a printer, either print your certificate to a .pdf file and save it to print later or come back to www.cmevillage.com at any time and print a copy of your educational transcript.

Credits are only available by book, not by individual unit within the books. Available credits for completion of each book exam are as follows: Book 1: 14.5 credits; Book 2: 16 credits; Book 3: 17 credits; Book 4: 9 credits.

For more details, navigate to the PCEP webpages at www.cmevillage.com.

Unit 5: Obstetric Risk Factors: Prior or Current Pregnancy

Objectives 178

Obstetric History

1. How does previous uterine surgery affect pregnancy? 181
2. How do you manage pregnancy with a history of a previous macrosomic newborn? 181
3. How do you manage pregnancy with a history of previous fetal or neonatal death? 183
4. How does a history of previous congenital malformation(s) or hereditary disease affect pregnancy? 183
5. What risks are associated with high parity (multiple previous births)? 184
6. What risks are associated with previous cesarean delivery? 184
7. How is red blood cell alloimmunization diagnosed and managed? 186

Current Pregnancy

8. What risks are associated with teen pregnancy? 189
9. What risks are associated with pregnancy in women of increased maternal age (≥35 years)? 190
10. What is genetic screening and how is it used in pregnancy? 190
11. How are multifetal gestations managed? 192
12. How is an abnormal amount of amniotic fluid diagnosed and managed? 194
13. How is fetal growth restriction diagnosed and managed? 199
14. What risks are associated with late term and post-term gestational age? 200

Tables and Figure

Table 5.1. Recommended Weight Gain in Pregnancy 182
Table 5.2. Delivery of Twins 193
Figure 5.1. Uterine Quadrants for Amniotic Fluid Measurements 195

Recommended Routines 204

PCEP BOOK 2: MATERNAL AND FETAL CARE

Objectives

In this unit you will learn

A. What obstetric conditions (factors identified in a previous pregnancy or present in the current pregnancy) place a woman or her fetus at risk

B. How to evaluate and monitor obstetric risk factors during pregnancy, labor, and the postpartum period

C. What implications obstetric conditions have for the baby after birth

D. How to evaluate and monitor the baby for possible complications from obstetric conditions

Note: Not all management and treatment details are presented in this unit. Obstetric hemorrhage, preterm labor, and prelabor rupture of membranes are covered in detail in other units in this book. The scope of this unit does not allow the inclusion of material on all obstetric risk factors and how they may affect pregnancy. The problems covered here are either relatively common, serious, or both, and each section provides an overview of the risks associated with that condition and the basic evaluation needed. Many of these high-risk conditions necessitate consultation with or referral to maternal-fetal medicine specialists. Several of these conditions may pose significant risk to the woman's health at delivery, or to fetal health and well-being. A woman needs to have specific, detailed, and current information about the risks and management options to make informed decisions.

Unit 5 Pretest

Before reading the unit, please answer the following questions. Select the *one best* answer to each question (unless otherwise instructed). Record your answers on the test and check them with the answers at the end of the book.

1. **True False** Women who are heavy smokers are much more likely than non-smokers to deliver babies who are large for gestational age.

2. **True False** A woman who delivered one stillborn baby has an increased risk of delivering another stillborn baby.

3. **True False** Placental function declines in post-term gestations, significantly increasing the risk for category II and category III fetal heart rate tracings during labor.

4. Which of the following are recommended for a 26-year-old woman who is pregnant with twins?

Yes	No	
___	___	Prenatal visit every week during the third trimester
___	___	Extra iron and folic acid supplementation
___	___	Amniocentesis for chromosomal analysis
___	___	Serial ultrasonographic evaluations of fetal growth

5. Which of the following conditions are associated with fetal growth restriction?

Yes	No	
___	___	Polyhydramnios
___	___	Systemic lupus erythematosus
___	___	Severe maternal hypertension
___	___	Multifetal gestation
___	___	Placenta previa

6. **True False** Twins in non-vertex (A) –vertex (B) presentation are generally delivered vaginally.

7. **True False** Growth-restricted fetuses are at increased risk for abnormal fetal heart rate patterns during labor.

8. Which of the following conditions is most likely to be associated with oligohydramnios?
   - **A.** Fetal growth restriction
   - **B.** Fetal gastrointestinal tract abnormality
   - **C.** Maternal diabetes mellitus
   - **D.** Multifetal gestation

9. Which of the following conditions is most likely to be identified in a post-term pregnancy?
   - **A.** Decreased volume of amniotic fluid
   - **B.** Cardiac defect in the fetus
   - **C.** Multiparity
   - **D.** Congenital infection

(continued)

Unit 5 Pretest (*continued*)

10. Vaginal birth after a cesarean delivery is usually contraindicated when
    A. Estimated fetal weight is more than 2,500 g (>5 lb 8 oz).
    B. Epidural anesthesia is planned.
    C. The woman has undergone a prior classical (vertical) cesarean delivery.
    D. Previous birth was preterm.

11. Polyhydramnios is associated with an increased risk for
    A. Umbilical cord compression
    B. Anencephaly
    C. Maternal hypertension
    D. Congenital infection

12. In general, pregnant teenagers are at increased risk for all of the following complications, except:
    A. Sexually transmitted infections
    B. Rapid labor
    C. Hypertensive disorders of pregnancy
    D. Preterm delivery

13. **True   False**   Polyhydramnios is associated with congenital infection.

UNIT 5: OBSTETRIC RISK FACTORS: PRIOR OR CURRENT PREGNANCY

For each condition presented in this unit, sections are given for *prenatal considerations, intrapartum considerations,* and *postpartum considerations, maternal* and *neonatal*. Lists within each section identify the procedures or tests that comprise the minimum basic evaluation for all women, fetuses, and babies with that particular risk factor. Women and their babies may each have several risk factors that may be the same or may be different from each other. Tests or procedures beyond those listed may also be needed. In addition, the lists do not include routine evaluation and care measures.

Obstetric History

It is important to obtain a thorough, detailed history during the first prenatal visit. Special attention should be given to eliciting a detailed obstetric and reproductive history, to be able to identify risk factors that may affect the current pregnancy. Attempt to obtain complete copies of a woman's earlier reproductive health care records. If fetal or neonatal death occurred, those records—including autopsy findings—can be extremely valuable in counseling the parents and providing future care.

1. How does previous uterine surgery affect pregnancy?

Uterine surgery, such as myomectomy, may increase the risk of uterine rupture in future pregnancies. Documentation of the depth of the incision into the myometrium is important in counseling women about the risk of uterine rupture and making a plan for delivery. Obtain the surgical report whenever possible.

A. Prenatal considerations
- Previous surgery may increase the risk of uterine rupture during labor.
- Consider cesarean delivery before the onset of labor and discuss the risks and benefits of this plan with the pregnant woman.

B. Intrapartum considerations
The risk of uterine rupture during labor is increased (see Section 6, What risks are associated with previous cesarean delivery? Intrapartum considerations, Signs of uterine rupture, later in the unit).

C. Postpartum considerations
Maternal
None specific to previous uterine surgery

Neonatal
In some cases, an early term delivery is recommended, which may be associated with more difficulties in neonatal transition.

2. How do you manage pregnancy with a history of a previous macrosomic newborn?

A. Prenatal considerations
- Many babies weighing more than 4,000 g (>8 lb 13 oz) are born to women without any medical complications. Gestational diabetes and preexisting diabetes mellitus are both associated with an increased risk of fetal macrosomia. Evaluate the woman for glucose intolerance early in the pregnancy and again at 24 to 28 weeks of gestation (see Unit 7, Gestational Diabetes, in this book).
- Counsel the woman to avoid excessive weight gain, as appropriate for her prepregnancy body mass index (Table 5.1).

Table 5.1. Recommended Weight Gain in Pregnancy		
Prepregnancy Weight Classification and BMI	**Weight Women Should Gain When Pregnant With One Baby**	**Weight Women Should Gain When Pregnant With Twins**
Underweight (BMI < 18.5)	28–40 lb	50–62 lb[a]
Normal weight (BMI of 18.5–24.9)	25–35 lb	37–54 lb
Overweight (BMI of 25.0–29.9)	15–25 lb	31–50 lb
Obese (BMI ≥ 30.0)	11–20 lb	25–42 lb

Abbreviation: BMI, body mass index.

[a] All recommendations are from the National Academy of Medicine, with the exception of underweight women with twins.

Adapted from https://www.cdc.gov/reproductivehealth/maternalinfanthealth/pregnancy-weight-gain.htm. Accessed May 15, 2020.

- Estimate fetal weight clinically, supplemented by ultrasonographic (US) examination as needed, near term. If an earlier delivery was complicated by shoulder dystocia with sequelae, consider cesarean delivery if the fetus is comparable in size to the previous baby.
- Vaginal delivery of a macrosomic fetus may be accompanied by shoulder dystocia, brachial plexus injury in the newborn, and vaginal lacerations in the mother. Shoulder dystocia is a serious and unpredictable complication.
  — Shoulder dystocia is encountered with 10% to 15% of babies weighing more than 4,000 g (>8 lb 13 oz).
  — When the estimated fetal weight is more than 4,500 g (>9 lb 15 oz) in a woman with diabetes, or 5,000 g (>11 lb) in a woman without diabetes, consider planned cesarean delivery.
  — *Brachial plexus injury:* Approximately 1 in 1,000 babies with shoulder dystocia will have *permanent* nerve damage (commonly called *Erb palsy*).
- Together with the patient, a decision about delivery route should be made on the basis of history, current pregnancy, and clinical judgment.

B. Intrapartum considerations
- Reevaluate fetal size and review delivery plans with the parent or parents.
- If vaginal delivery is the route planned, reevaluate the plan frequently on the basis of labor progress. Extra caution should be used when considering the use of operative vaginal delivery (forceps or vacuum).

C. Postpartum considerations

Maternal

If vaginal delivery, check for cervical, vaginal, and perineal lacerations.

Neonatal

If the baby is large, screen for hypoglycemia (see Book 1: Maternal and Fetal Evaluation and Immediate Newborn Care, Unit 8, Hypoglycemia) and check for brachial plexus injury (Erb palsy or paralysis).

3. How do you manage pregnancy with a history of previous fetal or neonatal death?

A. Prenatal considerations
- Review previous maternal and fetal records (including autopsy report, placental pathology report, and karyotype, whenever possible) to provide parents with the most accurate and complete information about the cause of the previous loss and risks in the current pregnancy.
- Evaluate the woman for syphilis, diabetes mellitus, thyroid disorders, red blood cell alloimmunization, and immunologic diseases (systemic lupus erythematosus and antiphospholipid antibody syndrome) because all are associated with an increased risk for fetal death.
- Begin daily fetal activity determinations at approximately 28 weeks of gestation.
- At a gestational age prior to when the previous loss occurred, begin regularly scheduled antenatal testing of fetal well-being, US for assessment of fetal growth, and frequent prenatal visits.

B. Intrapartum considerations
Continuous fetal heart rate monitoring is recommended.

C. Postpartum considerations
Maternal
The mother and/or father may continue to need support and counseling when dealing with the loss of a previous baby.
Neonatal
Evaluation of this baby depends on the cause of the previous perinatal death, as well as problems, if any, experienced during this pregnancy, labor, and delivery.

4. How does a history of previous congenital malformation(s) or hereditary disease affect pregnancy?

A. Prenatal considerations
- Some malformations and diseases have a predictable pattern of inheritance, but many do not. Parents need to know the cause, treatment, prognosis, and risk of recurrence. Arrange for genetic counseling before pregnancy or as early in pregnancy as possible. Discuss possible prenatal diagnosis of the fetus. Consultation with a maternal-fetal medicine specialist or geneticist is recommended.
- If the previous disorder was, or can be, clearly identified, use diagnostic tests specific for that malformation. Specific tests are not available for all malformations.
- The risk of neural tube defects (eg, anencephaly, meningomyelocele) has been shown to be reduced with folic acid supplementation. Folate (0.4 mg/d) is recommended for *all* women, beginning before conception or as early in pregnancy as possible. Women whose prior pregnancy was affected by a neural tube defect should take folate 4 mg/d beginning before conception until 10 weeks of gestation, then reduce the dose to 0.4 mg/d for the remainder of the pregnancy.

5. What risks are associated with high parity (multiple previous births)?

Traditionally, the definition of grand multiparity is 5 or more previous births.

A. Prenatal considerations
- Observe the woman closely for signs of hypertension and placenta previa.
- Risk for placental abruption is also increased, particularly if the woman smokes or has hypertension.

B. Intrapartum considerations
There is an increased risk for rapid labor and uterine rupture.

C. Postpartum considerations
Maternal
Women of high parity are at increased risk for postpartum hemorrhage owing to uterine atony.
Neonatal
None specific to high maternal parity

6. What risks are associated with previous cesarean delivery?

A. Repeat cesarean delivery
- If a repeat cesarean delivery is planned for a time prior to the onset of spontaneous labor, fetal maturity criteria should be fulfilled, as outlined in Book 1: Maternal and Fetal Evaluation and Immediate Newborn Care, Unit 2, Fetal Age, Growth, and Maturity.
- Most planned cesarean deliveries will be scheduled, as this will be the preference of most women. Another approach is to await the spontaneous onset of labor and perform the cesarean delivery at that time. This may be especially important if there is a question about the accuracy of a woman's estimated due date.

B. Trial of labor after cesarean delivery
Repeat cesarean deliveries account for approximately one-third of all cesareans. The overall success rate for trial of labor after cesarean delivery (TOLAC) is 60% to 80%. Successful TOLAC is more common for women who have had a previous vaginal birth and less common for women whose previous cesarean delivery was due to dystocia. Although they occur infrequently, serious risks are associated with TOLAC, including
- Uterine rupture (5–8 per 1,000 trials of labor after cesarean delivery), which can be life-threatening for the woman and the fetus
- Abnormal fetal heart rate patterns

C. Contraindications to TOLAC
- Previous vertical uterine incision
- Contracted pelvis
- Abnormal fetal heart rate patterns
- Lack of obstetric physician and anesthesia staff immediately available to provide emergency care (American College of Obstetricians and Gynecologists. ACOG Practice Bulletin No. 205: Vaginal Birth after Cesarean Delivery. 2019).

D. Prenatal considerations

Consider a trial of labor if all of the following conditions exist:
- One previous cesarean delivery with low transverse incision confined to the noncontractile lower uterine segment; no other uterine scars are present.
    Note: A trial of labor may be considered in women with 2 prior low-transverse cesarean deliveries. The risk of uterine rupture may be as high as double the rate for women with one prior cesarean delivery. A history of prior vaginal birth and 2 prior cesarean deliveries is associated with a higher success rate than in women without a history of vaginal birth.
- Clinically adequate maternal pelvis.
- Vertex presentation (some experts may offer TOLAC to women with breech presentation or twin pregnancy).
- No fetal contraindications to vaginal delivery.
- Availability of continuous fetal and uterine monitoring.
- Capability for immediate cesarean delivery and hysterectomy, if necessary.
- A woman who is well informed and well prepared.

 A trial of labor may not be appropriate for all women with a prior cesarean delivery, even if they meet all the conditions. Individual history must be carefully considered.

E. Intrapartum considerations
- Prostaglandins, such as misoprostol and dinoprostone, should not be used for third-trimester cervical ripening or labor induction in patients who have had a cesarean delivery or major uterine surgery. If indicated, cervical ripening may be performed with an intracervical balloon catheter.
- Oxytocin may be used for induction or augmentation of labor. No consistent relationship has been found between the use of oxytocin and an increased risk of uterine rupture, although some studies have indicated a relationship between high-dose oxytocin and uterine rupture.
- Epidural anesthesia does not seem to affect the success rate for vaginal birth after cesarean delivery, and its use rarely masks the signs of uterine rupture (if one occurs). However, it should be noted that with epidural anesthesia, maternal complaints of "shoulder strap" pain may be the first symptom of uterine rupture.

Signs of uterine rupture

Sudden cessation of labor progress, variable fetal heart rate decelerations that progress to late decelerations and bradycardia, uterine or abdominal pain, and loss of fetal station are the hallmarks of uterine rupture. Vaginal bleeding may not be present. Hypotension and signs of shock may develop and indicate intra-abdominal hemorrhage.

F. Postpartum considerations
Maternal
- Routine exploration of the uterus after a successful vaginal delivery is not recommended. Asymptomatic separation of an old scar generally heals well without surgical repair. There is no indication that surgical repair of an asymptomatic scar rupture improves future pregnancy outcome.

- If a woman experiences uterine rupture that can be repaired, she is not considered a candidate for TOLAC in a future pregnancy.

Neonatal
None specific to vaginal birth after cesarean delivery

7. How is red blood cell alloimmunization diagnosed and managed?

A. Prenatal considerations
- The presence of antibodies against a red blood cell antigen is known as *alloimmunization*. In pregnancy, antibodies against the Rh(D) antigen and several other antibodies can cross the placenta and lead to hemolysis of fetal red blood cells, resulting in anemia. If the anemia becomes severe, the fetus may develop hydrops or be stillborn. If a woman has a positive antibody screening result at her initial prenatal visit, several steps are taken to assess the risk to the fetus.
- Careful medical and obstetric history, including a history of blood transfusion at any time in the woman's life and a history of all prior pregnancies, including antepartum bleeding, early pregnancy losses, and ectopic pregnancies.
- For women with anti-Rh(D) antibodies, a history of having received Rh immunoglobulin in prior pregnancies.
- A determination of the titer of maternal antibody.
- Paternal history—is the current pregnancy with the same partner as prior pregnancies?
- Paternal testing—determination of the paternal genotype for the specific red blood cell antigen to which the woman has an antibody.
- If it is determined that the fetus is at risk for hemolytic anemia, in some cases, amniocentesis can be performed to test the fetal genotype for the specific red blood cell antigen.

Surveillance of a pregnancy with alloimmunization includes regular US monitoring of the fetus, including middle cerebral artery blood flow studies by using Doppler US. Fetal therapy may include one or several intrauterine fetal blood transfusions.
- Timing of delivery requires a balance between gestational age and the extent to which the fetus is being affected by anemia.
- The risk of preeclampsia is increased if fetal hydrops is present.
- If fetal hydrops is found before the onset of labor, delivery at a regional perinatal center is strongly recommended. Fetuses with fetal hydrops generally do not tolerate labor well, will require neonatal intensive care, and have a high mortality rate.

 Because of the high risk of fetal death or serious neonatal illness associated with red blood cell alloimmunization, co-management with or referral to maternal-fetal medicine specialists is strongly recommended for all Rh(D)-sensitized women.

B. Intrapartum considerations
- If hydrops is found during labor and transfer of the woman is unwise at that time, monitor the fetal heart rate continuously and be prepared for a cesarean delivery because fetuses with hydrops are more likely to have abnormal fetal heart rate tracings.

- If you plan a delivery with a woman with Rh alloimmunization electively in your hospital
  — If hydrops is not present, monitor the woman carefully and deliver vaginally, unless there are obstetric indications for cesarean delivery.
  — Plan to have blood ready in the delivery room for emergency transfusion if a seriously anemic newborn is anticipated. The blood volume of babies with Rh disease is often normal or even high. If transfusion is needed for anemia, it must be given cautiously and, perhaps, as an exchange transfusion. Blood that may be transfused includes
    - O Rh-negative red blood cells, *crossmatched against the mother's blood*
    or
    - Type-specific blood (same as fetal blood type)
    or
    - Maternal washed, packed red blood cells, donated and prepared in advance of delivery
- Anticipate and plan for intensive neonatal care.

C. Postpartum considerations

Maternal

Provide counseling on future pregnancies. Alloimmunization will be a concern for all future pregnancies.

Neonatal
- Consult with pediatric specialists and your hospital's blood bank.
- Be prepared to resuscitate the baby or provide continued respiratory support if hydrops is present.
- Check the baby's blood pressure, hematocrit level, bilirubin level, reticulocytes, peripheral smear, and antiglobulin (Coombs) test.
- Be prepared to start intensive phototherapy treatment for hyperbilirubinemia soon after delivery.
- Anticipate the need for exchange transfusion(s), as well as thoracentesis or paracentesis, if the baby has hydrops.

Self-test A

Now answer these questions to test yourself on the information in the last section.

A1. Match each condition in the left column with the most closely associated condition on the right.

_____ Shoulder dystocia   a. Cesarean delivery

_____ Brachial plexus injury   b. Macrosomia

_____ Neonatal hypoglycemia

_____ Previous uterine surgery

_____ Abnormal maternal glucose tolerance

A2. The risk of uterine rupture during labor is increased when previous uterine surgery entered the _____

A3. Soon after delivery, women who give birth vaginally to large babies should be checked for _____

A4.	True	False	The presence of fetal hydrops indicates that the fetus will tolerate labor poorly and the baby will need intensive care.
A5.	True	False	Vaginal birth is successful for 60% to 80% of women with a previous cesarean delivery.
A6.	True	False	When Rh disease is present, the baby may require a transfusion in the delivery room for severe anemia.
A7.	True	False	All congenital malformations have a predictable pattern of inheritance.
A8.	True	False	Vaginal birth after cesarean delivery is contraindicated when a previous classical (vertical) cesarean delivery was done.
A9.	True	False	Autopsy reports of a previous fetal or neonatal death are rarely useful in providing information to parents about future pregnancies.
A10.	True	False	Evaluation of fetal death may include testing of the woman for various medical illnesses.

A11. Large babies, especially those weighing more than 4,000 g (>8 lb 13 oz) at birth, should be screened for _____, whether or not their mothers were known to have abnormal glucose intolerance during pregnancy.

A12. A 27-year-old woman who has had 6 previous deliveries is at risk for which of the following complications?

Yes	No	
___	___	Post-term pregnancy
___	___	Uterine rupture
___	___	Postpartum hemorrhage
___	___	Placental abruption
___	___	Rapid labor
___	___	Fetal chromosomal abnormality

Check your answers with the list that follows the Recommended Routines. Correct any incorrect answers and review the appropriate section in the unit.

Current Pregnancy

Complications or risk factors may be identified in an ongoing pregnancy in several different ways. A woman without prior pregnancy complications may develop clinically significant complications during a subsequent pregnancy. This may occur in the antepartum period or during labor and may be preceded by the identification of warning signs or symptoms or occur suddenly. Various screening tests that are used during pregnancy may indicate the possibility of an abnormality in the fetus.

8. What risks are associated with teen pregnancy?

A. Prenatal considerations
- Pregnant teenagers are at increased risk for hypertensive disorders of pregnancy, poor nutrition, drug use, intimate partner violence, and sexually transmitted infections (STIs).
- Poverty, educational interruption, disruption of the teenager's own growth and development, and other adverse social or economic factors may be present. Provide social service consultation, psychological counseling, and family support services as appropriate to individual needs. Pregnant teenagers may want to receive information about pregnancy termination or adoption.
- Pregnancy is most often unplanned and may create additional family stress and social upheaval. Provide emotional support, pregnancy and childbirth information, parenthood preparation discussions, and other teaching or resources as appropriate to individual needs.
- Teenagers may benefit from counseling and prenatal care geared specifically toward them. Counseling, teaching, and discussions in peer groups, rather than one on one, may be valuable.
- The risk of preterm delivery is increased in teen pregnancy.
- Provide regular prenatal visits, dietary and drug counseling, contraceptive information, and information about transmission, consequences, and prevention of STIs.

B. Intrapartum considerations
- Consider the possibility of fetopelvic disproportion in pregnant teenagers with small stature.
- Support from family and friends takes on more than the usual importance.
- A combination of praise, patience, encouragement, and gentle guidance from health professionals is especially valuable.

C. Postpartum considerations
Maternal
- Provide parenting information and support.
- Provide child development and care instruction.
- Review contraceptive options and information about STIs. Long-acting reversible contraception methods, including intrauterine devices and subdermal contraceptive implants, are especially effective and are recommended as first-line agents in adolescents.
- Provide emotional support and praise; recognize the stress of parenting before the woman has herself achieved adulthood.

Neonatal
- Consult with social services.
- Establish a system of follow-up care.
- Assess the need for a support network for the woman or to oversee the welfare of the baby.

9. What risks are associated with pregnancy in women of increased maternal age (≥35 years)?

A. Prenatal considerations
- The proportion of pregnancies occurring in women over 35 has increased, because of delayed childbearing. Most women over 35 will have normal pregnancies, although the likelihood of complications is related to the existence of underlying medical conditions, such as diabetes mellitus, chronic hypertension, and obesity. Maternal death is more common after age 40 years and especially after age 45 years. Even healthy women age 35 years and older are more likely to have pregnancies affected by placenta previa, hypertensive disorders of pregnancy, and gestational diabetes.
- The risk of having a pregnancy affected by a fetal chromosomal abnormality is increased after age 35 years. The risk of a newborn delivered at term having trisomy 21, or Down syndrome, is 1 in 353 for women aged 35 years and 1 in 35 for women aged 45 years (American College of Obstetricians and Gynecologists. ACOG Practice Bulletin No. 162, May 2016. Invasive Prenatal Testing for Genetic Disorders). Offer genetic counseling, aneuploidy screening, and diagnostic testing, such as chorionic villus sampling or amniocentesis.
- The risk of preterm delivery is increased because of a higher frequency of medically or obstetrically indicated preterm birth.
- Consider screening for gestational diabetes early in pregnancy and again at 24 to 28 weeks of gestation (see Unit 7, Gestational Diabetes, in this book).
- Begin antenatal testing as indicated by a woman's preexisting or acquired clinical condition.

B. Intrapartum considerations
- Continuous electronic fetal monitoring is recommended, especially if the woman has a coexisting medical condition.
- The likelihood of cesarean delivery is increased.

C. Postpartum considerations
Maternal
Postpartum hemorrhage is more likely to occur.

Neonatal
- Evaluate and monitor the baby according to the mother's medical diseases, if any.
- Evaluate the baby for congenital malformations.

10. What is genetic screening and how is it used in pregnancy?

All pregnant women are at risk of having a fetus with a chromosomal abnormality. Screening tests are designed to identify the pregnancies most likely to be affected by any of a variety of abnormalities. These tests should be offered to *all* pregnant women. Each woman should make an informed choice about which screening test she would like to have, and each woman has the option to decline screening. (American College of Obstetricians and Gynecologists. ACOG Practice Bulletin No. 163: Screening for Fetal Aneuploidy, May 2016.)

While the risk of a chromosomal abnormality is higher in women aged 35 years and older, only about 20% of all births occur in this age group. Most babies, and thus most babies with chromosomal abnormalities, are born to women younger than 35 years. It is also important to remember that there are more babies born with birth defects and normal chromosomes than babies born with chromosome abnormalities.

- Early pregnancy dating is essential. For many screening tests, accurate determination of gestational age is necessary for interpretation of test results. Test values change with gestational age.
- Depending on test results, discuss the options available to the family during pregnancy, including diagnostic testing, such as amniocentesis or chorionic villus sampling. If a woman learns through diagnostic testing that a fetal chromosome abnormality is present, she should receive extensive counseling on the expected health outcomes of the specific abnormality, as well as her further management options, including continuation of the pregnancy, releasing the baby for adoption, and termination of the pregnancy. Consultation with experts is recommended.
- If a fetal abnormality is present, it may influence the route and location of delivery.
    A. Screening tests
    A screening test result that is reported as "low risk" or "negative" does not guarantee that a fetus is normal. Screening tests do not indicate the presence of abnormalities in the entire genetic code, but rather, they are used to screen for a limited number of more common abnormalities. Certain risk factors (eg, family history, advanced maternal age) may indicate the need for other diagnostic tests, even if initial screening results are within reference range. A screening test result that is reported as "high risk" or "positive" does not conclusively indicate that a fetus is abnormal. All screening tests are subject to the possibility of false-positive results. Certain tests, such as maternal serum α-fetoprotein and multiple marker tests, may yield abnormal results if the gestational age used in calculating test results is inaccurate.
    - *First-trimester nuchal translucency screening*: Measurement of the nuchal translucency (a specific measurement obtained at the back of the fetal neck by a certified ultrasonographer), in combination with serum concentrations of human chorionic gonadotropin and pregnancy-associated plasma protein A, will aid in the identification of approximately 85% of fetuses with trisomy 21 (Down syndrome) and a smaller proportion of fetuses with trisomy 18.
    - *Cell-free DNA screening*: A highly sensitive blood test performed after 10 weeks of gestation can be used to measure fragments of DNA from chromosomes 13, 18, and 21 and the X and Y chromosomes to screen for common trisomies.
    - *Maternal serum* α-fetoprotein can be measured at 15 to 20 weeks of gestation (most accurate at 16–18 weeks) to screen for open neural tube defects (and help detect about 85% of neural tube defects) and ventral wall defects (eg, gastroschisis, omphalocele). Most babies with neural tube defects (90%–95%) are born to families with no risk factors. All pregnant women should be informed of the availability of the test and its limitations. When increased maternal serum α-fetoprotein values are found, additional testing is recommended.

- *Multiple markers:* When interpreted in relation to maternal age, maternal serum α-fetoprotein, unconjugated estriol, inhibin-A, and human chorionic gonadotropin will help identify approximately 80% of fetuses with trisomy 21 (Down syndrome) and a smaller proportion of fetuses with trisomy 18.

Screening tests do not indicate a definitive diagnosis, nor do they allow a problem to be completely ruled out. In general, positive results can help identify patients who need to be offered diagnostic testing.

B. Diagnostic tests
- *Amniocentesis* can be performed any time after 15 weeks but usually before 20 weeks of gestation. Analysis of amniotic fluid obtained with amniocentesis can help detect fetal chromosomal, biochemical, and enzymatic abnormalities.
- *Chorionic villus sampling* is performed at 10 to 12 weeks of gestation. Analysis of placental villi obtained with chorionic villus sampling can help detect fetal chromosomal and genetic abnormalities.
- Comprehensive US is always performed in conjunction with amniocentesis or chorionic villus sampling. US alone cannot be used to diagnose or rule out a chromosomal or genetic abnormality.

11. How are multifetal gestations managed?

Women with twin gestation are at increased risk for preterm delivery, twin-twin transfusion, discordant growth or fetal growth restriction, placenta previa, placental abruption, abnormal presentation, non-reassuring fetal status, in utero death, and umbilical cord prolapse. One or both of the fetuses may be affected. The risk of all of these conditions is higher with a triplet pregnancy.

It is recommended that women who are pregnant with triplets, or any higher-order multiple gestation, be referred to regional perinatal center specialists for prenatal care, delivery, and neonatal care. The risk for fetal complications, extremely preterm birth, and neonatal illness is very high. Decreased activity, intensive fetal surveillance, and careful planning for delivery and neonatal care are generally required for optimal outcome.

A. Prenatal considerations
- Preterm birth is the most common risk in a multifetal gestation. Institute preterm labor precautions given in Unit 9, Preterm Labor, in this book. While aggressive management of preterm labor may be able to prolong gestation, the likelihood of delivery before term is high. It is recommended that this be discussed with the woman and plans made in advance for delivery at a hospital staffed and equipped to care for preterm newborns.
- Maternal risk for anemia is increased. Monitor the woman for anemia and treat it appropriately, with iron or other supplementation.
- Gestational diabetes is more common. Consider early glucose screening.
- The risk for development of hypertensive disorders of pregnancy is increased. Recommend low-dose aspirin to reduce the risk of preeclampsia.

- Schedule more frequent prenatal visits in the second half of pregnancy.
- Use serial US examinations to
  — *Evaluate each fetus for growth restriction.*
  — *Estimate the volume of amniotic fluid in each sac.* If either fetus has an abnormal amount of amniotic fluid, consultation with a maternal-fetal medicine specialist is recommended.
  — *Identify the number of placentas and amniotic sacs.* Complications are least common among dichorionic/diamniotic (2 placentas, separate amniotic sacs) twin gestations. Monochorionic/diamniotic (single shared placenta, separate amniotic sacs) twin pregnancies are at risk for twin-to-twin transfusion syndrome, which can result in death or neurological injury to one or both fetuses. Absence of a membrane separating the twins indicates monoamniotic twins. Monoamniotic twins are able to move around each other in the amniotic sac, which results in entanglement of the umbilical cords. The risk of fetal death is increased. Women with monoamniotic twins are typically admitted to the hospital in the third trimester for close fetal monitoring. Cesarean delivery is recommended for monoamniotic twins.
- Routine antepartum testing for dichorionic twin pregnancies has not been shown to be beneficial. If the woman has a high-risk condition, such as diabetes or hypertension, or if fetal growth restriction is diagnosed, initiate antepartum testing with nonstress tests and/or biophysical profiles. All monochorionic twin pregnancies require close surveillance throughout the pregnancy; consultation with a maternal-fetal medicine specialist is recommended.
- Near term, use US to determine
  — Fetal presentation
  — Placental location

B. Intrapartum considerations
- When the woman presents in labor, use US to document fetal presentations. Delivery route is usually determined by fetal presentation, gestational age, and training and experience of the health professional (Table 5.2).

Table 5.2. Delivery of Twins		
Fetal Presentation[a] (First Twin–Second Twin)	**Gestational Age**	**Recommended Route of Delivery**
Vertex-vertex	Term or preterm	Vaginal delivery[b]
Vertex–non-vertex	Term	Vaginal delivery[b]
Vertex–non-vertex	Preterm	Cesarean or vaginal delivery[b]
Non-vertex–vertex	Term or preterm	Cesarean delivery
Non-vertex–non-vertex	Term or preterm	Cesarean delivery

[a] If monoamniotic twins are present, cesarean delivery is the recommended route, regardless of fetal presentation.

[b] Acute fetal heart rate abnormalities and malpresentation of the second twin, requiring intrauterine fetal manipulation, occur often. Use the vaginal route only if the physician is experienced and skilled in the delivery of fetuses with abnormal presentation. If physician expertise for breech extraction is lacking, plan for cesarean delivery.

- Even when vaginal delivery is expected, anesthesia personnel and facilities should be *immediately* available throughout the second stage of labor, in case an emergency cesarean delivery becomes necessary. If anesthesia personnel and/or appropriate facilities are not available for the second stage of labor, cesarean delivery early in labor should be considered, regardless of fetal presentation.
- If vaginal delivery is planned, continuous fetal heart rate monitoring throughout labor is essential. Monitoring of the second twin should continue during and after delivery of the first twin because there is an increased likelihood of cord prolapse, placental separation, and cessation of uterine contractions during this time.
- Contractions may stop after delivery of the first twin. Oxytocin augmentation may be needed.
- Anticipate an increased likelihood of postpartum hemorrhage with vaginal or cesarean delivery. Insert a large-bore intravenous line for rapid fluid infusion and consider having blood crossmatched for the woman, in case transfusion or volume expansion is needed.
- Plan to have a neonatal team for each baby attend the delivery.

C. Postpartum considerations

Maternal

The risk of postpartum hemorrhage is increased. Check the woman's blood pressure and heart rate. Monitor the woman for excessive bleeding.

Neonatal
- Be prepared with a delivery room team for *each* baby.
- Check the babies' blood pressure and hematocrit values.

12. How is an abnormal amount of amniotic fluid diagnosed and managed?

Amniotic fluid volume varies with gestational age. It increases from 16 weeks of gestation until peaking at approximately 27 weeks of gestation, stays stable until approximately 33 weeks of gestation, and then decreases steadily through 42 weeks of gestation. Abnormal amounts of amniotic fluid, decreased (oligohydramnios) or increased (polyhydramnios), constitute a risk factor for adverse pregnancy outcome.

Amniotic fluid volume is assessed with US techniques, with several methods for assessment in wide use. Each requires a skilled sonographer using consistent technique, measuring pockets of amniotic fluid in a plane perpendicular to the examination table. All assessed pockets should be at least 1 cm in transverse diameter (parallel to the examination table). They should not contain loops of umbilical cord or fetal small parts in the middle of the pocket, but these may be present at the upper or lower border of the fluid pocket.

- *Maximum vertical pocket method:* The ultrasonographer identifies the deepest pocket of amniotic fluid in the uterus and measures its depth. Normal amniotic fluid is defined as a maximum vertical pocket measuring between 2 and 8 cm, regardless of gestational age.
- *Amniotic fluid index (AFI) method:* The ultrasonographer measures the deepest pocket of amniotic fluid in each of 4 uterine quadrants, using the umbilicus as the midpoint of the 4 quadrants (Figure 5.1). The sum of the 4 measurements is the AFI and is compared with standard tables that show the normal range of values for each week of gestation. Although values vary somewhat week by week, the lower limit of reference range is 7.9 to 9.8 cm, and the upper limit of reference range is 17.5 to 24.9 cm.

UNIT 5: OBSTETRIC RISK FACTORS: PRIOR OR CURRENT PREGNANCY

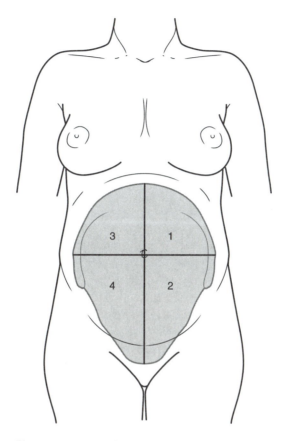

Figure 5.1. Uterine Quadrants for Amniotic Fluid Measurements

The maximum vertical pocket method has been shown to be superior to AFI in identifying decreased amniotic fluid, while neither method has been shown to be superior for identifying increased amniotic fluid.

A. Polyhydramnios (increased amniotic fluid)
   Common definitions include
   - Maximum vertical pocket of amniotic fluid of 8 cm and larger

   or
   - Free-floating fetus, not touching any uterine surface

   or
   - AFI of 25 cm and more, regardless of gestational age

   or
   - AFI greater than the 95th percentile for the specific gestational age of the fetus

Most cases of polyhydramnios have no identifiable cause. In more than one-half of cases, the fetus is normal. Nevertheless, polyhydramnios may be associated with
   - Multifetal gestation
   - Placental abnormalities
   - Red blood cell alloimmunization
   - Nonimmune hydrops
   - Maternal diabetes mellitus

- Fetus large for gestational age
- Fetal abnormalities, including
  — Anencephaly
  — Gastrointestinal tract abnormality
  — Chromosomal abnormality; in particular, Down and Turner syndromes

Prenatal considerations
- If fundal height is more than 3 to 4 cm *higher* than expected or if palpation of the uterus indicates excessive fluid, perform a US examination to assess the amniotic fluid volume.
- If polyhydramnios is found, evaluate the woman and the fetus for the conditions listed previously.
- Women with polyhydramnios, regardless of the cause, are at increased risk for development of premature rupture of membranes and preterm labor and delivery.
- Discuss findings, particularly those that might influence the route of delivery or plans for neonatal care, with pediatric practitioners.
- Perform serial US examinations to assess changes in amniotic fluid.
- If maternal respiratory compromise develops (from pressure on the diaphragm), amniocentesis to remove excess fluid may be helpful. Because fluid usually re-accumulates in a few days, symptomatic relief is transient, and the benefits of the procedure are short lived. Preterm labor, premature rupture of membranes, or placental abruption may occur with this degree of polyhydramnios, and repeated amnioceteses carry an increased risk for infection.

Intrapartum considerations
- When membranes rupture with polyhydramnios present, there may be a sudden loss of a large amount of fluid and a corresponding rapid decrease in intrauterine volume. Immediately
  — *Perform a vaginal examination:* A rush of excess fluid increases the risk for umbilical cord prolapse when the fetal presenting part is unengaged.
  — *Check fetal heart rate and maternal blood pressure:* Sudden decompression of an overdistended uterus may lead to placental abruption.
  — *Check uterine tone:* Tense, "boardlike" consistency suggests placental abruption with collection of blood between the placenta and uterine wall.
- An overdistended uterus generally does not contract well during labor or after delivery. Consider the use of an internal uterine contraction monitor to assess the strength of contractions; be prepared for the possibility of a postpartum hemorrhage. If contractions are poor, oxytocin augmentation of labor may be needed (see Unit 10, Inducing and Augmenting Labor, and Unit 11, Abnormal Labor Progress and Difficult Deliveries, in this book).

Postpartum considerations
Maternal
Check the woman's blood pressure and monitor her for excessive bleeding. Women with polyhydramnios often have poor progress during labor and are at increased risk for postpartum hemorrhage, owing to uterine atony.

Neonatal
- Evaluate the baby for abnormality of swallowing (ie, gastrointestinal obstruction or neurological malfunction).
- Consider evaluation for neurological, genetic, or chromosomal abnormality.

B. Oligohydramnios (decreased amniotic fluid)
Common definitions include
- The largest vertical pocket of amniotic fluid is less than 2 cm.

or
- The AFI is less than 5 cm, regardless of gestational age.

or
- The AFI is less than the fifth percentile for the specific gestational age of the fetus.

Oligohydramnios may be associated with
- Postmaturity
- Fetal growth restriction
- Fetal abnormalities, including
  — Pulmonary hypoplasia
  — Certain chromosomal abnormalities
  — Congenital infection
  — Genitourinary tract abnormalities
- Fetal death
- Unrecognized rupture of membranes
- Reduced fetal urine output due to chronic uteroplacental insufficiency

Prenatal considerations
- If fundal height is more than 3 to 4 cm *lower* than expected, or if palpation of the uterus suggests decreased fluid, perform a US examination to assess the amniotic fluid volume.
- If oligohydramnios is found, take the following actions:
  — Attempt to rule out rupture of membranes.
  — Reassess pregnancy dates, as the volume of amniotic fluid declines in post-term pregnancies.
  — Perform comprehensive US examination to evaluate genitourinary tract abnormalities or fetal growth restriction.
  — Perform nonstress tests or obtain a biophysical profile and include a Doppler study of umbilical arterial blood flow if the fetus is growth restricted.
  — Consider fetal chromosomal analysis, especially if fetal anomalies are present.
- Consultation with maternal-fetal medicine specialists is recommended to identify additional tests that may be indicated, as well as the place and timing of delivery. Certain genitourinary tract abnormalities require intervention soon after birth.

Intrapartum considerations
- Anticipate the likelihood of umbilical cord compression during labor.
- Because of the increased risk for abnormal fetal heart rate patterns, an emergency cesarean delivery may be needed.
- If abnormal fetal heart rate patterns develop and are thought to be due to cord compression (without prolapse) after membranes rupture, consider performing amnioinfusion. Amnioinfusion is the infusion of fluid (usually sterile saline or lactated Ringer solution) into the uterus through an intrauterine pressure catheter. Several protocols for amnioinfusion exist; know which protocol is in use at your center. Infusion of excessive amounts of fluid may result in overdistension of the uterus and should be avoided.

PCEP BOOK 2: MATERNAL AND FETAL CARE

Postpartum considerations
Maternal
None specific to oligohydramnios

Neonatal
- Be prepared for the possibility of a newborn with severe respiratory distress due to underdeveloped lungs (pulmonary hypoplasia) if oligohydramnios has been present since the early second trimester.
- Evaluate the baby for urinary tract obstruction or absent kidneys (fetal urine is a major source of amniotic fluid).
- Evaluate for positional limb deformities, which may occur as a result of uterine pressure on the fetus without the cushion of amniotic fluid.
- Evaluate the baby for congenital infection or genetic defect.

Self-test B

Now answer these questions to test yourself on the information in the last section.

B1. True   False   Maternal serum α-fetoprotein testing is used as a screening tool for the detection of a neural tube defect in the fetus.

B2. True   False   Prenatal diagnosis has become so precise that every fetal defect can be identified early in pregnancy.

B3. True   False   Gastrointestinal obstruction in the fetus is associated with polyhydramnios.

B4. True   False   Fetal growth restriction can affect one twin but not the other.

B5. True   False   Oligohydramnios is associated with an increased risk for umbilical cord compression and fetal heart rate decelerations during labor.

B6. True   False   Fetal genitourinary tract abnormality is associated with oligohydramnios.

B7. What is the single biggest threat to multifetal gestation?
_____

B8. What are 3 identifiable causes of polyhydramnios?
_____
_____
_____

B9. Multifetal gestation increases the risk for

Yes	No	
___	___	Preterm delivery
___	___	Hypertensive disorders of pregnancy
___	___	Fetal growth restriction
___	___	Placenta previa
___	___	Abnormal presentation
___	___	Fetal death
___	___	Umbilical cord prolapse
___	___	Postpartum hemorrhage

B10. When polyhydramnios is present and membranes rupture, what 2 things may happen?
_____
_____

B11. True   False   Twins in non-vertex–vertex presentation are an indication for cesarean delivery.

B12.	True	False	When long-standing oligohydramnios is present, you should be prepared for the possibility of a newborn with severe respiratory distress.
B13.	True	False	The second twin should be monitored during and after delivery of the first twin.
B14.	True	False	Most fetuses with polyhydramnios have a congenital malformation or chromosomal defect.
B15.	True	False	Oligohydramnios indicates the need for a thorough evaluation of fetal well-being.

B16. Which of the following risks are increased after delivery of the first twin?

Yes	No	
____	____	Umbilical cord prolapse
____	____	Arrest of labor
____	____	Placental abruption

B17. Which of the following risks are increased with polyhydramnios?

Yes	No	
____	____	Postpartum hemorrhage
____	____	Hypertensive disorders of pregnancy
____	____	Hypotonic uterus
____	____	Fetal positional limb deformities
____	____	Preterm labor

B18. Which of the following tests are used to screen for or detect chromosomal abnormalities in a fetus?

Yes	No	
____	____	Multiple markers: combination of maternal age, maternal serum α-fetoprotein, estriol, human chorionic gonadotropin, and inhibin-A
____	____	Fetal activity determinations
____	____	Analysis of amniotic fluid
____	____	Maternal serum α-fetoprotein levels
____	____	Biophysical profile

Check your answers with the list that follows the Recommended Routines. Correct any incorrect answers and review the appropriate section in the unit.

13. How is fetal growth restriction diagnosed and managed?

The ability to reliably diagnose fetal growth restriction depends on *accurate pregnancy dating*. The causes of fetal growth restriction vary widely and include placental insufficiency, genetic or chromosomal abnormalities, maternal smoking and substance abuse, maternal hypertension, congenital viral or parasitic infections, and severe maternal malnutrition. In an individual pregnancy, the cause cannot always be clearly identified.

Fetal growth restriction may be suspected if the fundal height measurements are lower than expected for gestational age. A US examination is then performed to assess fetal growth. The fetal weight can never be known precisely according to US measurements; it can only be estimated. If the estimated fetal weight or the fetal abdominal circumference is below the 10th percentile for gestational age, fetal growth restriction is diagnosed, and increased fetal monitoring is initiated. Growth-restricted fetuses are at increased risk for intrauterine death, and the risk of death increases with the severity of growth restriction.

A. Prenatal considerations
- Perform US examination.
  — Check for fetal anomalies (if found, consult with specialists).
  — Assess amniotic fluid (oligohydramnios is often found with growth restriction).
- Consider amniocentesis for chromosomal analysis if no other reason for severe growth restriction can be found or if fetal anomalies are seen at US examination. Consult with maternal-fetal medicine specialists.
- Conduct antenatal testing for fetal well-being, beginning at the time growth restriction is identified. Growth-restricted fetuses have an increased risk for stillbirth. Testing usually consists of a nonstress test and amniotic fluid measurement, or a biophysical profile, along with umbilical artery Doppler blood flow studies on a weekly basis. In some cases, testing twice a week may be recommended.
- The timing of delivery is determined by the results of antenatal testing and the coexistence of any additional risk factors, such as diabetes or hypertension. Full-term or early term delivery is most common, but preterm delivery may be indicated if fetal compromise is suspected.
- If growth restriction is severe or early onset, consider referral for delivery at a regional perinatal center.

B. Intrapartum considerations
- Placental function may be diminished, increasing the risk for fetal heart rate abnormalities during labor, such as late decelerations and minimal variability.
- Check for meconium-stained amniotic fluid when membranes rupture.
- Plan for vaginal delivery, but because the likelihood of abnormal fetal heart rate tracings during labor is high, be prepared for possible emergency cesarean delivery or forceps/vacuum extraction, depending on fetal condition and stage of labor. Anticipate the possible need for neonatal resuscitation.

C. Postpartum considerations

Maternal

Review the risk factors associated with growth restriction, especially smoking, substance use, and maternal medical disease.

Neonatal
- If resuscitation is needed, monitor the baby for possible post-resuscitation complications.
- Screen the baby for hypoglycemia (perform an initial blood glucose check 30 minutes after birth). Begin early feedings or intravenous fluids (see Book 1: Maternal and Fetal Evaluation and Immediate Newborn Care, Unit 8, Hypoglycemia).
- Check the baby's hematocrit value (polycythemia may be present).
- Evaluate the baby for congenital malformation, infection, or chromosomal abnormality.

14. What risks are associated with late term and post-term gestational age?

A pregnancy is late term from $41^{0/7}$ weeks to $41^{6/7}$ weeks, and post-term from $42^{0/7}$ weeks on. Complications associated with late term and post-term gestation include macrosomia, oligohydramnios, meconium-stained amniotic fluid, low Apgar scores, neonatal intensive care unit admission, neonatal seizures, postmaturity syndrome, and perinatal death. Diminished placental function and umbilical cord compression increase the risk of abnormal fetal heart rate tracings during labor.

The risk of fetal death and neonatal complications increases significantly at 41 weeks of gestation. By 42 weeks, the risks are increased to an extent that the risks of additional time in utero exceed the potential benefits of awaiting spontaneous labor.

A. Prenatal considerations
- If spontaneous labor does not occur by 41 weeks of gestation, discuss the risks and benefits of induction and the risks associated with a pregnancy lasting longer than 41 weeks of gestation.

It is prudent to verify the accuracy of the estimated due date (EDD) when making decisions about management of a late term or post-term pregnancy. However, do not use the US results in late pregnancy to change the EDD. Refer to Book 1: Maternal and Fetal Evaluation and Immediate Newborn Care, Unit 2, Fetal Age, Growth, and Maturity, for more information about correctly establishing the EDD.

- Consider comprehensive US investigation to assess
  — Fetal growth
  — Amniotic fluid volume
- Establish a management plan.

Discuss with the woman the risks associated with continued gestation beyond 41 weeks and the risks associated with induction of labor. Induction of labor may be scheduled any time after 39 weeks of gestation in an adequately dated pregnancy. With close monitoring, a woman who strongly prefers to await the spontaneous onset of labor and who has no associated medical or obstetric risk factors may elect to continue her pregnancy past 41 weeks of gestation.
  — *Initiate antenatal testing,* consisting of once- or twice-weekly fetal monitoring (nonstress test with amniotic fluid assessment and/or biophysical profile).
  — *Recommend induction of labor* no later than 42 weeks of gestation, owing to the increased risk of perinatal death.

B. Intrapartum considerations
- Plan for vaginal delivery, but be prepared for possible emergency delivery.
- If the fetus is determined to be macrosomic (estimated fetal weight >4,000 g [>8 lb 13 oz]), discuss with the patient the risk of shoulder dystocia, birth trauma, brachial plexus injury (Erb palsy/paralysis) and other palsies, and maternal birth canal lacerations.
- If meconium is seen in the amniotic fluid, a period of fetal stress *may* have occurred. Fetal stress can cause the rectal sphincter to relax and result in meconium passage. Functional maturation in a post-term fetus can also cause the fetus to pass meconium in utero, without any evidence of stress (natural emptying of a full rectum).
- If the amniotic fluid is meconium stained, be prepared for the possible need for neonatal resuscitation. (See Book 1: Maternal and Fetal Evaluation and Immediate Newborn Care, Unit 5, Resuscitating the Newborn.)

C. Postpartum considerations
Maternal
None specific to post-term pregnancy

Neonatal
- Anticipate the possible need for neonatal resuscitation.
- If meconium is present, follow the guidelines for management of meconium-stained amniotic fluid in Book 1: Maternal and Fetal Evaluation and Immediate Newborn Care, Unit 5, Resuscitating the Newborn. Management of meconium is determined by the baby's condition at birth, which will determine the need for routine newborn care or neonatal resuscitation.
- If resuscitation is needed, monitor the baby for possible post-resuscitation complications.
- If the baby is large, examine the baby for signs of birth trauma.
- Begin early feedings and screen the baby for hypoglycemia. (See Book 1: Maternal and Fetal Evaluation and Immediate Newborn Care, Unit 8, Hypoglycemia.)

Self-test C

Now answer these questions to test yourself on the information in the last section.

C1. True False Uteroplacental insufficiency is rarely a cause of fetal growth restriction.

C2. True False When a fetus is suspected of being post-term, it is valuable to obtain US measurement of the amniotic fluid volume.

C3. True False The likelihood of abnormal fetal heart rate tracings during labor is increased in post-term pregnancies.

C4. True False Intrauterine viral infection is one cause of fetal growth restriction.

C5. True False A baby born post-term is at increased risk for neonatal hypoglycemia.

C6. True False Because of their small size, newborns with growth restriction rarely develop hypoglycemia.

C7. True False A growth-restricted fetus at term is at increased risk for fetal heart rate abnormalities during labor.

C8. True False Serial US measurements of fetal size are usually needed to identify fetal growth restriction.

C9. True False Meconium in the amniotic fluid is always an indication of fetal stress.

C10. What are 2 identifiable causes of growth restriction?
_____
_____

C11. With an uncomplicated, low-risk pregnancy, the risk of fetal death begins to increase at
  A. 37 weeks of gestation
  B. 39 weeks of gestation
  C. 41 weeks of gestation

C12. Post-term newborns are at increased risk for all of the following complications, except:
  A. Anemia
  B. Macrosomia
  C. Meconium-stained amniotic fluid
  D. Hypoglycemia

C13. Match each condition on the left with the best choice from the right.
  _____ Positional deformities in the fetus   a. Polyhydramnios
  _____ Placental abruption   b. Oligohydramnios
  _____ Postpartum hemorrhage   c. Fetal growth restriction
  _____ Pulmonary hypoplasia
  _____ Chronic maternal medical illness
  _____ Neonatal hypoglycemia

Check your answers with the list that follows the Recommended Routines. Correct any incorrect answers and review the appropriate section in the unit.

OBSTETRIC RISK FACTORS: PRIOR OR CURRENT PREGNANCY

Recommended Routines

All the routines listed below are based on the principles of perinatal care presented in the unit you have just finished. They are recommended as part of routine perinatal care.

Read each routine carefully and decide whether it is standard operating procedure in your hospital. Check the appropriate blank next to each routine.

Procedure Standard in My Hospital	Needs Discussion by Our Staff	Recommended Routine
_____	_____	1. Establish a system of prenatal consultation and referral, as appropriate, for the • Evaluation and care of high-risk pregnant women • Evaluation and care of at-risk or sick fetuses • Anticipated care of at-risk or sick newborns
_____	_____	2. Attempt a trial of labor after prior cesarean delivery only when physician(s), anesthesia staff, and neonatal staff are immediately available to provide emergency care, possible hysterectomy, and neonatal resuscitation.

Self-test Answers

These are the answers to the Self-test questions. Please check them with the answers you gave and review the information in the unit wherever necessary.

Self-test A

A1. _b_ Shoulder dystocia   a. Cesarean delivery
     _b_ Brachial plexus injury   b. Macrosomia
     _b_ Neonatal hypoglycemia
     _a_ Previous uterine surgery
     _b_ Abnormal maternal glucose intolerance

A2. The risk of uterine rupture during labor is increased when previous uterine surgery entered the *endometrium*.

A3. Soon after delivery, women who give birth vaginally to large babies should be checked for *lacerations of the birth canal*.

A4. True

A5. True

A6. True

A7. False   *Reason:* Many congenital malformations are not related to a genetic disease or chromosomal defect. Sometimes, fetal deformities develop with no identifiable cause. Sometimes, they result from adverse fetal environment during embryogenesis. For example, high maternal blood glucose levels (and, therefore, high fetal blood glucose levels because glucose easily crosses the placenta) early in pregnancy are associated with congenital malformations. Maternal ingestion of some drugs considered unsafe for the fetus can also result in deformities.

A8. True

A9. False   *Reason:* Autopsy reports of a previous fetal or neonatal death can be extremely useful in providing information to parents about future pregnancies. The cause of the previous death may indicate therapy or surveillance measures that can be instituted to avoid another death.

A10. True

A11. Large babies, especially those weighing more than 4,000 g (>8 lb 13 oz) at birth, should be screened for *hypoglycemia*, whether or not their mothers were known to have abnormal glucose intolerance during pregnancy.

A12.

Yes	No	
	X	Post-term pregnancy
X		Uterine rupture
X		Postpartum hemorrhage
X		Placental abruption
X		Rapid labor
	X	Fetal chromosomal abnormality

Self-test B

B1. True

B2. False   *Reason:* Prenatal diagnosis can provide a tremendous amount of detailed and useful information but cannot be counted on to indicate 100% of fetal defects.

B3. True

B4. True

B5. True

B6. True

B7. Preterm birth

B8. Any 3 of the following causes:
- Multifetal gestation
- Rh isoimmune disease
- Maternal diabetes mellitus
- Fetal gastrointestinal abnormality
- Anencephaly
- Down and Turner syndromes
- Placental abnormalities

B9.
Yes	No	
X	___	Preterm delivery
X	___	Hypertensive disorders of pregnancy
X	___	Fetal growth restriction
X	___	Placenta previa
X	___	Abnormal presentation
X	___	Fetal death
X	___	Umbilical cord prolapse
X	___	Postpartum hemorrhage

B10. Possible umbilical cord prolapse with rush of excess fluid

Possible placental abruption with sudden uterine decompression

B11. True

B12. True

B13. True

B14. False   *Reason:* While some fetuses with hydramnios have a congenital malformation or chromosomal defect, most fetuses with hydramnios develop normally.

B15. True

B16.
Yes	No	
X	___	Umbilical cord prolapse
X	___	Arrest of labor
X	___	Placental abruption

B17.
Yes	No	
X	___	Postpartum hemorrhage
___	X	Hypertensive disorders of pregnancy
X	___	Hypotonic uterus
___	X	Fetal positional limb deformities
X	___	Preterm labor

B18.	Yes	No	
	X	___	Multiple markers: combination of maternal age, maternal serum α-fetoprotein, estriol, human chorionic gonadotropin, and inhibin-A
	___	X	Fetal activity determinations
	X	___	Analysis of amniotic fluid
	X	___	Maternal serum α-fetoprotein levels
	___	X	Biophysical profile

Self-test C

C1. False *Reason:* The reverse is accurate. Uteroplacental insufficiency is often a cause of fetal growth restriction.

C2. True

C3. True

C4. True

C5. True

C6. False *Reason:* Babies with fetal growth restriction have decreased stores of glycogen and fat to metabolize after delivery and are therefore at increased risk for developing hypoglycemia after birth.

C7. True

C8. True

C9. False *Reason:* Meconium in the amniotic fluid may or may not be an indication of fetal distress. In mature fetuses, the rectum may simply empty when it is full. If a fetus is in distress, the rectal sphincter may also relax and release meconium into the amniotic fluid.

C10. Any 2 of the following causes:
- Maternal hypertension
- Renal disease
- Lupus
- Antiphospholipid syndrome
- Smoking
- Severe maternal malnutrition

C11. C. 41 weeks of gestation

C12. A. Anemia

C13.
- b Positional deformities in the fetus
- a Placental abruption
- a Postpartum hemorrhage
- b Pulmonary hypoplasia
- c Chronic maternal medical illness
- c Neonatal hypoglycemia

a. Polyhydramnios
b. Oligohydramnios
c. Fetal growth restriction

Unit 5 Posttest

After completion of each unit there is a free online posttest available at www.cmevillage.com to test your understanding. Navigate to the PCEP pages on www.cmevillage.com and register to take the free posttests.

Once registered on the website and after completing all the unit posttests, pay the book exam fee ($15) and pass the test at 80% or greater to earn continuing education credits. Only start the PCEP book exam if you have time to complete it. If you take the book exam and are not connected to a printer, either print your certificate to a .pdf file and save it to print later or come back to www.cmevillage.com at any time and print a copy of your educational transcript.

Credits are only available by book, not by individual unit within the books. Available credits for completion of each book exam are as follows: Book 1: 14.5 credits; Book 2: 16 credits; Book 3: 17 credits; Book 4: 9 credits.

For more details, navigate to the PCEP webpages at www.cmevillage.com.

Unit 6: Psychosocial Risk Factors in Pregnancy

Objectives 210

1. **What are psychosocial risk factors?** 213

    A. **Limited or no prenatal care** 213

    B. **Screening, brief intervention, and referral for treatment and motivational interviewing** 214

2. **How do psychosocial risk factors affect pregnancy?** 214

    A. **Intimate partner violence** 214

    B. **Mental health disorders** 216

    C. **Substance use disorders** 218

Tables

    Table 6.1. Validated Alcohol Use Screening Questions 223

    Table 6.2. The 5 A's Intervention for Tobacco Use in Pregnancy 225

Recommended Routines 227

Objectives

In this unit you will learn

A. What psychosocial factors put a pregnant woman and her fetus at risk

B. How to screen a pregnant woman for intimate partner violence

C. How maternal mental health disorders may affect a woman's health during pregnancy and after birth

D. How a maternal substance use disorder may affect fetal development and well-being

E. How to screen for substance use disorders in pregnant women

Unit 6 Pretest

Before reading the unit, please answer the following questions. Select the *one best* answer to each question (unless otherwise instructed). Record your answers on the test and check them with the answers at the end of the book.

1. Which of the following psychosocial risk factors should be assessed and managed during pregnancy?
   A. Substance use disorders
   B. Intimate partner violence
   C. Mental health disorders
   D. All of the above

2. True False Women who are heavy smokers are much more likely than nonsmokers to deliver babies who are large for gestational age.

3. True False Any illicit substance use in pregnancy is a potential risk to the fetus.

4. True False Women who have not received prenatal care are more likely to have an adverse psychosocial condition.

5. True False A woman who actively uses cocaine should be advised not to breastfeed.

6. True False Electronic cigarettes are a safe alternative to smoking in pregnancy.

7. Which of the following are recommended for a pregnant woman with an opioid use disorder?

Yes	No	
___	___	Referral for medication-assisted treatment
___	___	Monitoring of the newborn for neonatal abstinence syndrome
___	___	Amniocentesis for chromosomal analysis
___	___	Monitoring for increased risk of preterm labor

8. Which of the following conditions are associated with fetal growth restriction?

Yes	No	
___	___	Bipolar disorder
___	___	Tobacco smoking
___	___	Alcohol use
___	___	Amphetamine use

9. True False A woman can drink alcohol occasionally during pregnancy without risk of fetal harm.

10. True False Women who smoke cigarettes should not breastfeed.

11. True False All women should undergo urine drug testing during pregnancy.

12. True False Postpartum psychosis is associated with an increased risk of suicide.

(*continued*)

Unit 6 Pretest (*continued*)

13. When used during pregnancy, which of the following substances is associated with placental abruption?
    A. Cocaine
    B. Methamphetamine
    C. Heroin
    D. Marijuana

14. **True   False**   Only women with low socioeconomic status should be screened for intimate partner violence.

1. What are psychosocial risk factors?

Psychosocial risk factors contribute significantly to adverse outcomes of pregnancy, including perinatal and maternal mortality. They include medical conditions, such as substance use disorders and mental health disorders, and the environment and conditions in which a woman lives during her pregnancy. These risk factors may interact unfavorably with each other, with the woman's coexisting medical conditions, and with the pregnancy itself, even among otherwise healthy women. The effect of psychosocial conditions on pregnancy outcome may be magnified if the pregnancy is undesired. The effect of psychosocial conditions on pregnancy may include denial, depression, anger, withdrawal, self-destructive or risk-taking behavior, and child abuse.

Examples of how psychosocial conditions may affect pregnancy and underlying medical problems include the following:

- Economic disadvantage affects all aspects of a woman's health and well-being. Economic disadvantage may be a result of unemployment, underemployment, insufficient public benefits, or lack of access to public benefits. It may contribute to homelessness, undernutrition, inability to access prenatal care, and inability to adhere to medication treatment regimens.
- A woman with a substance use disorder who is not in recovery treatment may choose not to receive prenatal care, often because of fear that her newborn or other children will be removed from her custody if her substance use becomes known. These women are additionally at risk for undernutrition, sexually transmitted infections (STIs), blood-borne infections such as HIV and hepatitis, and complications unique to the particular substance they are using.

All women can benefit from screening for psychosocial risk factors during their pregnancies. Screen at the initiation of prenatal care to identify conditions that will benefit from intervention and referral. In some populations, screening again later in the pregnancy may help to identify problems that have arisen but the woman has not disclosed, such as loss of employment, development of food insecurity, or homelessness. Ask each woman what she sees as adverse circumstances for herself, provide intervention for risk factors she can address during her pregnancy, and refer her to social services and other agencies. Effective psychosocial screening includes assessment of

- Whether the pregnancy was intended
- Whether the father of the pregnancy will be involved
- Custody of her prior children
- Other social supports
- Employment or occupational risks
- Adequacy of housing and/or living situation
- Current or past history of substance use disorder
- Current or past history of intimate partner violence (IPV)
- Current or past use of social services support

A. Limited or no prenatal care

A pregnant woman who has not been receiving prenatal care or who has received very little prenatal care may seek care at a hospital at any time during the course of her pregnancy, potentially even in labor. When screened, many women who have not received prenatal care will be found to have one or more of the psychosocial risk factors described in this unit. Women who have not received consistent prenatal care may miss recommended pregnancy screenings, such as testing for STIs and gestational diabetes. They may also not receive care for preexisting medical problems. All of the above place a pregnant woman at increased risk for one or more complications of pregnancy. It is important to approach the woman in a supportive and nonjudgmental way, to allow her to feel comfortable with disclosing sensitive information.

B. Screening, brief intervention, and referral for treatment and motivational interviewing
Screening, brief intervention, and referral for treatment (SBIRT) is a standardized approach to identifying individuals who engage in illicit drug use and/or at-risk drinking. The 3 elements of SBIRT are
- Screening: Assessment of a patient for drug use or at-risk drinking via the use of a standardized screening questionnaire in a health care setting. Screenings may be administered by the health professional or self-administered by the patient and subsequently reviewed by the health professional. Validated screening questionnaires are sensitive and specific for identifying and ruling out problem drug and alcohol use. They are most effective when applied universally to a population of patients; universal screening reduces the effect of implicit bias on the screening process. Selective screening will also reduce the ability of the health professional to identify patients with a drug or alcohol problem.
- Brief intervention: The health care team member provides feedback and advice to a person whose screening results indicate a possible drug or alcohol problem.
- Referral for treatment: The health professional initiates a referral to a drug or alcohol treatment program or other interventions, as needed.

Motivational interviewing is a technique that health care professionals can use to assist patients in identifying and acknowledging substance use problems by using reflective listening and supportive discussion to motivate behavior change. By assisting patients in identifying uncertainty and ambivalence about certain behaviors, the health care provider can help the patient move through the stages of readiness for change.
- Precontemplation: The patient does not believe that a problem exists.
- Contemplation: The patient recognizes a problem and has begun to think about change.
- Action: The patient has begun treatment or behavioral change.
- Maintenance: The patient makes new behavior part of her daily life.
- Relapse: The patient returns to the prior unfavorable behavior.

Several training programs provide health professionals with instruction on how to incorporate motivational interviewing into their practice.

2. How do psychosocial risk factors affect pregnancy?

A. Intimate partner violence
IPV is a public health problem defined as physical violence, sexual violence, stalking, or psychological aggression by a current or former intimate partner. An intimate partner is any person with whom someone has had a close personal relationship, characterized by emotional connection, regular contact, ongoing physical contact and/or sexual contact, identity as a couple or familiarity, and knowledge about each other's lives.

Investigate the possibility of intimate partner violence (IPV) with every pregnant woman. IPV can include physical, psychological, and sexual abuse.

The National Intimate Partner and Sexual Violence Survey was completed in 2017 and reported the following estimates of violence against women:
- Physical violence: 22.3%
- Sexual violence: 43.9%
- Rape: 19.3%
- Stalking: 9.2%

IPV also includes reproductive coercion, defined as behaviors aimed at controlling reproductive or sexual health. This may include refusal to use or sabotaging birth control, coerced conception, or coerced pregnancy termination. The true incidence of reproductive coercion is not known.

IPV may affect a woman of any income level, educational attainment, or race. Disparities appear to exist along socioeconomic and racial and/or ethnic lines, with reports of higher prevalence among teenagers, women with disabilities, women with lower levels of education, Black and Native American women, and immigrant women. However, the true prevalence of IPV in any population is not known, owing to underreporting. IPV may begin or accelerate during pregnancy and affects all members of the woman's family.

1. Prenatal considerations
   - Screen *all* women for IPV at the initiation of prenatal care, and consider repeat screening later in pregnancy, especially if a woman has unexplained gaps in her prenatal care.
   - Use a screening tool that has been validated for sensitivity and specificity in identifying IPV. A review of screening approaches and the sensitivity/specificity of various tools is available in *The American Journal of Obstetrics and Gynecology* (http://dx.doi.org/10.1016/j.ajog.2017.05.043).
   - Women may respond more openly about abuse on a self-administered questionnaire (computer-based or written) than in a face-to-face interview.
   - Provide support to the woman by validating her right not to be subjected to abuse and violence. Refer her to local resources, which may include an IPV helpline, a shelter, social services resources, and law enforcement.
   - Acknowledge that women who have experienced sexual or other physical trauma may express fear or hesitation with physical contact, especially regarding pelvic examinations. Provide additional support and always request specific consent before proceeding with a pelvic examination in any woman.

2. Intrapartum considerations
   - Emotional support from family and friends is especially important.
   - Support of the woman's self-esteem throughout labor and delivery by health professionals is also particularly important.
   - Acknowledge that women who have experienced sexual or other physical trauma may express fear or hesitation with physical contact, especially regarding pelvic examinations. Provide additional support and always request specific consent before proceeding with a pelvic examination in any woman.

- Assure that hospital safety protocols include the ability of the woman to restrict her assailant from attempting to visit her in the hospital.
3. Postpartum considerations
   Maternal
   Review the prenatal support plan and revise as necessary.
   Neonatal
   Consult with social services and other agencies, as appropriate.

B. Mental health disorders
   1. Chronic mental health disorders
   Women with chronic mental health conditions, including depression, bipolar disorder, and schizophrenia, are at risk for complications during pregnancy, including destabilization of their mental illness, hospitalization, and suicide attempts. A woman with mental illness who desires pregnancy should plan her pregnancy in conjunction with her mental health and obstetric care providers to optimize her medication management. However, many pregnancies will be unplanned.

   The woman should be encouraged to maintain regular appointments with her mental health provider, including individual and group therapy. Adherence to the woman's medication regimen during pregnancy is usually necessary to prevent acute changes in her mental illness. In most cases, the benefits to the woman (and indirectly to the fetus) of maintaining stability of her mental illness will exceed the potential risk of congenital anomalies related to medication. Despite this, many women will not be consistently adherent to their medication regimen or will intentionally discontinue it out of fear that the medications may cause harm to the fetus. Coordinate a care plan with the woman's mental health provider and use reference resources to address potential risks associated with medications during pregnancy and lactation. Resources include Hale's *Medications and Mothers' Milk*; Briggs' *Drugs in Pregnancy and Lactation*; the National Institutes of Health LactMed database (http://toxnet.nlm.nih.gov/newtoxnet/lactmed.htm); the *Breastfeeding Handbook for Physicians*, 3rd edition; and the Reprotox database (www.reprotox.org).

   Lithium increases the risk of certain congenital heart defects and is generally not prescribed during pregnancy; however, the risk of congenital heart defects is small, and the woman and her psychiatrist may opt to continue lithium if this medication is the most effective option for treatment of her bipolar disorder. Lithium concentrates in breast milk, and women who take lithium should be advised not to breastfeed. Valproate (sometimes used as a mood stabilizer) should be avoided during pregnancy, as this medication is associated with a high risk for structural anomalies and developmental delays.

   a. Prenatal considerations
      - Screen women with mental health disorders for psychosocial problems (see Section 1, what are psychosocial risk factors?). Screening a woman only once may not be sufficient because issues in a woman's life can change as the pregnancy progresses; consider repeat screening as the pregnancy progresses.
      - Provide emotional support. Women with mental health disorders may encounter difficulties during pregnancy related to fear and worry about pregnancy or problems with their financial, emotional, family, employment, or social circumstances.

- Involve family members, as appropriate, in establishing a support network during pregnancy and during the woman's adaptation to parenting after delivery.
- Provide social service and other consultation, if there are specific stressors that can be eliminated or alleviated.

b. Intrapartum considerations
- Emotional support from family and friends is especially important.
- Support of the woman's self-esteem throughout labor and delivery by health professionals is also particularly important.

c. Postpartum considerations

Maternal
- Continue to assess adaptation to parenting after delivery.
- Monitor the woman for exacerbation of her mental health condition or the development of coexisting postpartum depression, anxiety, or psychosis.
- Review the prenatal support plan and revise as necessary.

Neonatal
- Arrange for ongoing follow-up care.
- Consult with social services and other agencies, as appropriate.

2. Perinatal mood and anxiety disorders

Perinatal mood and anxiety disorders encompasses depression and anxiety that occurs during pregnancy or in the postpartum period. Postpartum depression is a well-recognized condition known to affect 10% to 20% of women after delivery. More recently, the scope of this spectrum of conditions has been expanded, in recognition that prenatal onset of depression is also common and that a woman with a pregnancy-associated mood disorder may manifest symptoms of anxiety and not purely depression. Perinatal mood and anxiety disorders may have severe and debilitating manifestations and may be associated with an increased risk of suicide and infanticide attempts.

a. Prenatal considerations
- Screen all women for perinatal mood and anxiety disorders at the initiation of prenatal care, and consider repeat screening in the third trimester.
- Use a screening tool that has been validated for identifying depression, such as the *Edinburgh Postnatal Depression Scale* or the *Patient Health Questionnaire-9*.
- Provide emotional support and referral to resources such as a support group or a mental health professional. Antepartum hospitalization is rarely needed.
- Involve family members, as appropriate, in establishing a support network during pregnancy.

b. Intrapartum considerations
- Emotional support from family and friends is especially important.
- Support of the woman's self-esteem throughout labor and delivery by health professionals is also particularly important.

c. Postpartum considerations

Maternal
- Screen all women at least once in the postpartum period for perinatal mood and anxiety disorders.
- Provide increased support for women with perinatal depression or anxiety. This may include more frequent visits, home visits, support group referral, mental health referral, or the support of a postpartum doula.

- Educate the mother regarding the compatibility of antidepressant medication with breastfeeding.
- Review the prenatal support plan and revise as necessary.

Neonatal
- Observe the newborn for signs of withdrawal from maternal antidepressant medication, if the mother took medication during pregnancy. The symptoms are short-lived and respond to supportive care. Encourage breastfeeding.
- Arrange for ongoing follow-up care.
- Consult with social services and other agencies, as appropriate.

3. Postpartum psychosis

Postpartum psychosis is a rare but serious condition that occurs in 1 to 2 per 1,000 births. Women with a prior history or a family history of a psychotic episode or bipolar disorder are at higher risk for postpartum psychosis, but it can also occur in a woman with no prior history of mental illness. A woman experiencing postpartum psychosis will have disordered thinking and judgment and may have hallucinations, rapid mood swings, paranoia, or other symptoms. The risk for suicide and/or infanticide is increased. Women who demonstrate signs of postpartum psychosis should undergo an urgent evaluation by a psychiatrist and will likely require hospitalization for treatment.

C. Substance use disorders

Approximately 7% to 8% of the U.S. population has a substance use disorder. *Addiction*, as defined by the American Society of Addiction Medicine, is characterized by craving, compulsive use, continued use despite harm (consequences), impaired control over drug use, and chronicity. Not all individuals who use drugs develop addiction, but the use of illicit substances always carries the risk of harm in pregnancy. The prevalence of substance use declines as pregnancy advances, but not all women will be able to stop substance use without medical assistance. It is important for health care providers to recognize that addiction is a biological illness that requires treatment and that women with addiction require compassion and support from their health care team.

All women should be screened for substance use disorders at the initial prenatal visit. Screening consists of the administration of a validated questionnaire, such as the National Institute on Drug Abuse (NIDA) Quick Screen, the 4 P's questionnaire, or the 5 P's questionnaire. Urine drug testing is not recommended as a universal screening tool or as the initial step in screening. In addition to being costly, urine drug testing has low sensitivity for detecting drug metabolites among infrequent users. Urine drug testing is most appropriately used to test women who had a positive questionnaire screening result or in the medical evaluation of a woman who appears acutely intoxicated, with unexplained decreased level of consciousness, or with symptoms of withdrawal.

 Routine screening for substance use disorders should be part of prenatal care for all *women.*

Illicit drugs may be consumed orally, by injection (intradermal, intramuscular, or intravenous), or through inhalation. Polysubstance use (use of more than one drug) may compound the effects of substance use on the woman and fetus. Women with a substance use disorder are more likely to also use tobacco or drink alcohol. Obstetric care providers should inform all pregnant women that tobacco, alcohol, and drugs are harmful to themselves and their babies.

Drug use in pregnancy is harmful, regardless of whether the woman is an infrequent or a frequent user.

Women with substance use disorders during pregnancy are at increased risk for a wide range of health problems. They are at risk for hepatitis and HIV via sexual transmission and via blood exposure when needles are shared. They are also at increased risk for STIs, particularly if they exchange sex for drugs. See Unit 3, Infectious Diseases in Pregnancy, in this book for more information about screening and diagnosis. They are at risk for IPV, poor nutrition, and encounters with law enforcement.

Women with substance use disorders may attend prenatal visits only sporadically or may not seek prenatal care, which reduces the opportunity for thorough assessment of maternal and fetal status. The first contact with the health care system may not occur until labor begins and sometimes not until labor is advanced. Conversely, some women with substance use disorders may consider pregnancy as a motivation to engage in treatment for their substance use disorder and to seek early and consistent prenatal care.

Overdose from any substance, or combination of substances, is an emergency. Maternal (and fetal) mortality is high with acute intoxication.

Most pregnant women with substance use disorders either use illegal drugs, or they use legal drugs illicitly—for example, prescription drug abuse. Obstetric care providers should know the laws in their own jurisdiction related to testing and reporting of positive results. In most cases, urine drug testing requires the consent of the person being tested, although it may not be possible to obtain consent in the setting of a medical emergency, such as an overdose. Some jurisdictions have enacted or have attempted to enact legislation that requires urine drug testing in pregnancy and reporting of positive results to law enforcement. These statutes tend to deter women with substance use disorders from seeking prenatal care because of fear of incarceration or other legal consequences. Federal and state law requires the development of a comprehensive plan of safe care for the newborn whenever a woman has been identified as having a substance use disorder during pregnancy, regardless of whether she is receiving treatment.

1. Opioids

    A pregnant woman with an opioid use disorder may use heroin or a legal drug such as oxycodone, hydromorphone, or morphine. Maternal opioid use disorder is associated with increased risk of fetal growth restriction, fetal death, and prematurity and may result in neonatal abstinence syndrome (also known as *neonatal opioid withdrawal syndrome*). Maternally consumed opioids cross the placenta and directly affect the fetus. It is not clear whether the risk of abnormal fetal growth is a consequence of

opioids directly or from coexisting medical conditions, tobacco use, or inadequate nutrition.
  a. Prenatal considerations
     - Use the SBIRT approach to educate the woman about the risks of opioid use and refer her to a substance use disorder treatment program. Medication-assisted therapy consists of either methadone, administered in a federally regulated methadone clinic, or buprenorphine, which may be administered as office-based opioid treatment by a licensed physician or allied health professional who has obtained additional training and receives authorization from the United States Drug Enforcement Administration to prescribe these medications.
     - Assess the woman's oral health and refer her to a dental care program.
     - Consider periodic ultrasonographic (US) evaluation of fetal growth in the third trimester.
  b. Intrapartum considerations
     - Acute opioid use, whether from prescribed pain medication or illicit drug use, can cause decreased fetal heart rate variability.
     - Be aware that the need for frequent or large doses of narcotic analgesia may indicate a previously unsuspected opioid use disorder.
     - Consider urine drug testing if use is suspected.
  c. Postpartum considerations
     Maternal
     - Consult social services and other agencies, as appropriate, to assist the woman with entering a substance use treatment program if she has not done so already and developing a plan of safe care for the newborn.
     - Breastfeeding is contraindicated with active maternal heroin use. Breastfeeding is usually *not* contraindicated for women in a methadone or buprenorphine maintenance program, unless another contraindication (eg, maternal HIV infection) is present.

     Neonatal
     - If the baby has respiratory depression at birth, provide assisted ventilation as necessary. Do *not* administer naloxone if maternal narcotic opioid use disorder is suspected. Naloxone will cause acute withdrawal in the baby, which may induce seizures.
     - Consider newborn drug testing according to your hospital's policy and practice.
     - Observe for signs of neonatal abstinence syndrome (see Book 3: Neonatal Care, Unit 11, Neonatal Abstinence Syndrome [Neonatal Opioid Withdrawal Syndrome]).
     - Involve social services in planning for the baby's care after discharge.
2. Amphetamines

Women who use amphetamines are more likely to engage in polysubstance abuse, to not receive prenatal care, to have poor nutrition, and to have oral health problems, including severe dental decay with tooth loss. Amphetamine use in early pregnancy has not been found to be associated with a specific syndrome or spectrum of congenital malformations. Maternal amphetamine use is associated with an increased risk for fetal growth restriction.

a. Prenatal considerations
- Use the SBIRT approach to educate the woman about the risks of amphetamine use and refer her to a substance use disorder treatment program. Owing to the intensive nature of treatment for amphetamine use, participation in a voluntary inpatient treatment program is ideal.
- Assess the woman's oral health and refer her to a dental care program.
- Monitor fetal growth with periodic US examinations in late pregnancy.

b. Intrapartum considerations
- A woman who is in labor and acutely intoxicated with amphetamines may pose challenges to safe intrapartum care. She may display disordered thinking and may not respond appropriately to verbal instructions or inquiries. She may also be physically combative. The use of physical restraints is controversial and may exacerbate combative behavior.
- Fetal heart rate abnormalities may occur more commonly.

c. Postpartum considerations

Maternal
- The mother's emotional state may remain unpredictable and irrational.
- Breastfeeding is contraindicated with maternal use of amphetamines.
- Consult social services and other agencies, as appropriate, to assist the woman with, for example, referrals to substance use treatment programs or parenting education.

Neonatal
- Consider newborn drug testing according to your hospital's policy and practice.
- Involve social services in planning for the baby's care after discharge.

3. Cocaine

Cocaine use during pregnancy is associated with an increased risk for premature rupture of membranes, preterm labor, placental abruption, fetal growth restriction, and fetal death. Fetal effects may result from cocaine crossing the placenta and directly affecting the fetus, as well as from the tachycardia, hypertension, and vasoconstriction that accompany maternal use, which may decrease placental perfusion.

a. Prenatal considerations
- Use the SBIRT approach to educate the woman about the risks of cocaine use and refer her to a substance use disorder treatment program.
- Monitor fetal growth with periodic US examinations in late pregnancy.

b. Intrapartum considerations
- Monitor the woman for hypertension, which may be caused by cocaine intoxication and may be difficult to distinguish from hypertensive disorders of pregnancy.
- Fetal heart rate abnormalities may occur more commonly.
- Consider that placental abruption may be present if fetal heart rate abnormalities such as fetal heart rate decelerations or fetal bradycardia are observed.

c. Postpartum considerations

Maternal
- The mother may have an increased need for pain medication.
- Breastfeeding is contraindicated with maternal cocaine use.

Neonatal
- Consider newborn drug testing according to your hospital's policy and practice.
- Involve social services in planning for the baby's care after discharge.

4. Alcohol

At-risk alcohol use in women is defined by the National Institute on Alcohol Abuse and Alcoholism as more than 3 drinks per occasion, more than 7 drinks per week, or any amount of alcohol consumption during pregnancy. Consumption of any amount of alcohol during pregnancy may result in manifestations of fetal alcohol spectrum disorder. The likelihood of fetal manifestations of maternal alcohol consumption is related in part to the amount and duration of maternal alcohol use; however, no "safe" amount of alcohol intake during pregnancy has been identified.

The fetal effects related to maternal alcohol consumption include abnormal development of the facial structures and central nervous system and abnormalities in fetal growth and intellectual development. Children who were exposed to alcohol before birth are more likely to have cognitive and behavioral problems. The most severe manifestations are known as *fetal alcohol syndrome*, which is characterized by facial and brain malformations, including shortened palpebral fissures, broad upper lip, flattened nasal bridge, small philtrum, small jaw, small eyes, fetal growth restriction, and intellectual disability. Congenital cardiac or other organ defects may also occur with this syndrome. The congenital anomalies, cognitive deficits, and behavioral problems associated with fetal alcohol exposure are completely preventable.

There is no known amount of alcohol that a woman can consume safely during pregnancy.

a. Prenatal considerations
- Screen all women for alcohol use at the first prenatal visit. Consider using a validated screening questionnaire, such as T-ACE (tolerance, annoyed, cut down, eye-opener) or the Alcohol Quantity and Drinking Frequency questions (see Table 6.1). However, any alcohol consumption during pregnancy is considered at-risk drinking.
- Give all pregnant women an unequivocal message that any alcohol intake should be avoided during pregnancy.
- For women with a positive screen for at-risk drinking, give an unambiguous message about the importance of stopping alcohol consumption. Provide a brief intervention and referral for treatment.
- Encourage good maternal nutrition, adherence to prenatal care, and participation in prenatal education and alcohol treatment support programs.
- If high alcohol intake occurs throughout the first trimester, the fetus is at increased risk for congenital anomalies. Order detailed fetal US for assessment for anomalies and discuss pregnancy options, including termination of pregnancy. Order serial US examinations if fetal growth restriction is suspected.

Table 6.1. Validated Alcohol Use Screening Questions		
Questionnaire	**Questions / Score**	**Interpretation**
T-ACE	Tolerance: How many drinks does it take to make you feel high? (More than 2 drinks = 2 points)	A score of 2 points or more indicates a positive screening result for at-risk drinking.
	Annoyed: Have people annoyed you by criticizing your drinking (Yes = 1 point)	
	Cut down: Have you ever felt you ought to cut down on your drinking? (Yes = 1 point)	
	Eye-opener: Have you ever had a drink first thing in the morning to steady your nerves or get rid of a hangover? (Yes = 1 point)	
Alcohol Quantity and Drinking Frequency questions	In a typical week, how many drinks do you have that contain alcohol?	Positive for at-risk drinking if more than 7 drinks
	In the past 90 days, how many times have you had more than 3 drinks on any one occasion?	Positive for at-risk drinking if more than one time

Abbreviation: T-ACE, tolerance, annoyed, cut down, eye-opener.
Derived from At-risk drinking and alcohol dependence: obstetric and gynecologic implications. American College of Obstetricians and Gynecologists Committee Opinion No. 496 (August 2011, reaffirmed 2013).

    b. Intrapartum considerations
    Monitor the woman for signs of alcohol withdrawal or surreptitious use of alcohol during labor.
    c. Postpartum considerations
    Maternal
- If not enrolled earlier, attempt to enroll the woman in an alcohol treatment program.
- Monitor the mother for signs and symptoms of withdrawal.

    Neonatal
- Examine the baby for physical features such as abnormal facial features, low body weight, and less than normal length, any of which may be evidence of fetal alcohol syndrome. Findings in the neonatal period, however, may be nonspecific or not detectable. Arrange longitudinal follow-up to assess the growing child for neurological, behavioral, or learning difficulties.
- In nearly all cases, acute maternal intake of alcohol will be eliminated from the baby by the time delivery occurs. In rare cases, a woman with a high blood alcohol level will deliver an intoxicated newborn. Provide resuscitation, as necessary; give supportive care; and monitor the baby until symptoms resolve.
- Involve social services in planning for the baby's care after discharge.

5. Marijuana
Marijuana has been legalized or decriminalized in many jurisdictions. Its use is reported by 2% to 5% of pregnant women overall, with higher rates in young urban residents with socioeconomic disadvantage. At least one-half of women who use marijuana will continue to do so throughout their pregnancy. Although its effects are difficult to separate from those caused by concurrent use of alcohol, tobacco, and other

drugs, there is evidence that marijuana adversely affects fetal brain development. Marijuana use alone does not appear to increase the risk of stillbirth. Heavier use (weekly or more often) appears to increase the risk of low birth weight, and concurrent use with tobacco appears to increase the risk of preterm birth.
   a. Prenatal considerations
      - Use the SBIRT approach to educate the woman about the risks of marijuana use and encourage her to make a plan to discontinue use. If chronic use and dependence is present, refer her to a substance use disorder treatment program.
      - Consider the use of marijuana and other substances when deciding on the need for US assessment of fetal growth in the third trimester.
   b. Intrapartum considerations
      None specific to marijuana use
   c. Postpartum considerations
      Maternal
      - The use of marijuana during breastfeeding is discouraged. Tetrahydrocannabinol (THC), the active compound in marijuana, is found in breast milk in concentrations 8 times that of maternal blood.

      Neonatal
      - Newborn exposure to THC through breast milk results in distribution and deposition of THC in the adipose tissue and the brain of the newborn. The long-term effects on infant development from exposure to THC during lactation is unknown.
      - Babies have an increased risk for pneumonia, bronchiolitis, and sudden infant death syndrome in the presence of secondhand smoke.
6. Tobacco products and electronic cigarettes
   Nicotine in all forms is the most commonly used substance in pregnancy. Use varies widely by geographic region, but nationally, more than 7% of women use tobacco products throughout pregnancy. Fetal risks associated with tobacco and nicotine include an increased risk of orofacial clefts, fetal growth restriction, low birth weight, preterm prelabor rupture of membranes, placenta previa, and placental abruption. Fetal effects result, at least in part, from uterine vasoconstriction caused by nicotine and from diminished oxygen delivery to the placenta, caused by carbon monoxide inhaled with cigarette smoke. In addition, the incidence of sudden infant death syndrome is significantly increased in babies born to women who smoked during pregnancy. The risks associated with tobacco and nicotine are not limited to pregnant women who smoke. Using smokeless tobacco or electronic cigarettes carries similar risks of fetal harm. Some users report using electronic cigarettes as a means to stop smoking, but many continue to smoke cigarettes while using electronic cigarettes, or users substitute electronic cigarettes without reducing total nicotine use.
   a. Prenatal considerations
      - Use the "5 A's" intervention approach to assess tobacco use and provide counseling (see Table 6.2).
      - Medication treatment (eg, nicotine patches or gum, bupropion) may be used to aid in smoking cessation. Varenicline has not been adequately assessed for use in pregnancy.

UNIT 6: PSYCHOSOCIAL RISK FACTORS IN PREGNANCY

Table 6.2. The 5 A's Intervention for Tobacco Use in Pregnancy

Step	Details
1. *Ask* about tobacco use at the initial prenatal visit and follow-up visits.	A. I have never used tobacco or nicotine or have used minimal amounts of tobacco or nicotine in my lifetime (eg, <100 cigarettes in my lifetime). B. I stopped using tobacco or nicotine before I found out I was pregnant, and I am not using tobacco or nicotine now. C. I stopped using tobacco or nicotine after I found out I was pregnant, and I am not using tobacco or nicotine now. D. I use some tobacco or nicotine now, but I have cut down on the amount of tobacco or nicotine I use since I found out I was pregnant. E. I use tobacco or nicotine regularly now, about the same as before I found out I was pregnant.
2. *Advise* the woman to stop.	Provide information about the risks of continued tobacco and nicotine use.
3. *Assess* her willingness to quit.	Give advice and assistance at each prenatal visit.
4. *Assist* women who are ready to quit.	Provide pregnancy-specific materials to assist the woman in quitting and provide a referral to the smoking cessation helpline (1-800-QUIT-NOW). Prescribe medication therapy as necessary.
5. *Arrange* follow-up visits.	Monitor and record progress toward cessation, while providing continued advice and encouragement.

Derived from Tobacco and nicotine cessation during pregnancy. American College of Obstetricians and Gynecologists Committee Opinion No. 807 (May 2020).

  b. Intrapartum considerations
   None specific to smoking
  c. Postpartum considerations
   Maternal
   - Provide additional counseling to assist the mother in stopping smoking or in remaining abstinent from tobacco if she has quit.
   - Tobacco smoking is not a contraindication to breastfeeding, but cessation efforts should continue.
   - Advise parents that no one should be allowed to smoke near the baby.

   Neonatal
   Babies have an increased risk for pneumonia, bronchiolitis, and sudden infant death syndrome in the presence of secondhand smoke.

Self-test

Now answer these questions to test yourself on the information in the last section.

1. What level of alcohol intake is considered safe for the fetus?
   _____
   _____

2. List at least 3 socioeconomic factors that may adversely affect pregnancy outcome.
   _____
   _____
   _____

3. **True / False** — Maternal cocaine use is associated with an increased risk of fetal cardiac defects.
4. **True / False** — Maternal use of illicit drugs may affect the fetus by interfering with placental function or directly by crossing the placenta.
5. **True / False** — Minimal or absent prenatal care increases the risk of pregnancy complications, regardless of a woman's socioeconomic status.
6. **True / False** — Maternal smoking increases the risk for fetal growth restriction.
7. **True / False** — Cocaine use during pregnancy is associated with placental abruption.
8. **True / False** — Women with no prior history of mental health disorders may develop a perinatal mood or anxiety disorder.
9. **True / False** — In states where marijuana has been legalized, women may be allowed to continue to use marijuana during pregnancy.
10. **True / False** — Acute opioid use may cause increased fetal heart rate variability.
11. **True / False** — Excessive need for pain medication during labor may indicate maternal opioid dependence.
12. **True / False** — Women who have difficulty adapting to pregnancy are much more likely to attempt suicide than women who do not have difficulty adapting to pregnancy.
13. **True / False** — Occasional recreational drug use is not as harmful to the fetus as chronic maternal addiction.

14. Which of the following risks are increased for women who inject illicit drugs?

Yes	No	
___	___	Becoming infected with HIV
___	___	Developing diabetes mellitus
___	___	Causing permanent fetal damage
___	___	Becoming infected with hepatitis B virus

Check your answers with the list that follows the Recommended Routines. Correct any incorrect answers and review the appropriate section in the unit.

UNIT 6: PSYCHOSOCIAL RISK FACTORS IN PREGNANCY

PSYCHOSOCIAL RISK FACTORS IN PREGNANCY

Recommended Routines

All the routines listed below are based on the principles of perinatal care presented in the unit you have just finished. They are recommended as part of routine perinatal care.

Read each routine carefully and decide whether it is standard operating procedure in your hospital. Check the appropriate blank next to each routine.

Procedure Standard in My Hospital	Needs Discussion by Our Staff	Recommended Routine
_____	_____	1. Establish a system of routine universal screening and referral for • Intimate partner violence • Psychosocial conditions • Mental health disorders
_____	_____	2. Establish a system for women with an opioid use disorder to receive • Referral for medication-assisted treatment • Monitoring for adherence to a treatment plan, including periodic urine drug testing • Monitoring at-risk newborns for neonatal abstinence syndrome

Self-test Answers

These are the answers to the Self-test questions. Please check them with the answers you gave and review the information in the unit wherever necessary.

1. There is no known amount of alcohol that a woman can consume safely during pregnancy.

2. Any 3 of the following socioeconomic factors:
   - Minimal or absent prenatal care
   - Low income
   - Poor housing
   - Nutritional deficiency
   - Obesity
   - Inadequate weight gain
   - Heavy manual labor
   - Hazardous work
   - Domestic violence

3. False   *Reason:* Maternal cocaine use does not appear to increase the risk of birth defects.

4. True

5. True

6. True

7. True

8. True

9. False   *Reason:* There is no known safe amount of fetal marijuana exposure.

10. False   *Reason:* Acute opioid use (pain medication or illicit use) is likely to decrease fetal heart rate variability.

11. True

12. False   *Reason:* Women who have difficulty adapting to pregnancy are not more likely to attempt suicide. Ongoing emotional stress is associated with a variety of problems during pregnancy (eg, greater risk for pregnancy-specific hypertension, preterm labor) and after birth (eg, depression, difficulty with parenting), but the risk for suicide is not increased.

13. False   *Reason:* The fetal effects of maternal drug use, especially cocaine, are unpredictable. Infrequent use has been associated with serious problems in the fetus, while, conversely, chronic use does not always cause injury to the fetus. That is the basis for any use being discouraged, particularly during pregnancy.

14.
Yes	No	
X	___	Becoming infected with HIV
___	X	Developing diabetes mellitus
X	___	Causing permanent fetal damage
X	___	Becoming infected with hepatitis B virus

Unit 5 Posttest

After completion of each unit there is a free online posttest available at www.cmevillage.com to test your understanding. Navigate to the PCEP pages on www.cmevillage.com and register to take the free posttests.

Once registered on the website and after completing all the unit posttests, pay the book exam fee ($15) and pass the test at 80% or greater to earn continuing education credits. Only start the PCEP book exam if you have time to complete it. If you take the book exam and are not connected to a printer, either print your certificate to a .pdf file and save it to print later or come back to www.cmevillage.com at any time and print a copy of your educational transcript.

Credits are only available by book, not by individual unit within the books. Available credits for completion of each book exam are as follows: Book 1: 14.5 credits; Book 2: 16 credits; Book 3: 17 credits; Book 4: 9 credits.

For more details, navigate to the PCEP webpages at www.cmevillage.com.

Unit 7: Gestational Diabetes

Objectives 232

1. Is management of pregestational diabetes mellitus in pregnancy included in this unit? 235
2. Why do some pregnant women develop gestational diabetes? 235
3. Why is it important to identify women with gestational diabetes? 236
4. Which women should be screened for gestational diabetes? 236
5. How is screening for gestational diabetes performed? 237
6. How is gestational diabetes diagnosed? 237
7. How do you care for women with gestational diabetes? 237
8. Are oral antidiabetic medications useful in the management of gestational diabetes? 239
9. How do you know when insulin therapy is needed to manage gestational diabetes? 239
10. What fetal monitoring is needed in pregnancies with gestational diabetes? 241
11. How do you prepare pregnant women with gestational diabetes for delivery? 242
12. What postpartum follow-up is needed for women who had gestational diabetes during their pregnancy? 242
13. What long-term care and advice should you give a woman with gestational diabetes? 243

Tables and Box

Table 7.1. Upper Limits of Reference Plasma Glucose Levels for the 3-hour (100-g) Oral Glucose Tolerance Test 237

Table 7.2. Recommended Capillary Blood Glucose Levels During Pregnancy 238

Table 7.3. Blood Test Results That Indicate Insulin Therapy May Be Needed During Pregnancy 239

Table 7.4. Postpartum Evaluation of Women With Gestational Diabetes Mellitus 243

Box 7.1. Criteria for Diagnosis of Pregestational (or Preexisting) Diabetes Mellitus During Pregnancy 235

Recommended Routines 245

Objectives

In this unit you will learn

A. How gestational diabetes mellitus (GDM) is defined and diagnosed

B. Which pregnant women should be screened for GDM

C. Why it is important to identify pregnant women with GDM

D. How to screen for GDM

E. How GDM is managed during pregnancy

F. How the fetus is monitored during pregnancy complicated by GDM

G. How GDM is managed during labor

H. What postpartum follow-up should be provided to women with GDM

Unit 7 Pretest

Before **reading the unit, please answer the following questions. Select the *one best* answer to each question (unless otherwise instructed). Record your answers on the test and check them with the answers at the end of the book.**

1. True — False — Pregestational diabetes can be diagnosed in the first trimester of pregnancy.
2. True — False — Gestational diabetes mellitus (GDM) develops because the hormonal changes of pregnancy make a pregnant woman more resistant to the insulin her body produces.
3. True — False — After diagnosis is confirmed, GDM should be treated with insulin therapy.
4. True — False — It is desirable to keep the maternal fasting blood glucose level above 120 mg/dL throughout pregnancy.
5. True — False — Black women are at increased risk for GDM.
6. True — False — Pregnant women with an early 1-hour (50-g) oral glucose tolerance test (OGTT) blood glucose level above 140 mg/dL should have a standard 3-hour (100-g) OGTT value obtained to diagnose GDM.
7. True — False — Women with pregestational diabetes mellitus and women with GDM have the same risk of having a baby with congenital malformation(s).
8. True — False — Nearly all women with GDM will develop diabetes mellitus later in life.
9. True — False — Pregnant women with gestational diabetes are at increased risk for developing preeclampsia.
10. True — False — GDM is diagnosed with a 3-hour (100-g) OGTT value when results from 2 or more testing periods (fasting, 1-hour, 2-hour, or 3-hour values) are above the reference range.
11. True — False — Generally, a planned delivery at 36 to 37 weeks of gestation is recommended when GDM is diagnosed.
12. True — False — Insulin therapy may be needed during labor for women with GDM, even if insulin was not needed earlier in pregnancy.
13. During the peripartum period, women with GDM should routinely receive all of these, except
    A. Postpartum glucose tolerance test
    B. Oral medications to control blood glucose level
    C. Dietary intake of 60 to 65 g of protein each day
    D. Capillary blood glucose home monitoring

(continued)

PCEP BOOK 2: MATERNAL AND FETAL CARE

Unit 7 Pretest (*continued*)

14. Increased neonatal risks from maternal GDM include

Yes	No	
___	___	Neonatal hypoglycemia
___	___	Birth trauma
___	___	Neonatal diabetes mellitus
___	___	Neonatal hyperbilirubinemia

15. Which of the following indicate that a woman might be at increased risk for the development of GDM?

Yes	No	
___	___	Prepregnancy weight of 200 lb (91 kg) or more
___	___	Eastern European heritage
___	___	GDM in a previous pregnancy
___	___	Maternal age of 35 years or older

16. Which of the following actions are recommended for pregnant women with GDM?

Yes	No	
___	___	Begin testing for fetal well-being with nonstress tests or biophysical profiles at approximately 28 weeks of gestation
___	___	Consider the use of insulin if the blood glucose level is consistently 80 to 100 mg/dL
___	___	Plan to deliver at 39 weeks of gestation with well-controlled GDM and reassuring fetal well-being
___	___	Estimate fetal weight prior to undertaking vaginal delivery

UNIT 7: GESTATIONAL DIABETES

1. Is management of pregestational diabetes mellitus in pregnancy included in this unit?

The subject of this unit is the diagnosis and management of *gestational diabetes mellitus* (GDM), defined as newly diagnosed glucose intolerance in pregnancy, and most commonly referred to as *gestational diabetes*. It is difficult to reliably diagnose preexisting diabetes during pregnancy (see Box 7.1). Refer to Unit 4, Other Medical Risk Factors in Pregnancy, in this book for more information about preexisting diabetes.

Box 7.1. Criteria for Diagnosis of Pregestational (or Preexisting) Diabetes Mellitus During Pregnancy

The diagnosis of pregestational diabetes may be established if any of the following is observed in the first trimester or early second trimester of pregnancy:

Hemoglobin A_{1c} level $\geq 6.5\%$

Fasting glucose level ≥ 126 mg/dL

2-hour (75-g) oral glucose tolerance test ≥ 200 mg/dL

---

2. Why do some pregnant women develop gestational diabetes?

The normal hormonal changes of pregnancy make pregnant women more resistant to insulin. For women with pregestational diabetes mellitus, these changes usually require a woman to increase her daily dose of insulin to maintain the same degree of control over her blood glucose level that she had before pregnancy.

Nondiabetic pregnant women must produce more insulin to overcome the normal physiological insulin resistance of pregnancy to be able to maintain reference blood glucose levels. Some nondiabetic pregnant women cannot produce sufficient insulin, which ultimately results in *hyperglycemia* (blood glucose levels higher than reference range) after meals. In women without a diagnosis of diabetes mellitus prior to pregnancy, new-onset glucose intolerance during pregnancy is called *gestational diabetes mellitus* (GDM). Normal glucose control usually returns after the pregnancy ends.

Maternal evaluation for GDM can be performed at any time during pregnancy. When GDM is diagnosed during pregnancy, it is not possible to know whether a woman has developed true diabetes mellitus or simply has abnormal glucose tolerance temporally related to pregnancy.

GDM is estimated to occur in 6% to 7% of pregnant women, on the basis of diagnostic criteria outlined in this unit. The prevalence of GDM varies according to ethnic group, personal and family history, and body mass index (BMI). The recurrence rate of GDM in a future pregnancy is as high as 50%.

For some nondiabetic women, the physiological changes of pregnancy may lead to the earliest stage of diabetes mellitus. After delivery, these women may continue to have increased blood glucose levels after meals. Some may require ongoing insulin therapy.

3. Why is it important to identify women with gestational diabetes?

A. Maternal risks from GDM
Continuous exposure to increased blood glucose levels in women with GDM leads to the same metabolic problems observed in women with pregestational diabetes mellitus. In this way, maternal health may be compromised by persistently increased blood glucose levels. In addition, women with GDM are more likely to develop preeclampsia and to require a cesarean delivery than women without GDM.

B. Fetal and neonatal risks from maternal GDM
Alterations of maternal glucose metabolism may lead to fetal hyperglycemia because maternal blood glucose readily crosses the placenta. The fetus has a normal physiological response to its hyperglycemia by secreting increased levels of insulin. The combination of fetal hyperglycemia and fetal hyperinsulinemia may result in excessive fetal growth.

When the pregnant woman has hyperglycemia at the time of labor and delivery, the newborn is at risk for postdelivery hypoglycemia. In this case, the newborn initially has increased serum glucose and circulating insulin levels at birth. Hypoglycemia occurs in the newborn because increased insulin levels persist after the umbilical cord is cut and the maternal source of excess serum glucose is removed. (See Book 1: Maternal and Fetal Evaluation and Immediate Newborn Care, Unit 8, Hypoglycemia.)

Fetal and neonatal risks from maternal GDM include large size for gestational age and macrosomia, surgical delivery, shoulder dystocia and subsequent adverse neonatal outcomes (eg, brachial plexus injury, clavicular fracture), neonatal hypoglycemia, and neonatal hyperbilirubinemia.

4. Which women should be screened for gestational diabetes?

The American College of Obstetricians and Gynecologists recommends all pregnant women be screened for gestational diabetes at or beyond 24 weeks of gestation (universal screening). Screening or testing for gestational diabetes (Box 7.1) should be considered before 24 weeks of gestation or at the initial prenatal visit for women with overweight or obesity (BMI > 25; Asian women BMI > 23) with any of the following risk factors:

- GDM in a previous pregnancy
- Previous baby who was large for gestational age or had a birth weight of 4,000 g (8 lb 13 oz) or more
- Family history of a first-degree relative with diabetes mellitus
- African American, Hispanic, Native American, South or East Asian, or Pacific Islander heritage
- Chronic hypertension
- History of cardiovascular disease
- Polycystic ovary syndrome
- Medical condition associated with insulin resistance or impaired glucose tolerance
- Prepregnancy high-density lipoprotein level less than 35 mg/dL or total triglycerides level greater than 250 mg/dL
- History of hemoglobin A_{1c} of 5.7% or more
- Physical inactivity

UNIT 7: GESTATIONAL DIABETES

5. How is screening for gestational diabetes performed?

Women at average risk for GDM should undergo laboratory screening for GDM at 24 to 28 weeks of gestation.

Women at increased risk for GDM should undergo laboratory screening as early in pregnancy as is practical. Even if screening results early in pregnancy are within reference ranges, women at increased risk for GDM should be screened *again* at 24 to 28 weeks of gestation. Women with gestational diabetes during the first half of pregnancy are more likely to demonstrate severe hyperglycemia later in pregnancy.

Screening for GDM is accomplished by administering a 1-hour (50-g) oral glucose tolerance test (OGTT). The woman is advised to fast for 2 hours before the test. The woman orally consumes a 50-g glucose solution within 5 minutes, and a blood sample is collected 1 hour later. The threshold for defining a positive (abnormal) 1-hour OGTT screening result is usually 130 to 140 mg/dL but varies by institution.

Women with an increased screening blood glucose level should undergo a standard 3-hour glucose tolerance test.

6. How is gestational diabetes diagnosed?

A standard 3-hour (100-g) OGTT is used to diagnose GDM. For at least 3 days before the test, the woman should follow an unrestricted diet, consuming at least 150 g (5 oz) of carbohydrates per day. However, for 8 to 14 hours overnight before the 3-hour OGTT, the woman should not eat anything and should drink only water.

The test is performed after the fasting period, with the woman in the sitting position. The woman is not permitted to smoke immediately before or during the test. After the fasting blood glucose level is determined, the woman drinks a 100-g glucose solution. Blood glucose levels are determined hourly for the next 3 hours (Table 7.1).

Table 7.1. Upper Limits of Reference Plasma Glucose Levels for the 3-hour (100-g) Oral Glucose Tolerance Test	
Fasting evening to morning (8–14 h)	95 mg/dL
1 h after glucose solution	180 mg/dL
2 h after glucose solution	155 mg/dL
3 h after glucose solution	140 mg/dL

When results from any 2 sampling periods reach or exceed the upper limit of the reference range, the 3-hour OGTT result is interpreted as abnormal, and GDM is diagnosed.

Example: If a woman's 3-hour OGTT results are 165 mg/dL at 2 hours and 150 mg/dL at 3 hours after drinking the glucose solution, she has GDM, even if her fasting and 1-hour glucose levels are within reference range limits.

7. How do you care for women with gestational diabetes?

The principal goal for women with GDM is to achieve reference blood glucose levels throughout the remainder of their pregnancy. When reference blood glucose levels are maintained, the complications and risks of gestational diabetes are reduced for the woman and the fetus (or newborn). Care is based on diet, exercise, and monitoring blood levels.

A. Diet

The goal of diet therapy for a woman with GDM is to achieve reference blood glucose levels, provide adequate nutrition for normal weight gain, and avoid ketosis.

For healthy normal-weight pregnant women (prepregnancy BMI of 19–24), the recommended diet during pregnancy contains 30 kcal/kg of nonpregnant body weight per day. No specific dietary changes are recommended for overweight women (prepregnancy BMI of 25–29). Underweight women (prepregnancy BMI ≤ 18) should consume an additional 200 kcal/d. Obese women (BMI ≥ 30) should restrict their intake slightly to approximately 25 kcal/kg per day of ideal nonpregnant body weight.

Example: For a woman with a prepregnancy weight of 54.5 kg and BMI of 23, the recommended caloric intake is approximately 1,635 kcal/d.

Example: Another woman, also weighing 54.5 kg but significantly underweight for her height (BMI of 18), should have an intake of approximately 1,835 kcal/d.

The caloric restriction for obese women has been associated with improved pregnancy outcome for the incidence of macrosomia but also carries the possibility of starvation ketosis.

For patients with GDM, the specific proportions of fat and carbohydrate in the diet may be varied, as long as a pregnant woman obtains 60 to 65 g of protein each day. Carbohydrate intake should be 33% to 40% of the total daily calories, with protein and fats contributing approximately 20% and 40%, respectively, of the remaining calories. Other dietary suggestions include avoiding concentrated sweets (candy, refined sugars, sweetened drinks) and consuming up to 4 to 6 smaller meals each day. These recommendations may be adjusted to individual dietary habits to foster compliance.

B. Exercise

Regular exercise metabolizes glucose in the blood, thus helping the body reduce the need for insulin production. Diet and exercise together have been shown to improve fasting blood glucose levels and response to a 50-g oral glucose challenge in women with GDM. Pregnant women should be encouraged to engage in moderate-intensity exercise a minimum of 150 minutes each week; this is often suggested to occur in episodes of 30 minutes, on 5 days. Exercise should not cause pain or involve significant impact forces. Walking, stretching, yoga, gardening, and swimming are examples of appropriate exercise during pregnancy.

C. Home blood glucose monitoring

Teaching should be provided about diet and exercise, and the woman should be afforded several days to adjust to her new regimen. After a few days of capillary blood glucose level monitoring, it will become clear whether reference blood glucose levels can be maintained with diet and exercise alone (Table 7.2).

Table 7.2. Recommended Capillary Blood Glucose Levels During Pregnancy	
Fasting evening to morning	60–90 mg/dL
1 h after a meal	<140 mg/dL
2 h after a meal	<120 mg/dL

The optimal glucose testing regimen has not been determined. It has been shown, however, that more intensively monitored women with GDM undergo fewer primary cesarean deliveries, have fewer macrosomic babies, and have fewer babies who develop newborn hypoglycemia.

The optimal timing of glucose testing has not been determined. It is believed, however, that the fetus may be at greatest risk when the maternal glucose levels are highest. Post-meal monitoring is therefore recommended, although it has not been determined whether 1-hour or 2-hour post-meal monitoring is superior.

Most women with gestational diabetes mellitus can achieve and maintain reference blood glucose levels with diet and exercise.

8. Are oral antidiabetic medications useful in the management of gestational diabetes?

Insulin is recommended as the first-line agent to treat GDM. Nevertheless, the orally administered antidiabetic medications metformin and glyburide are frequently used during pregnancy. Neither of these oral medications offer superior outcomes when compared to insulin, but they may be preferred for some patients and by some health professionals. Dosing of these medications is similar to that used for nonpregnant women. These oral antidiabetic medications cross the placenta and are detectable in cord blood at birth. The long-term effects of metformin and glyburide during pregnancy is not known. In about 25% to 45% of women, GDM will remain uncontrolled with oral antidiabetic medications alone and will require insulin for optimal management.

9. How do you know when insulin therapy is needed to manage gestational diabetes?

Persistent failure to maintain reference blood glucose levels with diet and exercise may necessitate insulin therapy to provide control. Table 7.3 indicates blood levels that should prompt consideration of insulin therapy.

Women with GDM who require insulin therapy to maintain reference blood glucose levels or who have complications (eg, hypertension) should be managed in the same way as women with prepregnancy insulin-dependent diabetes mellitus. Risks to maternal and fetal health increase dramatically whenever complications develop or glucose intolerance becomes severe enough to require insulin for blood glucose control.

Referral to care by experts is strongly recommended if a woman with gestational diabetes mellitus develops a complication or complications or a need for insulin therapy.

Table 7.3. Blood Test Results That Indicate Insulin Therapy May Be Needed During Pregnancy	
Fasting from evening to morning (8–14 h)	>95 mg/dL
1 h after a meal	>140 mg/dL
2 h after a meal	>120 mg/dL

Self-test A

Now answer these questions to test yourself on the information in the last section.

A1. True / False — Women at high risk for gestational diabetes mellitus (GDM) should be screened as soon as their risk status is identified and again at 24 to 28 weeks of gestation.

A2. True / False — Healthy pregnant women produce more insulin to maintain reference blood glucose levels.

A3. True / False — Fasting blood glucose levels that remain above 105 mg/dL, despite diet and exercise, are likely to require insulin therapy during pregnancy.

A4. True / False — Pregnant women with early pregnancy 1-hour oral glucose tolerance test (OGTT) results above reference range should undergo a standard 3-hour OGTT.

A5. True / False — Babies born to women with GDM diagnosed in the second trimester are more likely to have congenital malformation(s) than if diabetes is diagnosed before pregnancy.

A6. List at least 3 factors that suggest a woman may be at increased risk for GDM.
_____
_____
_____

A7. What are the 3 main components of GDM management?
_____
_____
_____

A8. What are 2 fetal or neonatal risks caused by maternal GDM?
_____
_____

Check your answers with the list that follows the Recommended Routines. Correct any incorrect answers and review the appropriate section in the unit.

10. What fetal monitoring is needed in pregnancies with gestational diabetes?

A. Fetal well-being

The risk of fetal death in utero is increased with GDM that requires treatment with medication; the risk is minimized in women with well-controlled GDM who do not require oral antidiabetic medication or insulin therapy.

Tests for fetal well-being include the nonstress test, biophysical profile, modified biophysical profile, and contraction stress test. Once started, antepartum fetal surveillance tests are usually repeated weekly until delivery. Since the optimal antepartum fetal surveillance strategy has not been determined for patients with diabetes in pregnancy, a pregnant woman's specific antepartum fetal surveillance plan should be consistent with local standards.

Recommendations for antepartum fetal surveillance for pregnant women with well-controlled GDM managed only with diet and exercise are as follows:
- There are no evidence-based recommendations for antepartum fetal surveillance for these pregnant women.
- Antepartum fetal surveillance may not be necessary prior to 40 weeks of gestation.
- If antepartum fetal surveillance is desired, it is usually initiated at a gestational age later than that for women with pregestational diabetes, GDM that requires treatment, or poorly controlled GDM.

Recommendations for antepartum fetal surveillance for prepregnancy diabetes mellitus, poorly controlled GDM, or well-controlled GDM that requires medical treatment (with oral antidiabetic medication or insulin) are as follows:
- All women should be advised to maintain a general awareness of fetal activity each day and to report decreased fetal movement promptly. Current evidence suggests that general awareness is as reliable as formal "kick counting."
- Antepartum fetal surveillance starting at 32 to 34 weeks of gestation. Antepartum fetal surveillance at earlier gestational ages may be considered if there are additional maternal-fetal comorbidities.

B. Fetal size

Because macrosomia is of concern in pregnancies complicated by GDM, serial ultrasonographic (US) measurements may be useful in demonstrating the rate of fetal growth and, hence, the likelihood of a large fetus. US, however, has *not* been shown to be more accurate than clinical measurements in estimating actual fetal weight during labor.

Early delivery to avoid the development of macrosomia and the possibility of associated shoulder dystocia is *not* recommended. Counseling for *cesarean delivery, at term* and before the onset of labor, is recommended by some experts if the fetal weight is estimated to be such that shoulder dystocia becomes a clinically significant concern.

C. Timing of delivery
- For pregnant women with well-controlled GDM managed only with diet and exercise, delivery prior to $39^{0/7}$ weeks of gestation is not recommended, and expectant management may be considered through $40^{6/7}$ weeks of gestation.
- For pregnant women with well-controlled GDM that requires treatment with oral antidiabetic medications or insulin, delivery is recommended from $39^{0/7}$ to $39^{6/7}$ weeks of gestation.

- For pregnant women with poorly controlled GDM, delivery from $37^{0/7}$ to $38^{6/7}$ weeks of gestation may be justified. Preterm delivery prior to $37^{0/7}$ weeks of gestation should be reserved for women with hyperglycemia refractory to treatment or abnormal antepartum fetal surveillance.

11. How do you prepare pregnant women with gestational diabetes for delivery?

Fetal size should be estimated near the time of delivery. Fetal size may be estimated according to recent US findings or clinically by an experienced clinician. The fetal size may affect patient counseling and may influence the route of delivery.

At the time of labor or in preparation for cesarean delivery, the maternal blood glucose level should be monitored hourly and kept between 80 and 120 mg/dL. Insulin therapy may be necessary to maintain this glycemic control.

If volume expansion is needed during labor or cesarean delivery, *avoid* the use of solutions that contain glucose.

12. What postpartum follow-up is needed for women who had gestational diabetes during their pregnancy?

Approximately 10% of women with gestational diabetes will continue to have fasting hyperglycemia after delivery. A random blood glucose level should be obtained in the immediate postpartum period. Any value less than 200 mg/dL is within reference range. Oral hypoglycemic agents or insulin should be prescribed to women who have postpartum random blood glucose values $\geq$ 200 mg/dL.

Women with GDM or postpartum hyperglycemia should be evaluated after pregnancy for diabetes mellitus. In addition, women who delivered a large-for-gestational-age baby should be considered for postpartum diabetes mellitus testing. The recommended postpartum evaluation for diabetes mellitus is the standard 2-hour (75-g) OGTT performed 4 to 12 weeks after delivery by using non-pregnancy screening criteria.

Women with gestational diabetes during pregnancy should be advised about the importance of glucose control before future conception and during early pregnancy. Hyperglycemia that occurs early in gestation, during the formation of fetal organs, is thought to be responsible for the higher incidence of congenital malformations in babies of women with diabetes.

13. What long-term care and advice should you give a woman with gestational diabetes?

Up to one-half of women with gestational diabetes will develop insulin-dependent diabetes mellitus within 20 years of the pregnancy in which GDM was discovered, even if their initial postpartum 2-hour (75-g) OGTT result was within reference range. Women should be advised about the increased likelihood of developing diabetes mellitus and what signs and symptoms to report, such as increased thirst, increased urination, and unexplained weight loss.

Advice on lifestyle, weight control, exercise, and diet may be helpful in delaying the onset of diabetes mellitus. Refer your patient to a registered dietitian or diabetes educator for individualized help with meal planning, exercise, and blood glucose management. Annual examination of fasting blood glucose levels is recommended (Table 7.4).

Table 7.4. Postpartum Evaluation of Women With Gestational Diabetes Mellitus			
	Plasma Glucose Levels		**Diabetes Mellitus**
	Reference	**Prediabetes**[a]	
Fasting	<110 mg/dL	110–125 mg/dL	126 mg/dL
2 h	<140 mg/dL	140–199 mg/dL	200 mg/dL

[a] High risk for future development of diabetes mellitus.

Based on ACOG Practice Bulletin No. 190. Gestational diabetes mellitus. *Obstet Gynecol*. 2018;131:e49–64; ACOG Practice Bulletin No. 201. Pregestational diabetes mellitus. *Obstet Gynecol*. 2018;132;e228–248; and American Diabetes Association. 14. Management of diabetes in pregnancy: Standards of Medical Care in Diabetes 2019. *Diabetes Care*. 2019;42(suppl 1):S165–S172.

Self-test B

Now answer these questions to test yourself on the information in the last section.

B1. True / False — Women with gestational diabetes mellitus (GDM) should have their blood glucose levels monitored throughout labor and maintained between 80 and 120 mg/dL.

B2. True / False — A woman who delivered a very large newborn should be evaluated for gestational diabetes in the postpartum period.

B3. True / False — Women with GDM will develop diabetes mellitus in the immediate postpartum period.

B4. True / False — Women with GDM should receive a glucose tolerance test in the postpartum period.

B5. True / False — Up to one-half of women with gestational diabetes go on to develop insulin-dependent diabetes within 20 years of the pregnancy in which gestational diabetes occurred.

B6. If volume expansion is needed during labor for a woman with GDM, what type of fluids should be used?

_____

B7. Which of the following actions are recommended for pregnant women with gestational diabetes?

Yes	No	
___	___	Begin testing of fetal well-being at approximately 28 weeks of gestation.
___	___	Consider the use of insulin if the blood glucose level is consistently above 80 mg/dL.
___	___	Plan to deliver at 35 to 36 weeks of gestation unless fetal well-being test results indicate the need for earlier delivery.
___	___	Estimate fetal weight prior to undertaking vaginal delivery.

Check your answers with the list that follows the Recommended Routines. Correct any incorrect answers and review the appropriate section in the unit.

GESTATIONAL DIABETES

Recommended Routines

All the routines listed below are based on the principles of perinatal care presented in the unit you have just finished. They are recommended as part of routine perinatal care.

Read each routine carefully and decide whether it is standard operating procedure in your hospital. Check the appropriate blank next to each routine.

Procedure Standard in My Hospital	Needs Discussion by Our Staff	Recommended Routine
_____	_____	1. Establish a protocol to screen all women for pregestational diabetes through the identification of risk factors followed by laboratory assessment, as early in pregnancy as possible.
_____	_____	2. Establish a protocol of laboratory screening of women at high risk for gestational diabetes early in pregnancy and again at 24 to 28 weeks of gestation, even if their earlier results were within reference range.
_____	_____	3. Establish a protocol for estimation of fetal weight on admission to the labor unit for women with gestational diabetes mellitus (GDM).
_____	_____	4. Establish a protocol for management of GDM during labor.

Self-test Answers

These are the answers to the self-test questions. Please check them with the answers you gave and review the information in the unit wherever necessary.

Self-test A

A1. True

A2. True

A3. True

A4. True

A5. False   *Reason:* Women with pregestational diabetes mellitus are at increased risk of having a baby with a congenital malformation, especially if blood glucose levels are uncontrolled at conception and shortly thereafter, during fetal organ formation. Hyperglycemia later in pregnancy does not carry the same risk for fetal malformation.

A6. Any 3 of the following factors:
- Gestational diabetes mellitus in a previous pregnancy
- Prepregnancy or early pregnancy weight greater than 200 lb (>90 kg)
- Family history of diabetes mellitus
- Previous baby who was large for gestational age or had a birth weight of 4,000 g (8 lb 13 oz) or more
- African American, Hispanic, Native American, South or East Asian, or Pacific Islander heritage
- Maternal age 35 years and older
- Previous babies with nonchromosomal congenital anomalies
- History of unexplained stillbirths or miscarriages beyond the first trimester

A7. Diet
Exercise
Capillary glucose monitoring

A8. Any 2 of the following risks:
- Macrosomia
- Cesarean delivery
- Shoulder dystocia (birth trauma)
- Neonatal hypoglycemia
- Neonatal hyperbilirubinemia

Self-test B

B1. True

B2. True

B3. False   *Reason:* About 10% of women with gestational diabetes mellitus (GDM) continue to have fasting hyperglycemia postpartum. Up to one-half of women with GDM will develop diabetes mellitus within 20 years of the pregnancy in which GDM occurred, even when their initial postpartum glucose tolerance test result was within reference range.

UNIT 7: GESTATIONAL DIABETES

B4. True

B5. True

B6. Fluids that do not contain glucose

B7. Yes   No
    _X_   ____   Begin testing of fetal well-being at approximately 28 weeks of gestation.
    ____   _X_   Consider the use of insulin if the blood glucose level is consistently above 80 mg/dL.
    ____   _X_   Plan to deliver at 35 to 36 weeks of gestation unless fetal well-being test results indicate the need for earlier delivery.
    _X_   ____   Estimate fetal weight prior to undertaking vaginal delivery.

Unit 7 Posttest

After completion of each unit there is a free online posttest available at www.cmevillage.com to test your understanding. Navigate to the PCEP pages on www.cmevillage.com and register to take the free posttests.

Once registered on the website and after completing all the unit posttests, pay the book exam fee ($15) and pass the test at 80% or greater to earn continuing education credits. Only start the PCEP book exam if you have time to complete it. If you take the book exam and are not connected to a printer, either print your certificate to a .pdf file and save it to print later or come back to www.cmevillage.com at any time and print a copy of your educational transcript.

Credits are only available by book, not by individual unit within the books. Available credits for completion of each book exam are as follows: Book 1: 14.5 credits; Book 2: 16 credits; Book 3: 17 credits; Book 4: 9 credits.

For more details, navigate to the PCEP webpages at www.cmevillage.com.

Unit 8: Prelabor Rupture of Membranes and Intra-amniotic Infection

Objectives 250

1. What is prelabor rupture of membranes (PROM)? 253
2. What factors increase the risk of PROM? 253
3. What maternal-fetal risks are affected by PROM? 253
4. How do you determine whether the membranes have ruptured? 254
5. How is PROM managed? 258
6. What should you do if there is evidence of intra-amniotic infection? 259
7. What should you do if there is *no* evidence of intra-amniotic infection? 261
8. What postdelivery care should be provided for women with PROM or intra-amniotic infection? 269

Table

    Table 8.1. Management of Preterm Prelabor Rupture of Membranes 268

Recommended Routines 271

Skill Units

Sterile Speculum Examination 275

Tests for Suspected or Proven Rupture of Membranes 281

Objectives

In this unit you will learn

A. What maternal, fetal, and neonatal risks are associated with
- Prelabor rupture of membranes (PROM)
- Intra-amniotic infection
- Prolonged rupture of membranes

B. How to determine whether the amniotic membranes are ruptured

C. The signs and symptoms of intra-amniotic infection

D. How to treat intra-amniotic infection

E. How to manage PROM when there are no signs of intra-amniotic infection in a
- Term fetus
- Preterm fetus

F. What postdelivery maternal and neonatal care to provide for patients with a history of PROM or infection of the amniotic membranes

Unit 8 Pretest

Before reading the unit, please answer the following questions. Select the *one best* answer to each question (unless otherwise instructed). Record your answers on the test and check them with the answers at the end of the book.

1. Which of the following complications are associated with prelabor rupture of membranes (PROM)?

Yes	No	
___	___	Amniotic fluid embolism
___	___	Umbilical cord compression
___	___	Neonatal sepsis
___	___	Placental abruption

2. **True False** If the amniotic fluid is foul smelling and maternal fever is present, you should begin treatment for intra-amniotic infection.

3. **True False** Rupture of membranes for 18 hours or longer increases the risk of neonatal infection for preterm babies but not for term babies.

4. **True False** Intra-amniotic infection can occur only after the membranes have ruptured.

5. **True False** When intra-amniotic infection develops in a preterm gestation, the early use of intravenous antibiotics usually allows the pregnancy to continue for at least another 1 to 2 weeks.

6. **True False** Intra-amniotic infection increases the risk for postpartum endometritis.

7. PROM has occurred at 32 weeks of gestation. There are no signs or symptoms of labor or infection, and the fetal heart pattern is reactive. For which of the following reasons should a sterile speculum examination be performed?

Yes	No	
___	___	Assess cervical dilation and effacement.
___	___	Obtain samples for group B β-hemolytic streptococcus, chlamydia, and gonorrhea testing.
___	___	Collect amniotic fluid from the vaginal pool to test for phosphatidyl glycerol.
___	___	Place internal fetal heart rate and uterine contraction monitoring devices.

8. A woman has PROM at 38 weeks of gestation, with foul-smelling amniotic fluid, maternal fever of 38.6°C (101.5°F), tender uterus, and fetal tachycardia. There is no other evidence of fetal distress; presentation is vertex. You should begin intravenous antibiotics and
   - **A.** Induce labor.
   - **B.** Perform a cesarean delivery.
   - **C.** Wait for spontaneous onset of labor.
   - **D.** Perform an amnioinfusion.

(continued)

Unit 8 Pretest (continued)

9. Which of the following actions may be appropriate for the management of preterm PROM at 30 weeks of gestation when a woman is not in labor and there are no signs of infection?

Yes	No	
___	___	Start antibiotics.
___	___	Use sterile speculum examination to check for a prolapsed umbilical cord.
___	___	Obtain urine for urinalysis and culture.
___	___	Periodically palpate the uterus.
___	___	Administer antenatal corticosteroids.
___	___	Perform digital cervical examination to assess cervical dilation.

10. **True** **False** When a woman is treated for intra-amniotic infection during labor, intravenous antibiotic therapy should be continued for 10 to 14 days after she becomes afebrile.

11. **True** **False** In the presence of asymptomatic maternal colonization with group B β-hemolytic streptococcus, there is no reason to use prophylactic antibiotics during labor.

12. **True** **False** Neonatal sepsis can follow PROM, even if the woman showed no sign of illness.

UNIT 8: PRELABOR RUPTURE OF MEMBRANES AND INTRA-AMNIOTIC INFECTION

1. What is prelabor rupture of membranes (PROM)?

The amniotic (fetal) membranes may rupture before, coincident with, or after the onset of labor. Rupture of the fetal membranes before the onset of labor is termed *prelabor rupture of membranes* (PROM) or *prelabor ROM*.

To eliminate possible confusion and misuse of the acronym PROM, some prefer to abbreviate rupture of membranes as ROM and then specify whether there is prelabor ROM, preterm ROM, or preterm prelabor ROM. Preterm ROM refers to ROM before 37 weeks' gestation. The acronym PPROM usually refers to preterm PROM. The term *prolonged ROM* refers to the duration of ruptured membranes, typically defined as being longer than 18 hours. For the purposes of this unit, PROM will refer to prelabor rupture of membranes.

2. What factors increase the risk of PROM?

The cause of PROM is not entirely understood. In most cases of PROM, there is no identifiable risk factor. Women with any of the following risk factors may be considered to have a higher risk for PROM or preterm labor:

- Prior preterm delivery, especially if associated with preterm PROM
- Cervical insufficiency
- Procedures involving the cervix, including cervical cerclage and conization
- Intra-amniotic infection (formerly termed *chorioamnionitis*)
- Maternal lower genital tract infection, especially *Trichomonas*, gonorrhea, chlamydia, or bacterial vaginosis
- Bacteriuria, with or without symptoms of urinary tract infection
- Uterine overdistension (polyhydramnios, multifetal gestation)
- Vaginal bleeding after 14 weeks of gestation
- Maternal smoking
- Lower socioeconomic status
- Amniocentesis (<1% risk for ROM to occur because of the procedure; if ROM occurs, the amniotic fluid leakage almost always stops spontaneously and the pregnancy continues)

3. What maternal-fetal risks are affected by PROM?

A. Maternal, fetal, or neonatal infection

While infection may be a *cause* of PROM, infection can also be a *consequence* of PROM. Ascending infections from the vagina to the uterus can be caused by normal vaginal flora or by pathogenic organisms. Intra-amniotic infection can develop even in the absence of maternal infection.

The intact membranes that surround the amniotic fluid and fetus and the thick cervical mucus provide a physical barrier to infection by organisms ascending from the vagina. When the membranes rupture, this protective barrier is broken. This increases the maternal risk for an intra-amniotic infection, sepsis, and postpartum endometritis. This also increases the fetal risk for in utero infection, preterm birth, and neonatal sepsis. Maternal and fetal infection is more common with earlier gestational age at membrane rupture and longer duration of pregnancy (latency period) after ROM has occurred. Although uncommon, intra-amniotic or fetal infection can also occur with intact membranes. The degree of maternal illness may not correlate with the degree of neonatal illness.

PROM is often followed by spontaneous labor and delivery. If preterm birth occurs, prematurity is the major risk for neonatal morbidity and death even in the absence of intra-amniotic infection. If intra-amniotic infection is present, the risk of neonatal morbidity or death is significantly increased.

B. Umbilical cord complications
1. Umbilical cord compression: Leakage of amniotic fluid from the uterus can result in oligohydramnios. When oligohydramnios is present, the umbilical cord can become compressed between the fetus and uterine wall, which may result in fetal hypoxia or fetal death in utero, whether or not labor is present.
2. Umbilical cord prolapse: PROM increases the risk of umbilical cord prolapse, especially if the fetus is breech or the presenting part is not engaged.

C. Oligohydramnios complications
Prolonged oligohydramnios, particularly if preterm PROM occurs during the second trimester, can result in pulmonary hypoplasia. The absence of fluid limits the growth and development of the terminal airways and alveoli that normally occur with fetal respiratory movements of a fluid-filled lung. Pulmonary hypoplasia may result in chronic lung disease or neonatal death because of respiratory insufficiency. Deformation of the fetus, with abnormal facies and limb positioning deformations, may also occur because of restriction of fetal growth and movement. These complications do not invariably occur after preterm PROM, even at very early gestational ages, and rarely develop when PROM occurs after 26 weeks of gestation.

D. Placental abruption
For reasons that are not clearly identified, PROM is associated with an increased risk for placental abruption. If blood (even a small amount) is passed vaginally, or if there are any other signs of a placental abruption, a careful maternal-fetal evaluation is indicated. The evaluation includes maternal vital sign assessment, physical examination, laboratory tests (complete blood count, blood type, Kleihauer-Betke test), tocometry, and fetal monitoring.

E. Fetal death
The risk of fetal death is increased in all cases of PROM. This risk increases with decreasing gestational age and is highest for fetuses of less than 26 weeks' gestation. The causes are not completely understood, but oligohydramnios, umbilical cord complications, and intra-amniotic infection all contribute to the risk of fetal death.

4. How do you determine whether the membranes have ruptured?

A. History
A pregnant woman will usually report an uncontrolled gush of fluid from her vagina as the first sign of ruptured membranes. Some women will report persistent but intermittent leakage of fluid instead of a gush, and the perceived quantity may be small. If the history includes a description of foul-smelling or cloudy amniotic fluid, clinical suspicion for intra-amniotic infection should be high.

Other causes of vaginal discharge in pregnancy may not be related to ROM. The amount of normal vaginal secretions typically increases during pregnancy. The vaginal discharge associated with bacterial vaginosis may be mistaken by the woman for fluid leakage. Spontaneous leakage of maternal urine may lead the woman to believe she is leaking amniotic fluid. Occasionally, painless cervical dilation in a woman with cervical insufficiency may be accompanied by a watery discharge without ROM.

B. Examination
1. Sterile speculum examination (See also the skill units that follow this unit.)

If membranes have ruptured and labor has not started, a digital examination should NOT be performed. Only sterile speculum examination(s) should be used to evaluate a woman with suspected ROM until a decision has been made to proceed promptly with delivery. This approach minimizes the risk of developing an intra-amniotic infection.

Perform a sterile speculum examination to
- Evaluate the patient for prolapse of the umbilical cord through the cervix.
- Assess cervical dilation and effacement with visual inspection.
- Evaluate whether there is leakage of fluid through the cervix.
- Evaluate whether there is pooling of amniotic fluid in the posterior fornix of the vagina.
- If pooling of fluid is observed, the fluid can be further evaluated.
  — Evaluate the fluid for its color, consistency, and odor.
  — If light microscopy is available, a fern test may be performed. A drop of the fluid may be spread and dried on a microscope slide (without coverslip) to evaluate whether there is salt-crystal arborization (ie, ferning).
  — Use a Nitrazine paper test to determine pH level. (See Skill Unit: Tests for Suspected or Proven Rupture of Membranes.)
  — Current recommendations do not include fetal lung maturity testing on pooled amniotic fluid for the purposes of delivery planning.
- Assess the patient for genital tract infection
  — Cervical culture or DNA probe test for gonorrhea and chlamydia
  — Vaginal and rectal cultures for group B β-hemolytic streptococcus (GBS)
  — Test for bacterial vaginosis

2. Assays for amniotic proteins in vaginal secretions

There are several commercial tests available to detect the presence of amniotic proteins in the vaginal secretions. These tests generally have high sensitivity for ruptured membranes but lower specificity, and false-positive rates as high as 30% have been reported. It is important to follow the manufacturer's instructions for sample collection and result interpretation. False-positive assay results may result from the presence of blood, seminal fluid, infection, soap, or other alkaline substances in the vagina. These assays may be used as an adjunct to other assessments for ROM and should be interpreted in the overall context of the patient's clinical history, physical examination, and ultrasonographic (US) assessment, if performed (see below).

3. US examination

If PROM is suspected but not confirmed, transabdominal obstetric US may be performed as a part of the woman's evaluation. A US evaluation can be conducted to evaluate the amniotic fluid and fetal presentation, estimate the fetal weight, and assess fetal well-being. Interpretation of images of the amniotic fluid is challenging, however, because no specific measurement of amniotic fluid can confirm ROM, even if oligohydramnios is present. While the presence of oligohydramnios is consistent with ROM, a low volume of amniotic fluid may be present for other reasons not related to ruptured membranes. Conversely, a patient who has PROM may have apparently normal amounts of amniotic fluid at US examination.

4. Amniocentesis

   When the diagnosis of PROM cannot be established with sterile speculum and abdominal US examination(s), and the diagnosis is critical for management decisions (eg, PROM before 34 weeks of gestation is suspected), consider amniocentesis and infusion of dye into the amniotic cavity.

Amniocentesis in the setting of possible PROM with decreased amniotic fluid volume requires special expertise. Consultation with maternal-fetal medicine specialists is strongly recommended.

If amniocentesis is appropriate, the following steps should be taken.

a. Withdrawal of amniotic fluid for analysis

   If analysis of amniotic fluid would be useful, fluid must be withdrawn *before* dye is injected. Useful amniotic fluid analyses include
   - Culture
   - Gram stain (for leukocytes or bacteria)
   - Glucose concentration (a low concentration indicates that glucose is being consumed by bacteria; intra-amniotic infection may be present)
   - Leukocyte (white blood cell) count
     Currently, tests for fetal lung maturity are not recommended.

b. Instillation of dye into the amniotic space

   A dye solution is created by using indigotindisulfonate sodium (indigo carmine). Typically, 1 mL of dye solution is diluted with 9 mL of sterile physiological (normal) saline solution. The dye solution is injected into the amniotic space after withdrawal of the amniotic fluid sample.

   Note: Methylene blue dye should *never* be used for this test because it can bind to fetal hemoglobin and cause methemoglobinemia.

c. Observation for leakage of the dye

   A sterile white gauze pad is placed high in the woman's vagina. The woman is encouraged to sit or ambulate, and the gauze pad is retrieved after 20 to 30 minutes. Blue dye on the gauze pad indicates ROM.

   Note: Indigo carmine dye in the amniotic cavity will be absorbed systemically by the fetus and pass across the placenta into the maternal circulation. Within a short period of time, the blue dye will be excreted in the maternal urine, making the woman's urine blue or green colored. Placing white gauze in the vagina, rather than placing a pad on the woman's perineum, will make certain any dye on the gauze pad is from amniotic fluid leakage through the cervix.

When the diagnosis of PROM is established, the pregnant woman should be admitted to a hospital for further evaluation and management. In most cases, maternal care will require hospitalization until delivery.

UNIT 8: PRELABOR RUPTURE OF MEMBRANES AND INTRA-AMNIOTIC INFECTION

Self-test A

Now answer these questions to test yourself on the information in the last section.

A1. **True** **False** The risk of prelabor rupture of membranes (PROM) is increased when gonorrhea or chlamydia infection is present.

A2. **True** **False** Ultrasonographic examination may be able to demonstrate a decrease in amniotic fluid, to help confirm suspected rupture of membranes (ROM).

A3. **True** **False** Intra-amniotic infection can occur with intact membranes.

A4. **True** **False** Life-threatening neonatal illness can develop after PROM, even when there is no evidence of intra-amniotic infection.

A5. **True** **False** Digital pelvic examinations should not be done when preterm PROM occurs and labor has not begun.

A6. **True** **False** Umbilical cord compression and cord prolapse are possible complications of PROM.

A7. **True** **False** Urinary tract infection increases the risk for PROM.

A8. **True** **False** After ROM, amniotic fluid obtained from a vaginal pool should be used to assess the fetus for lung maturity.

A9. List at least 3 complications associated with PROM.
_____
_____
_____

A10. The main risk associated with PROM is maternal or neonatal _____. (single word answer)

A11. After amniocentesis and infusion of dye to test for ROM, a sterile gauze pad should be placed where?
_____

Check your answers with the list that follows the Recommended Routines. Correct any incorrect answers and review the appropriate section in the unit.

5. How is PROM managed?

The period between ROM and onset of labor is called the *latency period*. In the absence of infection, approximately 75% of all women with PROM will deliver within 7 days. Earlier gestational age at ROM may be associated with longer latency.

Maternal treatment is primarily determined by the fetal gestational age and whether intra-amniotic infection is present.

A. Evaluation of the fetus

Fetal evaluation includes establishing or confirming the gestational age of the fetus. Fetal well-being is established by using standard tests, such as fetal heart rate monitoring with tocometry or a biophysical profile. If not done earlier (see Section 4B3, US examination), a transabdominal US examination should be performed to assess amniotic fluid volume, fetal size, and fetal presentation.

B. Evaluation for intra-amniotic infection

The maternal evaluation for intra-amniotic infection includes maternal vital sign assessment, physical examination, and laboratory testing (complete blood count with differential, urine analysis and culture, cultures for gonorrhea and chlamydia, and rectovaginal cultures for GBS).

An intra-amniotic infection is suspected when there is an increased maternal temperature not readily attributable to other sources on the basis of the following criteria:
- Single maternal temperature of 39.0°C (102.2°F) and higher, or
- Maternal temperature of 38.0°C to 38.9°C (100.4°F–102°F) lasting for at least 30 minutes with the presence of at least one of the following: maternal leukocytosis (>15,000 cells/mm^3), purulent cervical discharge, and/or fetal tachycardia (baseline heart rate > 160 beats/min).

Unexplained maternal temperature of 38.0°C to 38.9°C (100.4°F–102°F) lasting less than 30 minutes or without maternal leukocytosis, purulent cervical discharge, or fetal tachycardia is interpreted as an isolated maternal fever and should be closely followed.

Even without maternal temperature increase, uterine tenderness, low biophysical profile score (≤6 points), leukocytosis, and maternal malaise ("I just don't feel well") are associated with intra-amniotic infection.

If the clinical assessment for intra-amniotic infection is uncertain, amniocentesis is sometimes used to aid in the diagnosis. The following findings in amniotic fluid (obtained via amniocentesis) suggest infection.
- Amniotic fluid glucose concentration less than 15 mg/dL
- Positive Gram stain result (for leukocytes or bacteria)
  Note: By itself, a positive Gram stain result is a better test than a low glucose level, but, together, these tests provide stronger evidence for infection than either test alone.
- *Amniotic fluid* leukocyte count above 100/mm^3
- Positive amniotic fluid culture result

The diagnosis of intra-amniotic infection is confirmed only with positive amniotic fluid tests or by placental pathology findings consistent with infection. In some cases, the diagnosis of intra-amniotic infection is established only after delivery of the fetus. The histologic diagnosis of infection involving the placenta and membranes does not alter postpartum treatment of the mother.

6. What should you do if there is evidence of intra-amniotic infection?

When there is evidence of intra-amniotic infection, the woman and fetus may develop serious complications. The fetus must be delivered, regardless of gestational age. Antibiotic therapy should be started promptly, but antibiotics cannot completely treat an intra-amniotic infection while the woman remains pregnant. The obstetric management for suspected and confirmed intra-amniotic infection is the same.

 If intra-amniotic infection develops over time, the specific infectious organism and length of time until delivery are key factors in determining the severity of maternal illness. When intra-amniotic infection is present, the longer the fetus and placenta remain undelivered, the more serious the infection is likely to become.

A. Begin intravenous antibiotic therapy
   Promptly begin administration of broad-spectrum antibiotics. Antibiotics are continued until delivery occurs. Oral antibiotics are not effective for treatment of intra-amniotic infection.

   Primary antibiotic regimen
   - Ampicillin dose of 2 g administered initially, then 1 g administered every 6 hours until delivery

   and
   - Gentamicin, either 2-mg/kg loading dose followed by 1.5 mg/kg administered intravenously every 8 hours or 5 mg/kg administered every 24 hours

   The primary antibiotic regimen is altered for patients who are allergic to penicillin.
   - Mild allergy: Replace ampicillin with cefazolin, 2 g, every 8 hours
   - Severe allergy: Replace ampicillin with either clindamycin, 900 mg, every 8 hours or vancomycin, 1 g, every 12 hours

   If cesarean delivery is performed while the woman is receiving a primary antibiotic regimen, recommendations include adding a preoperative 500-mg intravenous dose of azithromycin and an additional postdelivery dose of the primary antibiotic regimen plus one dose of either of the following:
   - Clindamycin, 900 mg, administered every 8 hours
   or
   - Metronidazole, 500 mg, administered every 12 hours

   If the primary regimen is not selected, alternative intravenous antibiotic regimens include any of the following:
   - Ampicillin-sulbactam, 3 g, administered every 6 hours
   - Piperacillin-tazobactam, 3.375 g, administered every 6 hours or 4.5 g, administered intravenously every 8 hours
   - Cefotetan, 2 g, administered every 12 hours
   - Cefoxitin, 2 g, administered every 8 hours
   - Ertapenem, 1 g, administered every 24 hours

   If cesarean delivery is performed while the woman is receiving an alternative antibiotic regimen, current recommendations include adding an additional post-delivery dose of the alternative regimen. An additional clindamycin dose is not necessary when one of the alternative regimens is used.

B. Administer antenatal steroids

Currently, there is insufficient evidence on the administration of corticosteroids in the setting of overt intra-amniotic infection for women with preterm PROM before 34 weeks of gestation. Consultation with maternal-fetal medicine specialists is strongly recommended.

For women with preterm PROM between $24^{0/7}$ and $33^{6/7}$ weeks of gestation with a stable clinical presentation and suspected or confirmed intra-amniotic infection, a single course of antenatal corticosteroids is recommended. A course of corticosteroids may be administered as early as $23^{0/7}$ weeks of gestation on the basis of local standards and after appropriate counseling. The administration of antenatal corticosteroids in this context improves newborn survival and reduces newborn morbidity. Delivery should not be delayed to complete the steroid course, and tocolysis should not be administered to women with intra-amniotic infection.

Antenatal corticosteroids are NOT recommended for women at or beyond $34^{0/7}$ weeks of gestation who have suspected or confirmed intra-amniotic infection.

C. Deliver the fetus

Continuous fetal heart rate and uterine contraction monitoring is recommended. Internal monitoring should only be used as clinically indicated. If labor has not started or if the progression of labor is inadequate, augment uterine contractions with oxytocin as clinically indicated. Minimize digital pelvic examinations, but examine the mother frequently enough to verify progression of labor. Intra-amniotic infection increases the likelihood of dysfunctional labor.

Consider amnioinfusion if persistent variable decelerations occur. Amnioinfusion may provide sufficient intra-amniotic fluid to relieve cord compression. If variable decelerations cannot be corrected, cesarean delivery may become necessary.

Note: Amnioinfusion is described in Unit 5, Obstetric Risk Factors: Prior or Current Pregnancy, in this book.

Cesarean delivery should be performed for standard obstetric indications.

In addition, owing to ineffective uterine contraction observed in the context of intra-amniotic infection, postpartum hemorrhage due to uterine atony is more likely. The obstetric team should have an increased index of suspicion for this obstetric emergency and make appropriate preparations.

UNIT 8: PRELABOR RUPTURE OF MEMBRANES AND INTRA-AMNIOTIC INFECTION

7. What should you do if there is *no* evidence of intra-amniotic infection?

- When there is no suspected or confirmed intra-amniotic infection, the management of pregnant women with PROM depends on the gestational age and whether the woman is in labor.

A. Term fetus ($37^{0/7}$ weeks of gestation or more)
  1. Term gestation, woman **in labor**, no intra-amniotic infection
     - Evaluate the risk for early-onset neonatal GBS sepsis. (See also Unit 3, Infectious Diseases in Pregnancy, in this book.)
       — *Maternal rectovaginal or urine culture result positive for GBS or a history of having a prior child with early-onset GBS sepsis:* Initiate prophylaxis.
       — *Maternal rectovaginal or urine culture result negative for GBS or nucleic acid amplification (NAAT) result negative for GBS:* Prophylaxis not indicated.
       — *Maternal GBS status unknown:* Prophylaxis indicated in the presence of maternal intrapartum fever (>38.0°C [>100.4°F]), prolonged ROM (>18 hours), NAAT result positive for GBS, or history of GBS colonization in a prior pregnancy.
     - Delivery of the fetus
       Either continuous fetal heart rate and uterine contraction monitoring or intermittent fetal heart rate auscultation may be appropriate, depending on the presence of other risk factors. Internal monitoring should only be used as clinically indicated. If the progression of labor is inadequate, augment uterine contractions with oxytocin as clinically indicated. Minimize digital pelvic examinations, but examine the woman frequently enough to verify the progression of labor. Continue to evaluate the woman and the fetus for evidence of intra-amniotic infection.
     - Consider amnioinfusion if persistent variable decelerations occur. Amnioinfusion may provide sufficient intra-amniotic fluid to relieve cord compression. If variable decelerations cannot be corrected, cesarean delivery may become necessary.

     Note: Amnioinfusion is described in Unit 5, Obstetric Risk Factors: Prior or Current Pregnancy, in this book.
     - Cesarean delivery should be performed for standard obstetric indications.
  2. Term gestation, woman not in labor, no evidence of intra-amniotic infection
     More than 90% of pregnancies greater than 37 weeks of gestation will enter labor spontaneously and deliver within 24 hours of PROM.
     - Evaluate the risk for early-onset neonatal GBS sepsis. (See also Unit 3, Infectious Diseases in Pregnancy, in this book.)
       — *Maternal rectovaginal or urine culture result positive for GBS or a history of having a prior child with early-onset GBS sepsis:* Initiate prophylaxis.
       — *Maternal rectovaginal or urine culture result negative for GBS or NAAT result negative for GBS:* Prophylaxis not indicated.
       — *Maternal GBS status unknown:* Prophylaxis indicated in the presence of maternal intrapartum fever (>38.0°C [>100.4°F]), prolonged ROM (>18 hours), positive NAAT result positive for GBS, or history of GBS colonization in a prior pregnancy.

- Delivery of the fetus
  Management options should be discussed with the patient and family. There are 2 commonly followed approaches for delivery of the fetus: immediate induction of labor or a period of observation while awaiting spontaneous onset of labor.
  a. Immediate induction of labor
     This approach has a lower risk for intra-amniotic infection but may be associated with an increased risk for unsuccessful induction of labor, cesarean delivery, and operative vaginal delivery (forceps or vacuum extraction).
  b. Observation until spontaneous labor begins
     Observation carries a higher risk for intra-amniotic infection but is associated with a lower risk for surgical delivery. Generally, it is not advisable to wait longer than 24 to 72 hours for spontaneous labor to begin, owing to increasing risks of intra-amniotic infection. If labor does not begin spontaneously within this observation period, consider labor induction. This approach is associated with an increased rate of infections in women who are carriers of GBS.

     Continuous fetal heart rate and uterine contraction monitoring are recommended whenever contractions are being induced or augmented with medication. Intermittent auscultation of the fetal heart rate may be appropriate if contractions begin spontaneously and the woman does not have additional risk factors. Internal monitoring should only be used as clinically indicated. If the progression of labor is inadequate, augment uterine contractions with oxytocin as clinically indicated. Minimize digital pelvic examinations, but examine the woman frequently enough to verify the progression of labor. Continue to evaluate the woman and the fetus for evidence of intra-amniotic infection, and initiate induction of labor if infection is diagnosed.
- Consider amnioinfusion if persistent variable decelerations occur. Amnioinfusion may provide sufficient intra-amniotic fluid to relieve cord compression. If variable decelerations cannot be corrected, cesarean delivery may become necessary.

  Note: Amnioinfusion is described in Unit 5, Obstetric Risk Factors: Prior or Current Pregnancy, in this book.
- Cesarean delivery should be performed for standard obstetric indications.

B. Preterm fetus

 Consultation with maternal-fetal medicine specialists is recommended, especially when the pregnancy is extremely preterm or previable.

1. Preterm gestation, $23^{0/7}$ to $36^{6/7}$ weeks of gestation, woman **in labor**, no evidence of intra-amniotic infection
   a. Antibiotics
      In the absence of intra-amniotic infection, antibiotics other than for possible GBS prophylaxis are not recommended.
   b. Evaluate the risk for early-onset neonatal GBS sepsis
      Risk assessment for early-onset neonatal GBS is recommended if the woman is at $24^{0/7}$ to $36^{6/7}$ weeks of gestation. Antibiotics for GBS prophylaxis may be

considered as early as $23^{0/7}$ weeks of gestation, based on local standards and after appropriate counseling. (See Unit 9, Preterm Labor, in this book.)
(See also Unit 3, Infectious Diseases in Pregnancy, in this book.)
— *Maternal rectovaginal or urine culture result positive for GBS or a history of having a prior child with early-onset GBS sepsis:* Initiate prophylaxis.
— *Maternal rectovaginal or urine culture result negative for GBS or NAAT result negative for GBS:* Prophylaxis not indicated.
— *Maternal GBS status unknown:* Prophylaxis *indicated due to preterm gestational age*

c. Tocolysis
If the woman is at $24^{0/7}$ to $33^{6/7}$ weeks of gestation, tocolysis is recommended if there is an indication for antenatal corticosteroids or neuroprotection. Tocolysis may be considered as early as $23^{0/7}$ weeks of gestation, based on local standards and after appropriate counseling. Tocolysis should be continued only as long as necessary to complete the course of antenatal steroids or magnesium sulfate for neuroprotection (see Unit 9, Preterm Labor, in this book).

d. Antenatal corticosteroids (See Unit 9, Preterm Labor, in this book.)
The benefits of antenatal corticosteroids include reducing neonatal risks of respiratory distress syndrome, intraventricular hemorrhage, necrotizing enterocolitis, and death. When a pregnant woman presents in labor with PROM between $24^{0/7}$ and $36^{6/7}$ weeks of gestation with no evidence of intra-amniotic infection, the appropriateness of administering antenatal corticosteroids should be considered. All patients in this gestational age range who have not previously received corticosteroids should receive a first dose, even if it is thought that delivery will likely occur before the second dose is given. A partial course of corticosteroids can improve neonatal outcomes.

Administration of corticosteroids as early as $23^{0/7}$ weeks of gestation may be considered after appropriate counseling. In some centers, administration of corticosteroids before 23 weeks is considered an option. The decision to administer corticosteroids before $24^{0/7}$ weeks is best undertaken at a regional perinatal center, where the patient and her family can receive detailed counseling about risks and benefits from maternal-fetal medicine and neonatology specialists.

The role of a second course of corticosteroids is controversial but may be considered in patients in labor before $34^{0/7}$ weeks of gestation, if at least 7 days have passed since the first course. A second course is not recommended after $34^{0/7}$ weeks.

e. Neuroprotection
Magnesium sulfate is currently recommended for neuroprotection during anticipated delivery from 24 to 32 weeks of gestation. Magnesium sulfate may be considered as early as 23 weeks of gestation after appropriate counseling (see Unit 9, Preterm Labor, in this book).

f. Delivery of the fetus
Continuous fetal heart rate and uterine contraction monitoring is recommended. Use internal monitoring only as clinically indicated. If the progression of labor is inadequate, augment uterine contractions with oxytocin as clinically indicated. Minimize digital pelvic examinations, but examine the woman frequently enough to verify progression of labor. Continue to evaluate the woman and the fetus for evidence of intra-amniotic infection.

- Consider amnioinfusion if persistent variable decelerations occur. Amnioinfusion may provide sufficient intra-amniotic fluid to relieve cord compression. If variable decelerations cannot be corrected, cesarean delivery may become necessary.

  Note: Amnioinfusion is described in Unit 5, Obstetric Risk Factors: Prior or Current Pregnancy, in this book.

- Cesarean delivery should be performed for standard obstetric indications.

2. Preterm gestation, $23^{0/7}$ to $36^{6/7}$ weeks of gestation, woman **not in labor,** no evidence of infection

    a. Antibiotics

    Prophylactic (latency) antibiotics are recommended from $24^{0/7}$ to $36^{6/7}$ weeks of gestation. Prophylactic antibiotics may be considered as early as $23^{0/7}$ weeks of gestation on the basis of local standards and after appropriate counseling. Even in the absence of labor or clinical evidence of infection, antibiotics given prophylactically have demonstrated several benefits when used for patients with PROM before 35 weeks of gestation, including
    - Significantly prolonging pregnancy
    - Reducing the incidence of
        — Maternal infection (intra-amniotic infection and postpartum endometritis)
        — Neonatal sepsis
        — Neonatal intraventricular hemorrhage

    Evidence supports the use of a single course of the following 7-day antibiotic regimen:
    - Ampicillin, 2 g, administered intravenously every 6 hours and erythromycin, 250 mg, administered intravenously every 8 hours for 48 hours
    followed by
    - Amoxicillin, 250 mg, given orally every 6 hours and erythromycin base, 333 mg, given orally every 6 hours for an additional 5 days

    Azithromycin may be substituted for erythromycin in women with gastrointestinal sensitivity to erythromycin or during times of drug shortages.

    b. Evaluate the risk for early-onset neonatal GBS sepsis

    Risk assessment for early-onset neonatal GBS assessment is recommended if the woman is at $24^{0/7}$ to $36^{6/7}$ weeks of gestation. Antibiotics for GBS prophylaxis may be considered as early as $23^{0/7}$ weeks of gestation, on the basis of local standards and after appropriate counseling.

    If there is concern about labor and delivery, GBS prophylaxis should be managed according to the following:

    — *Maternal rectovaginal or urine culture result positive for GBS or a history of having a prior child with early-onset GBS sepsis:* Initiate prophylaxis.
    — *Maternal rectovaginal or urine culture result negative for GBS or NAAT result negative for GBS:* Prophylaxis not indicated.
    — *Maternal GBS status unknown:* Prophylaxis *indicated, owing to preterm gestational age*

    If the course of prophylactic (latency) antibiotic therapy is completed before the onset of labor, the need for intrapartum antibiotic therapy for prevention of neonatal GBS disease should be reassessed when labor begins.

UNIT 8: PRELABOR RUPTURE OF MEMBRANES AND INTRA-AMNIOTIC INFECTION

c. Tocolysis

The administration of a tocolytic medication will not prevent the onset of labor and is therefore not indicated in women with preterm PROM who are not in labor at the time of presentation. If labor begins after preterm PROM has occurred between $24^{0/7}$ weeks and $33^{6/7}$ weeks of gestation and before the woman has received a complete course of antenatal corticosteroids, short-term tocolysis may be initiated. Tocolysis may be considered as early as $23^{0/7}$ weeks of gestation, on the basis of local standards and after appropriate counseling. (See Unit 9, Preterm Labor, in this book.)

d. Antenatal corticosteroids (See Unit 9, Preterm Labor, in this book.)

When there is PROM with no evidence of intra-amniotic infection or labor, a single course of antenatal corticosteroid therapy is recommended for patients at $24^{0/7}$ to $33^{6/7}$ weeks of gestation. Administration of corticosteroids as early as $23^{0/7}$ weeks of gestation may be considered after appropriate counseling. The benefits of antenatal corticosteroids include reducing neonatal risks of respiratory distress syndrome, intraventricular hemorrhage, necrotizing enterocolitis, and death. A recent study demonstrated neonatal benefit from a single first course of antenatal steroids for women with PROM from $34^{0/7}$ to $36^{6/7}$ weeks of gestation who have no evidence of intra-amniotic infection. A repeat course of steroids is not recommended from $34^{0/7}$ to $36^{6/7}$ weeks of gestation if the woman had received a prior course of steroids in the pregnancy.

e. Neuroprotection

Magnesium sulfate for neuroprotection may be initiated if labor begins after preterm PROM at gestational ages less than $32^{0/7}$ weeks. (See Unit 9, Preterm Labor, in this book.)

f. Expectant management and delivery options

Management of women with PROM from $23^{0/7}$ to $36^{6/7}$ weeks of gestation depends on the current gestational age and the gestational age at the time of PROM. Consultation with maternal-fetal medicine specialists for the care of the woman and fetus is strongly recommended, particularly if the fetus is extremely preterm. The onset of labor may occur at any time and is likely to progress rapidly, so transfer for continued inpatient observation and delivery at a regional perinatal center should be considered for preterm pregnant women.

Note: The optimal management of preterm PROM when a *cervical cerclage* is in place has not yet been established.

The following options, including the associated risks and benefits, should be reviewed with the pregnant woman.

- *Expectant management (prolonged hospitalization):* If the gestational age is between $23^{0/7}$ and $33^{6/7}$ weeks, hospitalization with frequent reassessment of maternal and fetal condition may be required for weeks or months. Women with preterm PROM should receive fetal surveillance. While a daily nonstress test or daily biophysical profile testing is typically used to assess fetal status, the optimal testing scheme and frequency of testing is not known. Any abnormal test results, however, should prompt further investigation. Delivery is recommended when the pregnant woman reaches $34^{0/7}$ weeks of gestation to as late as $37^{0/7}$ weeks.

- *Labor induction:* Labor induction is recommended when preterm PROM occurs from $34^{0/7}$ to $36^{6/7}$ weeks of gestation. Antenatal steroids may be considered as noted earlier, but tocolysis and magnesium sulfate for neuroprotection are not indicated. It is not recommended to delay delivery for completion of the antenatal steroids.

  For labor induction, continuous fetal heart rate and uterine contraction monitoring is recommended. Internal monitoring should only be used as clinically indicated. If the progression of labor is inadequate, augment uterine contractions with oxytocin as clinically indicated. Minimize digital pelvic examinations, but examine the woman frequently enough to verify progression of labor. Continue to evaluate the woman and the fetus for evidence of intra-amniotic infection.

  Consider amnioinfusion if persistent variable decelerations occur. Amnioinfusion may provide sufficient intra-amniotic fluid to relieve cord compression. If variable decelerations cannot be corrected, cesarean delivery may become necessary.

  Note: Amnioinfusion is described in Unit 5, Obstetric Risk Factors: Prior or Current Pregnancy, in this book.

  Cesarean delivery should be performed for standard obstetric indications. There is limited evidence to indicate that cesarean delivery for fetal indications before $24^{0/7}$ weeks of gestation improves neonatal outcomes.

3. Preterm gestation, fetus less than $22^{0/7}$ weeks of gestation, woman **in labor**, no evidence of intra-amniotic infection
   Women with PROM and labor prior to $22^{0/7}$ weeks of gestation are expectantly managed. There is no indication for tocolysis, antibiotics, antenatal steroids, or neuroprotection for these patients. In this case, the pregnant woman should be counseled that the newborn is not expected to survive.

4. Preterm gestation, fetus less than $22^{0/7}$ weeks of gestation, woman **not in labor**, no evidence of infection
   Optimal management of PROM prior to $22^{0/7}$ weeks of gestation has not been established. Delivery *prior* to 22 to 23 weeks' gestation is associated with high neonatal mortality, but some pregnant women can be expectantly managed to achieve a gestational age at which intact newborn survival is more likely. In many cases, early PROM results in pulmonary hypoplasia and musculoskeletal abnormalities that can be life-limiting or fatal to the newborn. Consultation with a maternal-fetal medicine specialist is recommended for the management of these patients.
   a. Antibiotics
      There is no recommendation for prophylactic (latency) antibiotics prior to $23^{0/7}$ weeks of gestation, due to insufficient data or no evidence of improved or worse obstetric outcomes. However, prophylactic (latency) antibiotics may be administered prior to $23^{0/7}$ weeks of gestation, after appropriate counseling, especially if resuscitation of the newborn is planned. If prophylactic (latency) antibiotics have not been given, and the pregnant woman reaches 23 to 24 weeks of gestation, prophylactic (latency) antibiotics should be recommended at that time.
   b. Evaluate the risk for early-onset neonatal GBS sepsis
      Although GBS cultures may be collected, GBS prophylaxis is not recommended for the pregnant woman prior to $23^{0/7}$ weeks of gestation.
   c. Tocolysis
      Tocolysis is not recommended prior to $23^{0/7}$ weeks of gestation for the pregnant woman with PROM.

UNIT 8: PRELABOR RUPTURE OF MEMBRANES AND INTRA-AMNIOTIC INFECTION

d. Antenatal corticosteroids (see Unit 9, Preterm Labor, in this book)
Antenatal corticosteroids are not recommended prior to $23^{0/7}$ weeks of gestation. If, after appropriate counseling, a family has decided that they wish for an attempt at resuscitation to be made for a baby at $22^{0/7}$ weeks' gestation or older, then antenatal corticosteroids may be considered appropriate.

e. Neuroprotection
Magnesium sulfate for neuroprotection is not recommended prior to $23^{0/7}$ weeks of gestation. If, after appropriate counseling, a family has decided that they wish for an attempt at resuscitation to be made for a baby at $22^{0/7}$ weeks' gestation or older, then magnesium for neuroprotection during labor may be considered appropriate.

f. Expectant management and delivery options
Consultation with a maternal-fetal medicine specialist is recommended for women with PROM prior to $22^{0/7}$ weeks of gestation. The options of delivery and expectant management, including the associated risks and benefits, should be reviewed with the pregnant woman.

- *Delivery:* Delivery of the fetus by labor induction or a surgical procedure (dilation and extraction) may be considered for pregnant women with early PROM before 20 weeks, owing to ongoing maternal pregnancy risks combined with the high risk of newborn morbidity and mortality. Induction of labor is appropriate for most women and is accomplished by using oxytocin or prostaglandins (misoprostol or dinoprostone), with or without cervical ripening. Transcervical surgical extraction of the fetus from the uterus requires special training; consultation with physicians trained in the procedure is recommended. Hysterotomy (cesarean delivery) is performed only for maternal indications.

  For labor induction, fetal heart rate monitoring is not performed. Uterine contraction monitoring may be performed as clinically appropriate. Minimize digital pelvic examinations, but examine the woman frequently enough to verify progression of labor. Continue to evaluate the woman and the fetus for evidence of intra-amniotic infection and treat with antibiotics as clinically indicated. Amnioinfusion is not indicated.

- *Expectant management:* In the absence of bleeding, labor, and intra-amniotic infection, inpatient hospitalization is not necessary but may be considered for women with PROM prior to $22^{0/7}$ weeks of gestation. At a minimum, a brief hospitalization may be required to assess the pregnant woman to verify that she remains stable. In the outpatient setting, frequent outpatient visits are recommended to assess the woman for signs and symptoms of intra-amniotic infection and for fetal viability. While an outpatient, the pregnant woman should monitor her temperature at least once or twice per day and immediately report any symptoms that are concerning for infection. Once the pregnant woman reaches 22 to 24 weeks of gestation, hospitalization is recommended, at which time antenatal steroids should be administered. The woman may require a prolonged hospitalization for weeks or months. Delivery due to PROM is recommended at or after 34 weeks of gestation.

Note: The optimal management of preterm PROM when a *cervical cerclage* is in place has not yet been established. Consultation with a maternal-fetal medicine specialist is recommended.

The management recommendations for preterm PROM are summarized in Table 8.1.

Table 8.1. Management of Preterm Prelabor Rupture of Membranes

Variable	<22 wk[a]	22^0/7 to 23^6/7 wk[a]	24^0/7 to 31^6/7 wk[a]	32^0/7 to 33^6/7 wk	34^0/7 to 36^6/7 wk	≥37^0/7 wk
Delivery plan	Expectant vs IOL[a]	Expectant	Expectant	Expectant	Delivery / IOL	Delivery / IOL
GBS prophylaxis	No[a,b]	Evaluate and treat[c]	Evaluate and treat[c]	Evaluate and treat[c]	Evaluate and treat[c]	Evaluate and treat[c]
Antenatal steroids	Situational[a,b]	Consider; consultation advised[a]	Yes; consult for repeat course[a]	Yes; consult for repeat course[a]	Yes; repeat courses NOT advised[d]	No
Tocolysis	No[a,b]	Yes (during steroid course or transport)	Yes (during steroid course or transport)	Yes (during steroid course or transport)	No	No
Latency antibiotics	Consider if ≥20 wk[a,b]	Yes	Yes	Yes	No	No
Magnesium for neuroprotection	Situational[a,b]	Yes	Yes	No	No	No

Abbreviations: GBS, group B streptococcus; IOL, induction of labor.

[a] Consultation is recommended with maternal-fetal medicine and/or neonatology specialists regarding plans for newborn resuscitation, antenatal steroids, repeat steroid courses, and/or magnesium for neuroprotection.

[b] Not recommended before viability.

[c] GBS prophylaxis should be provided on the basis of standard protocols. If gestational age is <34 weeks and there is no evidence of labor, perform rectovaginal GBS cultures if no culture has been conducted within the past 4 to 5 weeks. At any gestational age, if there is labor or concern about labor, GBS prophylaxis is indicated (1) when there are positive maternal rectovaginal or urine GBS culture results (or positive nucleic acid amplification test results); (2) when there is a history of having a prior child with early-onset GBS sepsis; or (c) if GBS status is unknown, there are additional risk factors, such as rupture of membranes > 18 hours, maternal intrapartum fever, or gestational age less than 37 weeks. See Unit 3, Infectious Diseases in Pregnancy, in this book for complete GBS prophylaxis recommendations.

[d] A single steroid course is recommended only if the pregnant woman has not received any prior antenatal corticosteroids in the pregnancy. Delivery should not be delayed to await completion of the steroid course.

8. What postdelivery care should be provided for women with PROM or intra-amniotic infection?

A. Maternal care
   1. PROM without clear evidence of intra-amniotic infection
   Continue to observe the woman for evidence of infection. Endometritis, if untreated, can progress to life-threatening maternal sepsis (see Unit 3, Infectious Diseases in Pregnancy, in this book).

   If antibiotics were started during labor but there is no evidence of infection, antibiotic therapy may be stopped at or shortly after delivery.

   2. Suspected or proven intra-amniotic infection (with or without PROM)
   Current postdelivery recommendations for women with intra-amniotic infection are to discontinue antibiotics at the time of vaginal delivery. If a cesarean delivery is performed, one additional dose of the selected antibiotic regimen is provided after delivery. If a primary antibiotic regimen was chosen and a cesarean delivery is performed, then at least one 900-mg dose of clindamycin administered intravenously is recommended after delivery. Continued antibiotic therapy beyond this point should be individualized on the basis of ongoing maternal fever or other objective evidence of infection.

B. Neonatal care
   Prolonged ROM is defined as ROM for 18 hours or longer. Prolonged ROM can occur with or without PROM. Sometimes membranes rupture after the start of labor, but a lengthy labor then creates the situation of prolonged ROM by the time the baby is born.

   Prelabor or prolonged ROM increases the risk for neonatal sepsis. Although many babies do not become sick, some can become infected and gravely ill, even when there is no evidence of maternal infection. Even if a woman does not appear to be ill, a complete obstetric history should be conveyed promptly to neonatal care practitioners.

   Neonatal management after prelabor or prolonged ROM requires consideration of several factors, including obstetric history, gestational age, the woman's intrapartum treatment and current clinical condition, and the baby's clinical condition. This issue is addressed in Book 3: Neonatal Care, Unit 8, Infections.

Self-test B

Now answer these questions to test yourself on the information in the last section.

B1. Rupture of membranes occurs in a pregnancy at 29 weeks of gestation. There is no evidence of infection or preterm labor. Which of the following actions should be taken?

Yes	No	
____	____	Conduct urinalysis
____	____	Check maternal vital signs
____	____	Administer corticosteroids
____	____	Consider transfer to a regional perinatal center
____	____	Begin antibiotics

B2. A 28-year-old woman pregnant with her third baby presents with prelabor rupture of membranes and a temperature of 39.0°C (102.2°F) at 36 weeks of gestation. Her uterus is very tender, but labor has not started and there have been no other pregnancy complications. What should you do?

Yes	No	
____	____	Obtain specimens to test for group B β-hemolytic streptococcus, gonorrhea, and chlamydia
____	____	Begin intravenous broad-spectrum antibiotics
____	____	Obtain a complete blood cell count with differential
____	____	Notify pediatrics staff of maternal condition
____	____	Perform cesarean delivery
____	____	Begin oxytocin induction of labor

B3. List at least 4 signs of intra-amniotic infection (chorioamnionitis).

_____
_____
_____
_____

B4. In which of the following situations might it be appropriate to use amniocentesis with instillation of dye into the amniotic cavity to confirm suspected rupture of membranes?

Yes	No	
____	____	32 weeks of gestation with no evidence of infection
____	____	40 weeks of gestation with maternal fever and fetal tachycardia
____	____	30 weeks of gestation with uterine tenderness and a fetal biophysical score of 4
____	____	38 weeks of gestation with maternal hypertension

B5. Prelabor rupture of membranes occurred in a pregnancy at 39 weeks of gestation. Membranes ruptured 8 hours earlier, but labor has not yet started. There is no evidence of infection. The fetus has a cephalic presentation. Which of the following actions are appropriate?

Yes	No	
____	____	Begin induction of labor
____	____	Observe; begin induction if labor does not start spontaneously in 24 to 72 hours
____	____	Perform a cesarean delivery

B6. **True** **False** With an intra-amniotic infection, the specific infectious organism and length of time until delivery are the key factors in determining the severity of maternal illness.

Check your answers with the list that follows the Recommended Routines. Correct any incorrect answers and review the appropriate section in the unit.

UNIT 8: PRELABOR RUPTURE OF MEMBRANES AND INTRA-AMNIOTIC INFECTION

PRELABOR RUPTURE OF MEMBRANES AND INTRA-AMNIOTIC INFECTION

Recommended Routines

All the routines listed below are based on the principles of perinatal care presented in the unit you have just finished. They are recommended as part of routine perinatal care.

Read each routine carefully and decide whether it is standard operating procedure in your hospital. Check the appropriate blank next to each routine.

Procedure Standard in My Hospital	Needs Discussion by Our Staff	Recommended Routine
_____	_____	1. Establish a system for consultation and referral of women with preterm, prelabor rupture of membranes.
_____	_____	2. Establish a system to notify nursery personnel of women whose babies are at risk for infection, including women • With evidence of intra-amniotic infection • Who received antibiotics during labor and the indication for their treatment • With prelabor rupture of membranes • With prolonged rupture of membranes

_____	_____	3. Establish a protocol for the care of all women with prelabor rupture of membranes that includes
		• Evaluation for umbilical cord prolapse and compression
		• Evaluation for infection
		• Minimization of digital cervical examinations
		  — None for women not in labor or not expected to have immediate induction of labor
		  — As few as necessary for women in labor
		• As appropriate, administration of
		  — Antibiotics
		  — Corticosteroids
		  — Magnesium sulfate for neuroprotection

Self-test Answers

These are the answers to the Self-test questions. Please check them with the answers you gave and review the information in the unit wherever necessary.

Self-test A

A1. True

A2. True

A3. True

A4. True

A5. True

A6. True

A7. True

A8. False *Reason:* Fetal lung maturity testing is not recommended for management of patients with prelabor rupture of membranes (PROM).

A9. Any 3 of the following complications:
- Infection (intra-amniotic infection, maternal sepsis, puerperal endometritis, fetal or neonatal sepsis)
- Preterm birth
- Prolapsed umbilical cord
- Umbilical cord compression
- Oligohydramnios
- Placental abruption
- Fetal death

A10. The main risk associated with PROM is maternal or neonatal *infection*.

A11. High in the vagina

Self-test B

B1.
Yes	No	
X	___	Conduct urinalysis
X	___	Check maternal vital signs
X	___	Administer corticosteroids
X	___	Consider transfer to a regional perinatal center
X	___	Begin antibiotics

B2.
Yes	No	
X	___	Obtain specimens to test for group B β-hemolytic streptococcus, gonorrhea, and chlamydia
X	___	Begin intravenous broad-spectrum antibiotics
X	___	Obtain a complete blood cell count with differential
X	___	Notify pediatrics staff of maternal condition
___	X	Perform cesarean delivery
X	___	Begin oxytocin induction of labor

B3. Any 4 of the following signs:
- Maternal fever of 39.0°C (102.2°F) or higher on one occasion
- Maternal fever of 38.0°C (100.4°F) to 38.9°C (102°F) for 30 minutes or longer
- Increased white blood cell count
- Uterine tenderness
- Cloudy or foul-smelling amniotic fluid
- Maternal malaise
- Fetal tachycardia
- Biophysical profile score of 6 or lower

B4.
Yes	No	
X		32 weeks of gestation with no evidence of infection (If all other means to determine whether the membranes are ruptured are inconclusive, and knowing that is essential to clinical decision-making, an amniocentesis and dye test is likely to be helpful to determine whether membranes are ruptured and to show the presence or absence of bacteria in the amniotic fluid. Consultation with or referral to a regional perinatal center is recommended.)
	X	40 weeks of gestation with maternal fever and fetal tachycardia (A term newborn with findings suggestive of infection; induction of labor is indicated; a dye test is unlikely to add useful information because the baby needs to be delivered; assess fetal well-being and consider consultation with a regional perinatal center.)
	X	30 weeks of gestation with uterine tenderness and a fetal biophysical score of 4 (Evidence of an ill fetus and infection; delivery is needed; amniocentesis with a dye test is an invasive procedure unlikely to add useful information in this situation; consultation with or referral to a regional perinatal center is recommended.)
	X	38 weeks of gestation with maternal hypertension (Term fetus; dye test is unlikely to add useful information in this situation; assess fetal well-being and consider consultation with a regional perinatal center. If adequate amniotic fluid cannot be obtained with a sterile speculum examination, amniocentesis may be appropriate to collect fluid for culture and sensitivities and Gram stain.)

B5.
Yes	No	
X		Begin induction of labor
X		Observe; begin induction if labor does not start spontaneously in 24 to 72 hours
	X	Perform a cesarean delivery

B6. True

Unit 8 Posttest

After completion of each unit there is a free online posttest available at www.cmevillage.com to test your understanding. Navigate to the PCEP pages on www.cmevillage.com and register to take the free posttests.

Once registered on the website and after completing all the unit posttests, pay the book exam fee ($15) and pass the test at 80% or greater to earn continuing education credits. Only start the PCEP book exam if you have time to complete it. If you take the book exam and are not connected to a printer, either print your certificate to a .pdf file and save it to print later or come back to www.cmevillage.com at any time and print a copy of your educational transcript.

Credits are only available by book, not by individual unit within the books. Available credits for completion of each book exam are as follows: Book 1: 14.5 credits; Book 2: 16 credits; Book 3: 17 credits; Book 4: 9 credits.

For more details, navigate to the PCEP webpages at www.cmevillage.com.

UNIT 8: PRELABOR RUPTURE OF MEMBRANES AND INTRA-AMNIOTIC INFECTION

SKILL UNIT

Sterile Speculum Examination

This skill unit will teach you how to perform a sterile speculum examination. *Not everyone* will be required to learn and practice this skill. *All staff members,* however, should read this unit and attend a skill session to learn the equipment needed and the sequence of steps to be able to assist with a sterile speculum examination.

Study this skill unit, and then attend a skill demonstration and practice session. To master the skill, you will need to demonstrate correctly each of the steps listed below. You may be asked to demonstrate your proficiency with a mannequin or a patient (who requires the procedure).

1. Explain the procedure and be able to answer questions a pregnant woman might ask about the examination (in particular, why it is needed, what is involved, and how she can help during the examination).
2. Collect and prepare the equipment, including supplies for anticipated tests.
3. Position the woman for the examination.
4. Insert a sterile speculum.
5. Position the speculum so the cervix is clearly visible.
6. Withdraw the speculum and complete the examination.
7. Describe your findings accurately and completely for color, consistency, and odor of fluid; leakage of fluid; cervical dilation and effacement; and any other pertinent findings.

PERINATAL PERFORMANCE GUIDE

Sterile Speculum Examination

ACTIONS	REMARKS
Deciding When to Use a Sterile Speculum Examination	
1. What are the indications for an examination? • Is there doubt as to whether the membranes are ruptured? • Do cervical or vaginal samples need to be obtained for culture (whether or not the membranes are ruptured)? • Is visual inspection for a prolapsed umbilical cord or cervical dilation and effacement needed? **Yes:** Perform a sterile speculum examination if the answer is "yes" to any of these questions. **No:** A sterile speculum examination may not be needed.	These are the common indications for a sterile speculum examination. A sterile speculum examination may be indicated for other reasons in individual clinical situations. A sterile speculum examination, rather than a digital examination, is preferable whenever there is an increased risk of intra-amniotic infection. If labor is not present, *only* sterile speculum examination(s) should be used until a decision about whether to proceed with delivery has been made.

Preparing the Woman for the Examination

2. Talk to the woman about the examination.
   - Explain the procedure.
     — Why it is needed
     — What is involved
     — What she can do to help during the examination
   - Ask the woman to empty her bladder.

This is an intrusive procedure. Understanding the purpose of the examination and how it will be performed may help a woman to relax and cooperate more fully during the procedure.

The examination is easier to perform and is more comfortable when the woman's bladder is empty.

Collecting and Preparing the Equipment

3. Collect the necessary equipment.
   - Sterile speculum
   - Sterile gloves
   - Moveable, adjustable lamp
   - Stool for the examiner to sit on

   - Equipment for anticipated tests (gonorrhea, chlamydia, and group B β-hemolytic streptococcus); Nitrazine paper; containers for specimens to test amniotic fluid proteins as appropriate

Select the size and type of speculum according to the woman's history. A Pederson speculum (flatter and more narrow blades) may be more comfortable for primigravidae and very tense women than the more common Graves speculum, which has wider blades and comes in 2 sizes (standard and large).

Check to be sure you know the specific specimen containers needed for these tests in your hospital.

4. Set up a sterile tray. Open the packages of sterile supplies onto the tray.

Take care to maintain strict aseptic technique.

5. Position the tray so it is within easy reach of where the examiner will be sitting on the stool at the end of the examining table.

Be sure the tray and equipment are protected from contamination while you position the woman.

Positioning the Woman

6. Ask the woman to remove the clothes below her waist and then to lie on the examining table with
   - A pillow under her head
   - Her legs in stirrups before you begin the examination
   - Her arms at her sides or across her abdomen or chest

Be sure she is as comfortable as possible.

Abdominal muscles are more likely to be tense when a woman puts her arms and hands above or behind her head.

7. Drape the woman's legs with a sheet so her knees are covered but the pubic area is exposed.

Be sure you will be able to see her face when you are seated on the stool.

UNIT 8: PRELABOR RUPTURE OF MEMBRANES AND INTRA-AMNIOTIC INFECTION

Positioning the Woman (continued)

8. Position the lamp so the perineum and the anticipated visual field will be well lit, once the speculum is positioned properly.

   Be sure the light does not shine directly in the woman's eyes when she is looking toward you at the end of the table.

9. Position the stool so you will be comfortable performing the examination.

10. If the woman is tense, encourage her to use relaxation breathing techniques or slow, deep breathing.

    Relaxed abdominal and perineal muscles make insertion of the speculum easier and more comfortable.

Inserting and Positioning a Sterile Speculum

11. Wash your hands and put on the sterile gloves.

    Talk with the woman and help her relax.

12. Sit comfortably on the stool and ask the woman to open her legs.

    Cleansing the perineum is not necessary, and antiseptics such as povidone-iodine can interfere with test results.

13. Touch the inside of the woman's leg with the *back* of the hand *not* holding the speculum before you touch the perineum.

    This helps to avoid startling the woman when you touch the more sensitive perineum.

14. With this same hand, place your index and middle finger on either side of the vaginal opening. Exert gentle downward pressure with your fingers and spread the opening slightly.

15. With the other hand (the hand holding the speculum), tip the speculum slightly to one side and keep the blades closed as you pass them over your spread fingers and into the vagina.

    Turning the speculum blades 45° off midline prevents the urethra from getting pinched.

    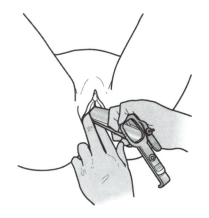

    Avoid use of lubricants. Antiseptics and lubricants can cause test results to be inaccurate. In addition, a lubricant is usually not needed because vaginal secretions or amniotic fluid provide adequate moisture.

    If a patient is very dry and a lubricant seems essential, use only sterile water. When the amount of amniotic fluid is small, however, even water may dilute it enough to provide misleading results.

Inserting and Positioning a Sterile Speculum (continued)

16. Maintain a slight downward pressure until the blades are fully inserted into the vagina.

    Take care to ensure that no tissue is caught between the blades as they are being inserted.

    Downward pressure will prevent pressing on the sensitive urethra.

    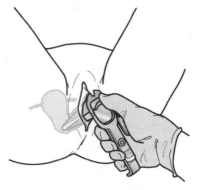

17. After the blades are fully inserted, remove your fingers from the vaginal opening, rotate the handle so it is vertical, and lift the tip of the blades to a more horizontal position.

    Let the woman know what you are doing and that she may feel some pressure.

18. Use the thumb piece on the speculum to open the blades and look for the cervix.

    Beware: **Prelabor rupture of membranes—especially preterm, prelabor rupture of membranes—carries an increased risk for umbilical cord prolapse. If the cord is seen, withdraw the speculum carefully and proceed to management of a prolapsed cord.**

    If you cannot see the cervix, reposition the speculum more anteriorly, posteriorly, or laterally until the cervix is completely in view.

    Tell the woman she may feel more pressure as the blades are opened and positioned.

    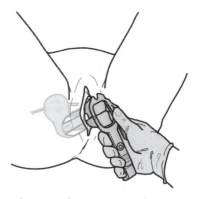

19. Once the cervix is clearly in view, tighten the thumbscrew to hold the blades open to that position.

    When the speculum is properly positioned, the cervix will be between the upper and lower blades.

UNIT 8: PRELABOR RUPTURE OF MEMBRANES AND INTRA-AMNIOTIC INFECTION

Obtaining Information From the Examination

20. Look at the cervix and determine if any fluid is leaking through it. If fluid is leaking, assess its color, consistency, and odor.

    - Is the fluid clear or very pale yellow?

      Second-trimester amniotic fluid is pale yellow, similar to the color of dilute urine. Near term, the fluid becomes less yellow and has vernix floating in it.

    - Is the fluid dark yellow?

      This indicates passage of meconium sometime in the past.

    - Is the fluid dark greenish brown and thick?

      This indicates recent passage of meconium.

    - Is the fluid bloody? If it is bloody, is the blood bright red or dark red? What is the volume of blood?

      A small amount of blood might be from normal bloody show late in labor. It might also be due to one of the causes of obstetric hemorrhage. There is an increased risk of placental abruption with prelabor rupture of membranes.

    - Is there a foul odor?

      Normal amniotic fluid has an odor, but it is not unpleasant. A foul odor suggests infection.

21. Look at the cervix and determine if there is any evidence of dilation or effacement.

22. Obtain specimens for testing (see Skill Unit: Tests for Suspected or Proven Rupture of Membranes).

23. When you have completed visual inspection of the cervix and collection of test samples, begin to withdraw the speculum.

    Having an assistant nearby will make specimen collection and proper handling of the specimens easier.

    - Release the thumbscrew but continue to hold the blades open.
    - Hold the blades open until the cervix is no longer visible between the upper and lower blades.
    - Allow the blades to close as the speculum is being withdrawn, so that they close completely just before reaching the vaginal opening.

24. If appropriate, obtain additional specimens from the lower blade (see Skill Unit: Tests for Suspected or Proven Rupture of Membranes).

Removing the Speculum and Completing the Examination

25. Remember, once the sterile speculum has been inserted, it is contaminated by body fluids and should be handled accordingly.

26. Wipe any fluid from the perineum and help the woman assume a more comfortable position.

27. Finish preparation of the collected specimens (see Skill Unit: Tests for Suspected or Proven Rupture of Membranes).

28. Record
    - Observations made
        — Absence or presence (and degree) of cervical dilation and effacement.
        — Absence or presence of leakage of fluid.
        — If leakage present, note color, consistency, and odor of fluid
    - Specimens obtained
        — Those sent for laboratory analysis
            ■ Those with results available at the bedside

Proceed to additional evaluation of maternal condition or fetal well-being, as warranted by your findings.

UNIT 8: PRELABOR RUPTURE OF MEMBRANES AND INTRA-AMNIOTIC INFECTION

SKILL UNIT

Tests for Suspected or Proven Rupture of Membranes

This skill unit will teach you how to obtain test specimens during a sterile speculum examination. *Not everyone* will be required to learn and practice this skill. *All staff members*, however, should read this unit and attend a skill session to learn the equipment needed for each test and the sequence of steps to be able to assist with collection and correct handling of the specimens.

Study this skill unit, and then attend a skill demonstration and practice session. To master the skills, you will need to demonstrate correctly each of the steps listed below. You may be asked to demonstrate your proficiency with a mannequin or a patient (who requires the test[s]), at the same time that you perform a sterile speculum examination.

pH Test (also known as *phenaphthazine or Nitrazine paper test*)
1. Moisten the test device with fluid in the vagina.
2. Interpret the results.
3. Identify possible causes for inaccurate results.

Amniotic Protein Assays
Several commercially available tests are available for ruptured membranes. The procedure for performing these tests is described in the package insert. Specimen collection generally does not require a speculum examination but may be completed during a speculum examination.

Tests for Gonorrhea, Chlamydia, and Group B β-Hemolytic Streptococcus
1. Collect the correct specimen containers.
2. Obtain specimens.
3. Prepare the specimens for laboratory analysis.

PERINATAL PERFORMANCE GUIDE

pH Test

ACTIONS	REMARKS
Deciding When to Obtain a pH Test	
1. Is rupture of membranes suspected but not confirmed? Yes: A pH test can help confirm or rule out rupture of membranes but cannot provide a definitive diagnosis. No: There is no reason to perform a pH test.	When moistened with a fluid, Nitrazine paper changes color in response to the fluid pH level. Different colors indicate different pH values. Results are unreliable when blood, mucus, semen, and certain vaginal infections are present, which have pH values close to that of amniotic fluid. Contamination with urine may also result in inaccurate results.
2. Is it appropriate to perform a sterile speculum or digital pelvic examination? Yes: Perform a pH test. No: Wait to conduct the test until an examination is done.	Nitrazine paper can be used during a sterile speculum examination or a digital examination, although there is greater risk of contamination and false values when it is tested as part of a digital examination.
Performing the Test During a Sterile Speculum Examination	
3. Collect the equipment and prepare the patient for a sterile speculum examination.	In addition to the equipment needed for a sterile speculum examination, you will need a piece of Nitrazine paper.
4. During a sterile speculum examination, fluid may be applied to Nitrazine test paper. • Grip a piece of test paper with sterile forceps, and then dip the paper in fluid that has collected in the posterior fornix. or • Moisten the Nitrazine paper with fluid collected in the hollow area of the lower speculum blade, immediately after the speculum is withdrawn. or • Place a sterile cotton-tipped swab deep in the vagina and moisten it with fluid collected there. Then touch the swab to a piece of Nitrazine paper, making sure the paper is wet thoroughly.	If an assistant is not available, tear a piece from the spool of test paper when you prepare for the examination. The paper is not sterile, so it should not be put on the sterile tray, but it can be placed in a convenient location where you can reach it with sterile forceps that have been placed on the sterile tray. 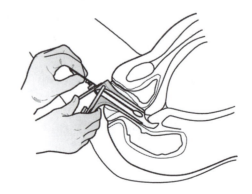

UNIT 8: PRELABOR RUPTURE OF MEMBRANES AND INTRA-AMNIOTIC INFECTION

Interpreting the Test Results

5. Compare the color of the moistened section of Nitrazine paper with the color chart on the Nitrazine paper box.

   The membranes are *probably intact* if the test paper is
   - Yellow, pH = 5.0
   - Olive yellow, pH = 5.5
   - Olive green, pH = 6.0

   The membranes are *probably ruptured* if the test paper is
   - Blue-green, pH = 6.5
   - Blue-gray, pH = 7.0
   - Deep blue, pH = 7.5

6. Record your findings.

   Be sure to note if you suspect there was an inadequate amount of amniotic fluid for accurate results or if contamination with other fluids may have occurred.

What Can Go Wrong?

1. The test paper may be contaminated
   - With other body fluids (eg, blood, mucus, semen)
   - From lubricants or antiseptics used previously

   Results may be falsely positive or falsely negative, depending on the source of the contamination.

2. There may be too little amniotic fluid to obtain an accurate result.

   If you think membranes are ruptured but fluid is not apparent during a sterile speculum examination, ask the woman to cough or bear down. This action usually causes fluid to leak through the cervix if the membranes are ruptured.

3. The Nitrazine paper may be outdated.

   Periodically check the expiration dates on the boxes of paper and discard any that have expired. Make it a habit to check the date again each time you use Nitrazine paper.

4. The Nitrazine paper may have been stored improperly.

   Exposure to light for long periods or to moisture can interfere with the accuracy of the paper.

PERINATAL PERFORMANCE GUIDE
Collecting Specimens for Gonorrhea, Chlamydia, and Group B β-Hemolytic Streptococcus Testing

ACTIONS	REMARKS
Deciding When to Perform These Tests	
1. Consider • Should cultures for group B streptococcus (GBS) and tests for gonorrhea and chlamydia be performed?	Consider cultures for GBS and testing for gonorrhea and chlamydia in all women with prelabor rupture of membranes.
Collecting the Equipment	
2. Collect the necessary equipment. • *Culture:* One sterile culture tube with swab for GBS culture. • *Gonorrhea and chlamydia:* Collect specimen container specific to the test used in your hospital.	Transport media and protocols for specimens vary. Check the requirements of the laboratory in your hospital. Various tests can be used to detect gonorrhea and chlamydia. Learn which one is used in your hospital.
Collecting the Specimens	
3. Group B streptococcus Use the sterile swab to sample the lower vagina and then the rectum, and then place the swab into the transport medium.	The area sampled is important to the accurate determination of the presence or absence of GBS. Omitting the rectal swab will fail to identify some women who carry this harmful bacterium. Clinical management is the same, regardless of the reservoir of GBS, so only one swab is needed.
4. Gonorrhea and chlamydia Use a sterile swab to swab the endocervix or vagina as appropriate in your hospital's testing procedure, and then place the swab in the appropriate transport container or medium.	
5. Label the specimens and send to the appropriate laboratories for culture and analysis.	

Unit 9: Preterm Labor

Objectives **286**

1. What are the risks of preterm labor? 289
2. What are the causes of preterm labor and delivery? 289
3. What interventions can reduce the risk of preterm delivery? 291
4. What should be offered to women known to be at risk for preterm labor? 295
5. How is possible preterm labor evaluated? 296
6. How is preterm labor treated? 302
7. How is preterm delivery managed? 306

Table

    Table 9.1. Tocolytic Medications Commonly Used to Treat Preterm Labor 304

Recommended Routines 310

Objectives

In this unit you will learn

A. The definition of preterm labor

B. The effect preterm birth has on neonatal morbidity and mortality

C. What factors increase the risks for preterm labor

D. What you can do to avoid preterm labor and delivery

E. How to evaluate preterm labor

F. How to treat preterm labor

G. How to manage a preterm delivery

H. What you should anticipate for the care of a preterm baby

Unit 9 Pretest

Before reading the unit, please answer the following questions. Select the *one best* answer to each question (unless otherwise instructed). Record your answers on the test and check them with the answers at the end of the book.

1. **True** **False** Fluid restriction may stop preterm uterine contractions if true labor has not developed.

2. **True** **False** Maternal hyperglycemia (high blood glucose level) is a possible side effect of magnesium sulfate.

3. **True** **False** Cervical cerclage at 12 to 14 weeks of gestation is recommended for women who are known to have cervical insufficiency.

4. **True** **False** The risk of preterm delivery is increased with multifetal gestation.

5. **True** **False** Tocolysis may be appropriate for a woman with intact membranes and preterm labor, even when the cervix is dilated 4 cm or more.

6. **True** **False** Optimal benefits from antenatal steroid administration are achieved when treatment is administered 24 to 48 hours before delivery.

7. Corticosteroids are administered to a pregnant woman to help (select one best answer)
   A. Prevent preterm labor
   B. Mature the fetal lungs when preterm delivery is unavoidable
   C. Treat genital herpes infection
   D. Ripen the cervix when induction of labor is planned

8. In which of the following situations is tocolysis most appropriate? (select one best answer)
   A. Preterm labor at 32 weeks of gestation with worsening maternal preeclampsia
   B. Preterm labor at 32 weeks of gestation with 2-cm cervical dilation and 80% effacement
   C. Preterm labor at 34 weeks of gestation with uterine tenderness and maternal fever
   D. Preterm labor at 36 weeks of gestation with prelabor rupture of membranes

9. Which of the following conditions increase the risk for preterm labor and delivery?

Yes	No	
___	___	Hypertension
___	___	Urinary tract infection
___	___	Cigarette smoking
___	___	Previous cesarean delivery
___	___	Maternal cocaine use
___	___	Uterine malformation

(continued)

Unit 9 Pretest (*continued*)

10. All of the following signs may indicate the onset of preterm labor, except (select one best answer)
    A. Decreased fetal movement
    B. "Ballooning" of the lower uterine segment
    C. Pelvic pressure
    D. Softened, anterior position of the cervix

11. True False When β-mimetic tocolytic medications are used, the maternal heart rate should be maintained above 140 beats per minute.

12. True False One indication to provide tocolysis is to allow time for administration of corticosteroids.

13. True False A negative fetal fibronectin test result indicates that delivery is unlikely to occur within the next 2 weeks.

14. True False Asymptomatic bacteriuria should not be treated in pregnancy.

15. True False Administration of corticosteroids should be considered only when the membranes are intact.

16. True False Vaginal delivery of a 2,000-g (4-lb 6½-oz) preterm fetus in breech presentation carries the same degree of risk to the fetus as a cesarean delivery.

1. What are the risks of preterm labor?

Preterm labor is defined as labor that occurs prior to $37^{0/7}$ weeks of gestation. The most serious threat from preterm labor is the risk of preterm birth. Approximately 10% of babies born in the United States are born preterm. Preterm labor does not necessarily result in preterm delivery. With early recognition, prompt intervention, and aggressive management, it may be possible to stop or delay preterm labor and prolong a pregnancy.

Preterm birth is the most common cause of neonatal morbidity and mortality and costs the U.S. health system more than $25 billion each year. It accounts for approximately 75% of neonatal deaths that are not caused by congenital malformations. Preterm birth is also a leading cause of long-term neurological disabilities in children. Although *most* preterm babies who survive *do not* develop physical or mental impairment, preterm babies are much more likely to have some degree of impairment than are babies born at term. The younger the gestational age at birth, the greater the risk of death or long-term problems. Some problems that a preterm baby may face include breathing problems, feeding difficulties, cerebral palsy, developmental delays, vision problems, and hearing impairment. Preterm births may also cause emotional and economic burdens for families.

In some cases, the cause for preterm labor can be identified, and that factor (eg, maternal medical illness, infection, multifetal gestation) may pose additional risks to the woman, fetus, or neonate. The specific risks posed by conditions are described in other units within this book.

2. What are the causes of preterm labor and delivery?

For most pregnant women who experience preterm labor, a cause for the preterm labor cannot be clearly identified. There are many factors, however, that are known to increase the risk of preterm labor and delivery. These risk factors have an additive effect, and the presence of several risk factors can dramatically increase a pregnant woman's risk of preterm birth. Interventions to reduce or eliminate any of these risk factors may help improve the outcome of a pregnancy.

   A. Maternal medical conditions

      Any serious medical disease increases the risk for preterm delivery either because the risk of spontaneous preterm labor is increased or because preterm delivery may become necessary to preserve maternal or fetal health. The following conditions are among the most likely to be associated with preterm birth:
- Hypertension, chronic or pregnancy related
- Pregestational diabetes mellitus
- Severe anemia
- Hemoglobinopathy
- Systemic lupus erythematosus
- Upper urinary tract infection, symptomatic or asymptomatic
- Substance use (especially cocaine use)

   B. Socioeconomic and lifestyle conditions

      All of the following conditions are associated with an increased risk for preterm labor:
- Maternal age of 18 years or younger or 40 years and older
- Non-Hispanic Black race
- Little or no prenatal care
- Inadequate nutrition, poor weight gain, or low prepregnancy body mass index
- Poverty, poor housing

- Heavy manual labor or very long work hours with extreme fatigue
- Severe emotional stress
- Trauma (fall, motor vehicle accident, domestic violence)
- Maternal smoking

C. Obstetric conditions

Risk factors may be related to obstetric history or to the current pregnancy. Some factors may recur from pregnancy to pregnancy, while others are a threat only in the present pregnancy. In the following lists, factors identified with an asterisk (*) are associated with a particularly high risk for preterm labor. However, only about 20% to 30% of women with any risk factor(s) for preterm labor will actually experience preterm labor. Preterm labor and birth occur in many pregnancies that have no recognizable risk factors. Some risk factors are present only because of events that occurred in a previous pregnancy and therefore cannot be identified during a first pregnancy.

1. Obstetric history
   - Cervical insufficiency
   - Uterine malformations, such as unicornuate or bicornuate uterus
   - Uterine fibroids
   - Spontaneous *second*-trimester miscarriage(s)
   - Multiple first-trimester dilation and curettage procedures
   - Previous preterm delivery*: The risk of preterm labor is *significantly* increased for women who have experienced a previous preterm delivery. The risk increases with the number of previous preterm births and decreases with the number of term births.

2. Current pregnancy
   - Assisted reproduction (in vitro fertilization or other fertility treatments)
   - Uterine overdistension
     — Polyhydramnios
     — Multifetal gestation*: Multifetal gestation occurs in about 1% to 2% of all pregnancies but accounts for about 15% of all preterm births. In the absence of additional risk factors: Singletons, twins, and triplets have approximately 10%, 60%, and 95% risk for preterm birth, respectively.
   - Antepartum obstetric bleeding
   - Short or dilated cervix
   - Intra-amniotic infection*
   - Preterm prelabor rupture of membranes*

Predicting which women will experience preterm labor and preterm birth is very difficult. Care aimed at early recognition of preterm labor and prevention of preterm delivery should be routinely provided to all women.

3. What interventions can reduce the risk of preterm delivery?

A. Educate all patients

All pregnant women should be educated about the signs and symptoms of preterm labor. Women may believe that only painful contractions indicate labor. Cervical dilation can occur even with relatively painless contractions.

The presence of any one of the following findings may indicate preterm labor:
- Abdominal cramping (may feel like gas pains or menstrual cramps)
- Increase in vaginal discharge; onset of watery, mucoid, or bloody discharge
- Low backache, intermittent or constant
- Pelvic pressure, sense of heaviness in the vagina

The earlier an intervention to stop preterm labor is started, the more likely it is to be successful. Any indication of preterm labor should be reported as soon as a woman becomes aware of her symptoms. Pregnant women should be given information about how to contact health professionals and report symptoms, 24 hours a day, 7 days a week.

Instruct all pregnant women in the signs and symptoms of preterm labor.

B. Recognize and address risk factors

A thorough history should be obtained at the first prenatal visit, including a comprehensive review of maternal medical conditions, socioeconomic and lifestyle risk factors, obstetric factors, and, for multigravida pregnancies, any changes since the previous pregnancy.

1. Medical conditions

   Maternal medical conditions and current treatments should be evaluated. In some cases, treatments may need to be modified to alternatives safer for pregnancy. For women with medical conditions during pregnancy, a plan should be created to monitor maternal and fetal health. Consultation with other medical specialists may be appropriate for the pregnant woman.

   The use of illicit and recreational drugs and other substances should be reviewed with *all* patients. Substance use occurs across all socioeconomic boundaries. Substance and drug use includes cigarette smoking, smokeless tobacco products, caffeine, alcohol consumption, and the use of illicit or prescription drugs. For pregnant women with substance use concerns, specialized counseling and treatment programs may be necessary.

2. Socioeconomic and lifestyle risk factors

   Socioeconomic and lifestyle risk factors can be extremely difficult to change. Alleviating any one risk factor, however, may improve pregnancy outcome.
   - *Help ensure compliance with the prenatal visit schedule:* Offer assistance with transportation or child care. Consider arranging appointments to see the same health professional at each visit.

- *Improve nutritional status:* Provide education about diet and normal weight gain and body changes during pregnancy; consider consultation with a registered dietician; offer to help make connections with social services and other community resources that offer food assistance.
- *Improve living conditions:* Assist the patient in connecting with community resources that provide housing assistance.
- *Reduce demanding physical labor or extreme fatigue:* Consider modification of employment activities or living conditions.
- *Modify an abusive situation:* Provide assistance to the woman in locating a support person or group or a safe living environment. Offer referral to legal aid or other assistance or interventions.
- *Relieve extreme emotional stress:* Offer interventions to alleviate the most pressing social, economic, or other problems.

Sometimes, a medical provider identifies a problem of which the patient is unaware. Also, the patient may attempt to communicate a problem that a medical provider does not recognize. Every effort should be made to involve the pregnant woman in decisions that affect her and her fetus. Involvement of the woman in identifying adverse conditions and in planning for change, including what she can do without outside assistance and what outside help she would accept, is essential for change to occur. Appropriate involvement of social services, counselors, educators, and other resources as early as possible can improve the health of the pregnant woman and improve pregnancy outcomes.

3. Obstetric factors
   a. History of a prior preterm birth

   The history of a prior preterm birth is the most reliable predictor of the risk of preterm birth in the current pregnancy. Some early studies involving weekly administration of 17-α-hydroxyprogesterone caproate (17-OHPC, 250-mg intramuscular injection), beginning as early as 16 weeks' gestation, indicated that a pregnant woman's risk for recurrent preterm birth could be reduced in a current pregnancy. However, a more recent, larger international study involving 17-OHPC did not show a benefit of using 17-OHPC for this purpose (*Am J Perinatol.* 2019;37[2]:127–136). It is currently recommended to seek consultation or other expert advice on the use of 17-OHPC for the purpose of recurrent preterm birth risk reduction.

   Indications for pregnant women who may consider the use of 17-OHPC during their current pregnancy include having a prior delivery at less than 37 weeks of gestation as a result of spontaneous preterm labor or preterm prelabor rupture of membranes. Therapy should ideally start from 16 to 20 weeks of gestation, but treatment may be started as late as 20 to 22 weeks of gestation. Cervical length screening may also be recommended for pregnant women with a history of a prior spontaneous preterm birth; in some cases, a shortened cervix may be treated with cerclage placement, in addition to 17-OHPC treatment.

b. Short cervix

Routine cervical length screening is not universally recommended for all pregnant women. It may be recommended that women with a history of prior preterm birth undergo serial ultrasonographic (US) measurement of cervical length between 16 and 24 weeks of gestation. Vaginal progesterone supplementation may be recommended to asymptomatic women with an incidentally identified short cervical length and no prior history of preterm birth.

c. Establish pregnancy dates

An estimated due date should be determined for every pregnancy as early as possible. If problems develop later in a pregnancy, this information is useful when deciding an appropriate course of action.

d. Treat all infections

Urinary tract infections (including asymptomatic bacteriuria), symptomatic vaginal infections, and sexually transmitted infections are associated with the occurrence of preterm labor and should be treated. Providers should routinely screen all women at the first prenatal visit for infections and treat, retest, and re-treat as necessary.

e. Reassess risk throughout pregnancy

The pregnant woman's risk factors for preterm birth can change, and new risk factors may develop during pregnancy. Prenatal care should be adapted to the changing needs of the pregnant woman as appropriate.

Self-test A

Now answer these questions to test yourself on the information in the last section.

A1. Preterm labor is defined as labor occurring before _____ weeks _____ days of gestation.

A2. Prematurity accounts for approximately _____% of neonatal deaths that are not caused by congenital malformations.

A3. Approximately _____% of babies born in the United States are born preterm.

A4. True False Preterm labor rarely occurs in women who do not have at least one risk factor.

A5. True False Routine screening for and treatment of asymptomatic bacteriuria may help prevent preterm labor.

A6. True False The earlier intervention to stop preterm labor is started, the more likely it is to be successful.

A7. What symptoms of preterm labor would you tell a pregnant woman to report?
_____
_____
_____
_____

A8. Which of the following conditions increase the risk for preterm labor and delivery?

Yes	No	
___	___	Intra-amniotic infection
___	___	Severe anemia
___	___	Gonorrhea
___	___	Maternal age of 18 years or younger
___	___	Cocaine use
___	___	Cervical insufficiency
___	___	Absence of prenatal care
___	___	Preterm, prelabor rupture of membranes

A9. List at least 3 conditions that put a pregnancy at particularly high risk for preterm labor.
_____
_____
_____

Check your answers with the list that follows the Recommended Routines. Correct any incorrect answers and review the appropriate section in the unit.

4. What should be offered to women known to be at risk for preterm labor?

A. Address risk factors for which treatment or intervention is available
   1. Cervical insufficiency

      The cause of cervical insufficiency is often unknown but may result from trauma from obstetric or gynecological procedures in the past or from in utero exposure to diethylstilbestrol. Diethylstilbestrol was in use from 1940 to 1971; most women who were exposed in utero have now completed their childbearing. Most women who receive a diagnosis of cervical insufficiency will not have a history of trauma or DES exposure.

      If a woman is known to have cervical insufficiency, cerclage is often effective when placed before cervical dilation occurs. A US examination should be performed to confirm fetal viability and to rule out major anomalies. If there are no fetal contraindications, prophylactic cerclage is generally performed at 12 to 14 weeks of gestation. Vaginal examinations or cervical US examinations may be performed as needed on the basis of symptoms to assess whether the cerclage is supporting the cervix and not causing erosion.

      The cerclage remains in place until 36 to 37 weeks of gestation, until labor begins, or until the time of planned cesarean delivery. If the cerclage remains in place during labor, heavy bleeding, along with cervical injury or uterine rupture, may occur. Cerclage removal by 37 weeks minimizes the risk that the woman will begin labor with the cerclage still in place.

   2. Suspected cervical insufficiency

      Cervical insufficiency may be suspected from a previous pregnancy that ended spontaneously between 16 and 20 weeks of gestation. If cervical insufficiency is suspected, but the diagnosis is not clear enough to warrant cerclage placement at 12 to 14 weeks of gestation, cervical US examinations are scheduled beginning at 16 weeks of gestation and are continued every 1 to 2 weeks until 24 weeks of gestation. Evidence of shortening or funneling of the cervix in a woman with a prior history of preterm birth may be treated with placement of a cerclage in some circumstances.

   3. Urinary tract infection (see Unit 3, Infectious Diseases in Pregnancy, in this book). Preterm labor may be associated with the presence of a urinary tract infection, whether or not the infection is symptomatic. In some cases, a urinary tract infection may progress to pyelonephritis with sepsis, which significantly increases the risk of preterm labor. The apparent mechanism for this is the release of toxins from the infecting organism into the bloodstream.

      All pregnant women should be screened for bacteriuria at the first prenatal visit. A positive screening test should be confirmed with a urine culture. Whether symptomatic or asymptomatic, bacteriuria should be treated promptly. Until antibiotic sensitivities are known, treatment with trimethoprim-sulfamethoxazole, nitrofurantoin, or cephalexin is recommended. Once antibiotic sensitivities are known, the choice of antibiotics can be adjusted as appropriate. A follow-up urine culture may be performed later in the pregnancy to assess the urine for recurrent bacteriuria.

      Pregnant women treated for bacteriuria should be periodically rescreened until delivery. If bacteriuria recurs, suppressive antibiotic therapy is usually recommended for the remainder of the pregnancy.

B. Increase surveillance of the pregnancy
If a woman is at high risk for preterm labor, a plan should be developed to closely follow the pregnant woman during her pregnancy.
1. Increase the frequency of prenatal visits
Women at high risk for preterm delivery should be assessed every 1 to 2 weeks, beginning at approximately 20 weeks of gestation.
2. Examine the cervix
Consider a baseline physical examination of the cervix (speculum and/or bimanual) at 18 to 24 weeks of gestation. As with measurements of fundal height, accuracy of the cervical examination is improved when the same examiner performs all subsequent examinations. Future examinations are usually prompted by maternal symptoms such as contractions, pelvic pressure, or a change in discharge.
3. Provide patient education
Review the symptoms of preterm labor and the importance of seeking prompt medical care if any symptoms occur.

5. How is possible preterm labor evaluated?

Any evidence of preterm labor should be investigated promptly to determine if labor is present. If labor is present or highly suspected to be present, all efforts should be made to stop or slow the progression of labor unless otherwise contraindicated.

The treatment of the pregnant woman with preterm labor includes
- Assessment of the condition of the pregnant woman and her fetus
- Consideration of consultation and referral to a regional perinatal center
- Consideration of tocolysis to stop or slow the progression of labor

A. Assessment of the condition of the pregnant woman and her fetus
An outpatient evaluation in an antenatal testing or triage area is recommended because some women will not be in labor and can safely go home after appropriate observation and assessment. For patients who require further treatment, hospital admission can be arranged after this period of outpatient evaluation.

 The cause of preterm labor symptoms may not be obvious. Maternal and fetal well-being should be carefully evaluated before deciding to attempt to slow or stop the progress of labor. This evaluation should indicate whether continuation of the pregnancy may significantly jeopardize the health of the woman or the fetus.

1. Physical examination
A physical examination and evaluation of the pregnant woman's vital signs should be performed. In some cases, there may be evidence of prelabor rupture of membranes or intra-amniotic infection (see Unit 8, Prelabor Rupture of Membranes and Intra-amniotic Infection, in this book). If not previously performed, a complete medical and obstetric history should be obtained.

2. Intravenous hydration
   Because dehydration can initiate uterine contractions, intravenous (IV) hydration of the pregnant woman is often recommended, with an initial bolus of 500 mL of an isotonic crystalloid solution. Rehydration usually inhibits contractions that are caused by maternal dehydration. Administration of IV fluids to a normally hydrated woman, however, has not been shown to have an effect on preterm labor. If IV tocolytic medications are administered with additional IV fluids, caution must be used to avoid fluid overload and minimize the risk of pulmonary edema.
3. Fetal monitoring
   - Fetal monitoring should include continuous external fetal heart rate monitoring and abdominal tocodynamometry to evaluate uterine activity.
4. Maternal urine evaluation
   - Urinalysis and urine culture should be performed.
5. Sterile speculum examination
   A sterile speculum examination should be performed to evaluate
   - Cervical dilation, effacement, consistency, and position.
   - Presence of ballooning of the lower uterine segment. This finding is present if there is clinically significant bulging of the anterior vaginal wall.
   - Whether amniotic membranes are ruptured or intact.
   - Collect samples to evaluate for infections and likelihood of preterm birth.
     — Cultures for group B streptococcus (GBS) (vaginal and rectal)
     — Samples to test for chlamydia and gonorrhea (cervical/vaginal)
     — Samples to test for bacterial vaginosis
     — Consider collection of cervicovaginal secretions for a fetal fibronectin test

Do not perform a digital examination if the amniotic membranes are ruptured (to avoid introducing infectious organisms into the uterus) or if vaginal bleeding is present and the location of the placenta is unknown. If placenta previa has been ruled out and the amniotic membranes are intact, digital examination may be performed.

6. Fetal fibronectin
   Fetal fibronectin is present in maternal tissue and appears in cervicovaginal secretions as the cervix is remodeled in preparation for labor. Evaluation of fetal fibronectin in the cervicovaginal secretions may help determine if preterm delivery is likely (or not). The test should only be used for pregnant women from 22 to 35 weeks of gestation who have intact amniotic membranes and no vaginal bleeding.

   A sample of cervicovaginal secretions should be obtained *before* a digital examination is performed because a digital examination may cause increased fetal fibronectin in the cervical mucus and a false-positive test result. For an accurate result, the secretions must be free of blood and amniotic fluid (membranes must be intact). Any manipulation of the cervix, including a pelvic examination or vaginal intercourse within 24 hours prior to sample collection, increases the risk of a false-positive test result. If a lubricant or antiseptic is used, sampling should be delayed by 6 to 8 hours because those compounds may cause false-negative results. Cervical dilation should be less than 3 cm.

Positive fetal fibronectin test results are associated with an increased risk of preterm delivery, but most women with a positive test result will not deliver preterm. Negative test results are more useful, however, and negative fetal fibronectin test results indicate that delivery is unlikely to occur within the next 2 weeks.

The fetal fibronectin test is not recommended for routine screening of pregnant women. It is most useful in the evaluation of pregnant women who have signs or symptoms of preterm labor with intact membranes or in women who are at high risk for preterm birth.

7. Evaluation of the pregnancy to include confirmation of the pregnancy dates, fetal size, and gestational age
8. Determination of the presence of preterm labor
Preterm labor is commonly defined by
   - Cervical changes that occur during the observation period
   or
   - Contractions that persist despite adequate hydration and sedation, and either
     — Cervical dilation of at least 2 cm
     or
     — Cervical effacement of at least 80%

There is no indication for the woman to stay in the hospital for continued observation if she does not have cervical change or persistent contractions, if the membranes are not ruptured, and if there are no other concerning symptoms. If the amniotic membranes are ruptured or if there is concern for intra-amniotic infection, refer to Unit 8, Prelabor Rupture of Membranes and Intra-amniotic Infection, in this book. US examination may be conducted to obtain additional information about the likelihood of preterm labor occurring in the future.

9. US examination
If the membranes are intact, vaginal probe US examination may be used to assess cervical length and funneling of the lower uterine segment. Cervical funneling refers to the shape created by the thinning and softening of the lower uterine segment and widening of the adjoining upper cervix. These changes allow the membranes to bulge into the upper cervix.

If cervical funneling is *not* present and the closed cervical length is longer than 3 cm, there is a less than 5% chance the woman will deliver before 35 weeks of gestation. Less than 1% of women who have an *absence* of funneling and an *absence* of fetal fibronectin in vaginal secretions will deliver preterm during the week after the examination. The *absence* of a short cervix and cervical funneling is predictive of a low chance for preterm birth. Conversely, the *presence* of funneling or cervical shortening does not reliably predict the occurrence of preterm birth but is associated with an increased likelihood of preterm labor and birth.

B. Consider consultation and referral
If an appropriate level of care is not available for the pregnant woman, the fetus, or the expected neonatal condition at the facility where the pregnant woman is being evaluated, a maternal-fetal transfer to a regional perinatal center should be conducted. A transfer of care is especially important if the fetus is 34 weeks of gestation or younger or if there are any other maternal-fetal complications. Delivery at a medical center with the appropriate level of neonatal care is consistently associated with better neonatal

outcomes than delivery followed by neonatal transfer. A transfer of care also prevents geographic separation of the mother and baby after birth.

If a maternal-fetal transfer is indicated, it should be accomplished *early* in the evaluation of preterm labor, well before labor has progressed to the point where en route delivery might occur. Delivery in the referring hospital with a neonatal transfer is preferable to delivery while en route between hospitals. Generally, therapy is started before transfer and continued during transport, as appropriate to individual circumstances.

C. Decide whether stopping or slowing the progression of labor should be attempted

 Consider consultation with maternal-fetal medicine specialists at any time, especially if the fetus is significantly preterm or if other maternal-fetal complications are present.

1. Contraindications to tocolysis
   a. Tocolysis *should not* be used with
      - Abnormal fetal heart rate patterns
      - A dead fetus or lethal fetal anomaly
      - Confirmed or suspected intra-amniotic infection. Intra-amniotic infection—even subclinical infection—is often associated with preterm labor, and the presence of infection should be evaluated very carefully.
      - Maternal myasthenia gravis (magnesium sulfate is contraindicated)
      - Severe fetal growth restriction
      - Preeclampsia with severe features or eclampsia (in this case, magnesium sulfate may be administered for seizure prophylaxis; tocolysis may be considered for some pregnant women with preeclampsia with severe features if the only severe feature of preeclampsia is hypertension)
      - Maternal physiological instability (eg, hemorrhage, sepsis, or other severe medical illness)
      - Any other condition in which prolonging a pregnancy may jeopardize fetal or maternal health
   b. Tocolysis *may be contraindicated* with
      - Maternal illness of mild or moderate severity, such as hypertension, heart disease, hyperthyroidism, or diabetes mellitus
      - *Pregnant women with contractions but without cervical change:* Reduced activity, adequate hydration, and close observation are recommended
      - Pregnant women who have received a course of antenatal corticosteroids earlier in the pregnancy
2. Indications for tocolysis
   The primary indication for tocolysis is treatment of preterm labor to allow for completion of antenatal steroids and/or transfer to a facility with higher-level care for the mother and the fetus or newborn. Tocolysis has only been demonstrated to be associated with short-term effectiveness; women treated with tocolysis are less likely to deliver within 72 hours after the initiation of treatment than women treated with a placebo. Repeated, recurrent, and prolonged courses of tocolytic medications have not been shown to improve pregnancy outcomes or reduce the rate of delivery before 37 weeks.

Generally, all pregnancies with preterm labor at 34 weeks of gestation or less are treated with tocolytic medication (unless there are specific contraindications) to allow for administration of antenatal corticosteroids. Tocolysis, however, is usually *not* used for preterm labor that occurs after $34^{0/7}$ weeks of gestation or after a prior course of antenatal steroids has been administered.

In cases in which cervical dilation is advanced (≥4 cm), tocolytic therapy may still be used in an attempt to administer magnesium sulfate for neuroprotection, to gain time for the administration of corticosteroids and, if appropriate, for safe transfer to a regional perinatal center.

In general, the use of tocolytic medications is most appropriate when
- Uterine contractions with cervical dilation and/or effacement are present.
- The fetus is preterm before $34^{0/7}$ weeks and can be assumed to have not achieved pulmonary maturity.
- Antenatal corticosteroids are being administered to the pregnant woman.
- The pregnant woman requires transfer to another higher-level facility.
- The pregnant woman is healthy.

When gestational age is 34 weeks of gestation or less, prolonging a pregnancy for even a brief period can be beneficial to fetal maturation and, thus, to neonatal survival and well-being.

D. Develop a plan of care

In the absence of other complications, the main risks of preterm labor are the neonatal risks associated with preterm delivery. If maternal-fetal complications are present, the obstetric care provider and the patient should decide together if the balance of risks to the mother and fetus favor delivery or tocolysis.

None of the drugs and other interventions used to treat preterm labor have been shown to be completely effective. In addition, tocolytic medications used to stop or slow the progress of labor may pose risks to maternal and fetal health, particularly when tocolytics are administered for a prolonged length of time. Clinically significant fetal and neonatal benefits, however, may be obtained from tocolysis when it slows the progression of labor long enough to allow administration of antenatal corticosteroids.

Pediatric and obstetric physicians should discuss the diagnosis of preterm labor and its treatment options with the pregnant woman and her family. The patient and her family should be involved in the deliberations about the use of tocolytics and have a thorough understanding of the purpose, possible risks, potential benefits, and limitations of the therapy. If the decision is made to attempt to stop or delay the progress of labor and continue the pregnancy, tocolysis should be started *immediately*.

Self-test B

Now answer these questions to test yourself on the information in the last section.

B1. If a woman is known to have cervical insufficiency, cerclage should be performed at _____ weeks of gestation.

B2. List 3 cervical changes that indicate possible preterm labor.
_____
_____
_____

B3. True False An attempt to stop labor should be made for all women who go into preterm labor.

B4. True False Preterm uterine contractions, without cervical changes, may stop with rehydration and rest.

B5. True False Every woman who goes into preterm labor should be checked for evidence of intra-amniotic infection.

B6. True False Tocolysis is of no value when delivery is likely to occur within 24 hours.

B7. True False The main risk of preterm delivery is the risk to the newborn of preterm birth and the subsequent risks associated with prematurity.

B8. True False Prenatal care for women with a history of a previous preterm delivery should include ultrasonographic examination of the cervix every 1 to 2 weeks during the second trimester.

B9. What is a common definition of preterm labor?
_____
_____
_____

B10. Which of the following actions should be included in the evaluation of preterm labor?

Yes	No	
____	____	Urinalysis
____	____	Discussion of treatment options and risks and benefits with the woman and her family.
____	____	Consideration of maternal-fetal referral for delivery at a regional perinatal center.
____	____	Internal monitoring of fetal heart rate and uterine activity
____	____	Physical examination
____	____	Sterile speculum examination
____	____	Vaginal/rectal cultures

Check your answers with the list that follows the Recommended Routines. Correct any incorrect answers and review the appropriate section in the unit.

6. How is preterm labor treated?

Ideally, treatment of preterm labor will provide tocolysis that stops or slows the progress of cervical dilation and allows the pregnancy to continue. However, patients with preterm labor rarely reach term. Therefore, the goal of preterm labor treatment is to delay delivery at least long enough to allow time for optimal administration of antenatal corticosteroids and to transfer the pregnant woman to a facility with an appropriate level of care in anticipation of preterm birth. Antenatal corticosteroids given to a pregnant woman facing the possibility of preterm birth have been shown to accelerate fetal maturity and reduce the frequency of certain serious complications of prematurity.

A. Stop or slow contractions

Tocolysis is most likely to be successful when there is rapid identification of preterm labor and prompt intervention provided to the pregnant woman.

Regardless of the drug used, tocolysis therapy is guided by the following principles:
- The minimum amount of medication to stop the contractions should be used.
- The woman and fetus should be monitored for possible medication side effects.
- The fetal heart rate and uterine activity should be monitored continuously.
- The medication dosage should be reduced or stopped if clinically significant side effects develop.
- If contractions continue after 12 to 18 hours of tocolytic therapy, the pregnant woman should be reassessed. A decision should be made about whether a different medication should be considered or if labor should be allowed to continue.

Magnesium sulfate is a commonly used tocolytic agent. Calcium channel blocking agents may also be used. β-mimetics may also be considered but are used less often than in the past, largely because of their side effects, including clinically significant maternal cardiac side effects. Prostaglandin synthesis inhibitors and other tocolytic medications are also available. Sometimes, one medication will not control uterine contractions, but switching from that drug to another tocolytic agent may prove to be effective.

All tocolytic agents have potentially serious side effects.

Table 9.1 lists commonly used tocolytic medications and how the woman and fetus should be monitored during their administration.

B. Accelerate fetal pulmonary maturity
 1. Indications and benefits of antenatal corticosteroids
    Antenatal corticosteroids are indicated whenever preterm delivery is determined to be likely to occur within the next 7 days because of spontaneous onset of labor or if there are other complications that require early delivery (ACOG Committee Opinion No. 713. Antenatal corticosteroid therapy for fetal maturation. *Obstet Gynecol.* 2017;130:e102–e109). The benefits of corticosteroid administration outweigh the

potential risks, even when preterm prelabor rupture of membranes has occurred. These benefits include a reduction in
- The risk or severity of respiratory distress syndrome
- The incidence of intraventricular hemorrhage
- Mortality

Treatment with a single course of antenatal corticosteroids should be considered for all pregnant women with fetuses between 24 and 34 weeks of gestation whenever preterm delivery is a strong possibility. Administration as early as 22 to 23 weeks may be considered after appropriate counseling with the woman and her family. In the case of preterm labor, a first course of antenatal corticosteroids may be provided for women from 34 weeks through $36^{6/7}$ weeks.

2. Timing of corticosteroid administration

    Optimal benefits begin 24 hours after corticosteroid therapy is started and last for at least 7 days.

    While the greatest benefits are achieved if delivery occurs more than 24 hours after treatment is started, treatment with corticosteroids for less than 24 hours is also associated with a reduction in neonatal mortality, respiratory distress syndrome, and intraventricular hemorrhage. Unless imminent delivery is anticipated, antenatal corticosteroids should be given for all women as early as possible when labor is suspected or diagnosed. Even an abbreviated course of corticosteroids is likely to be beneficial to neonatal outcome.

    When the use of antenatal steroids is appropriate, corticosteroids should be administered unless immediate delivery is expected.

3. Contraindications

    There are relatively few contraindications to the administration of antenatal corticosteroids. For pregnancies between $34^{0/7}$ and $36^{6/7}$ weeks of gestation with prelabor rupture of membranes, suspected intra-amniotic infection, or pregestational diabetes, antenatal corticosteroid treatment is currently NOT recommended. Consultation with maternal-fetal medicine or other obstetric specialists should be considered if there is uncertainty about administering antenatal steroids to the woman in preterm labor.

4. Repeated doses of corticosteroids

    The routine use of repeated doses of corticosteroids is not universally recommended. Although there is some evidence that repeated doses may be beneficial for improving lung function in babies born preterm, concerns have been raised about possible adverse effects on maternal and neonatal health, including possible inhibition of neurological and physical growth in preterm fetuses. Repeat courses of steroids are not administered to women after $34^{0/7}$ weeks of gestation. Until more evidence becomes available, repeated doses should be used cautiously in individual cases and only after weighing the relative risks to the woman and the fetus, the degree of immaturity of the fetus, and the perceived likelihood of early delivery.

Table 9.1. Tocolytic Medications Commonly Used to Treat Preterm Labor

Medication	Contraindications	Dosage	Administration	Side Effects	Monitoring

Magnesium sulfate[a]	1. Myasthenia gravis
	2. Hypocalcemia
	3. Impaired renal function
	4. Concurrent use with nifedipine
		Loading dose: 4–6 g
		Continuous infusion: 2–4 g/h
		Adjust dose, as needed, to inhibit uterine activity and keep serum magnesium (Mg^{2+}) level 6–8 mg/dL. For women with imminent preterm birth <32 weeks of gestation, antenatal magnesium sulfate administration should be considered for fetal neuroprotection. It should be administered as a 4-g loading dose, over 30 minutes, followed by a 1–2 g/h maintenance infusion until birth. It should be discontinued if delivery is no longer imminent or a maximum of 24 hours of therapy has been administered.
			Loading dose: Intravenously over 20 minutes
			Maintenance: Use piggyback intravenous infusion with pump to control rate.
			Duration: In general, intravenous therapy is used for approximately 24 hours.
			CAUTION: Use with nifedipine can cause significant hypotension.
				Maternal
				Transient flushing, headache, nystagmus, nausea, lethargy, dizziness, and blurred or double vision are common, especially during loading dose.
				1. *Pulmonary edema risk is reduced with*
				  • Careful monitoring of intake/output
				  • Serum level kept at 6–8 mg/dL
				2. *Hypocalcemia* (low serum calcium level)
				Signs of toxicity: Loss of deep tendon reflexes at serum level of 10–12 mg/dL
				At a higher serum Mg^{2+} level:
				  • Respiratory depression
				  • Severe hypotension
				  • Tetany or paralysis
				  • Cardiac arrest
				Neonatal
				Transient decrease in muscle tone, drowsiness in newborns may occur.
					Check
					• *Urine output*: Mg^{2+} excreted only by kidneys.
					• *Toxicity*: risk increased when output <30 mL/h.
					• Record intake and output.
					• Check vital signs every hour.
					• Check deep tendon reflexes every hour.
					• Measure serum Mg^{2+} levels if deep tendon reflexes diminish.
					• If there are signs of pulmonary edema, check breath sounds.
					• Monitor fetal heart rate and pattern.
					Keep calcium gluconate available.
					Administer calcium gluconate if signs of toxicity develop.

(continued)

UNIT 9: PRETERM LABOR

Table 9.1. Tocolytic Medications Commonly Used to Treat Preterm Labor (continued)

Medication	Contraindications	Dosage	Administration	Side Effects	Monitoring
Calcium channel blocker nifedipine	1. Liver disease 2. Concurrent use with magnesium sulfate	*Loading dose:* 10 mg may be repeated 1–2 times, at 20-min intervals, if contractions persist. *Maintenance:* 10–20 mg, every 4–6 h	*Route:* Oral *CAUTION:* Use of calcium channel blockers with magnesium sulfate can cause clinically significant hypotension.	**Maternal** Vasodilatation: flushing, headache, transient heart rate increase, transient hypotension	**Check** • Blood pressure • Fetal heart rate and pattern
β-Mimetic agent terbutaline	1. Cardiac disease or rhythm disturbance 2. Poorly controlled • Hypertension • Diabetes mellitus • Thyrotoxicosis *Note:* Because of the risk of fluid retention, use dextrose 5% in water and avoid salt-containing intravenous fluids. For women with diabetes mellitus, however, 0.25% saline (one-quarter normal) should be used to reduce the risk of hyperglycemia.	Obtain baseline information before first dose: maternal weight, complete blood cell count, electrolytes, blood glucose level, and urinalysis. *Dose:* 0.25 mg. Dose may be repeated 2 or 3 times at 30-min intervals. If contractions stop, administer 0.25 mg as a maintenance dose every 3–4 h.	*Route:* Subcutaneous, by intermittent dosing only, and for a maximum of 72 hours. Should be given in-hospital only and under close observation because of potential complications, including arrhythmia and death.	**Maternal** 1. *Pulmonary edema risk is reduced with* • Intake limited • Intravenous fluids without salt • Maternal heart rate kept <130 beats/min *Risk increased with* • Multifetal gestation • Cardiac disease • Maternal infection 2. *Cardiac ischemia,* arrhythmias, or severe hypotension 3. *Hyperglycemia* (high blood glucose level) 4. *Hypokalemia* (low serum potassium level) 5. *Maternal death* **Fetal** 1. *Tachycardia* 2. *Increased fetal heart rate variability*	**Check** • *Intake/output:* Limit fluid to 2,500 mL/d. • If there are signs of pulmonary edema, check breath sounds, use a pulse oximeter to check SpO$_2$. • *Check vital signs* every hour. • *Check serum potassium* levels every 4 h. • *Check blood glucose level* — Every 4 h in nondiabetic women, especially if giving an infusion for 12 h or longer — Frequently in women with diabetes mellitus or abnormal glucose tolerance • Monitor fetal heart rate and pattern.

[a] Magnesium sulfate is on the Institute for Safe Medication Practices high-alert medication list of drugs creating a heightened risk of causing clinically significant patient harm when used in error. Special precautions and protocols for administration can decrease the risk for error. (See www.ismp.org.)

5. Medication and dosage
   Betamethasone, 2 doses, each 12 mg, administered intramuscularly, 24 hours apart
   or
   Dexamethasone, 4 doses, each 6 mg, administered intramuscularly, 12 hours apart (used less commonly, but it is an alternative when betamethasone is not available)

7. How is preterm delivery managed?

If preterm labor cannot be stopped or is allowed to continue because of maternal or fetal condition, maternal-fetal transfer to a regional perinatal center for delivery is often indicated. If maternal-fetal transfer is not appropriate or if time does not allow safe transport, preparations should be made for preterm delivery and care of a preterm baby.

A. Discontinue tocolytics

Other than magnesium sulfate in some cases, tocolytic drugs should be discontinued, as their continued use provides no benefit and may increase the risk of postpartum hemorrhage.

For pregnant women in preterm labor prior to 32 to 34 weeks of gestation, magnesium sulfate is continued at 1 to 2 g/h until delivery because evidence suggests its use may reduce the risk of fetal-neonatal neurological injury leading to cerebral palsy.

B. Administer intrapartum antibiotics according to the presence of risk factors

Antibiotic therapy for GBS prophylaxis is recommended for women who have a history of a prior pregnancy affected by early-onset GBS disease or an episode of GBS bacteriuria during the current pregnancy. The recommendation for antibiotic therapy for GBS prophylaxis for these indications supersedes all other recommendations related to GBS culture or screening results.

For women with preterm labor prior to 37 weeks of gestation without the aforementioned history, antibiotic therapy is guided by GBS culture or screening test results in the current pregnancy. In this case, antibiotic therapy for GBS prophylaxis is recommended for either of the following:
- A positive or unknown vaginal-rectal culture result for GBS in the current pregnancy
- The results of a vaginal-rectal culture for GBS that are negative but were obtained more than 5 weeks prior

Antibiotic therapy for GBS prophylaxis is NOT recommended for women with preterm labor prior to 37 weeks of gestation who have negative GBS culture or screening results within 5 weeks of the current presentation.
- If a woman with prior positive or unknown GBS culture results is found to have negative GBS culture or screening results at the time of her evaluation for preterm labor, antibiotics for GBS prophylaxis should be discontinued.

Antibiotics used for GBS prophylaxis
- *Preferred antibiotic* regimen is IV penicillin G, 5.0 million units administered initially, then 2.5 million or 3.0 million units administered every 4 hours until delivery. The 2.5 million-unit and 3.0 million-unit doses are considered equivalent, and it is acceptable to use whichever your hospital pharmacy stocks.
- *Alternative antibiotic* is IV ampicillin, 2 g administered initially, then 1 g administered every 4 hours until delivery.
- For women who are allergic to penicillin, see the GBS section in Unit 3, Infectious Diseases in Pregnancy, in this book.

If an intra-amniotic infection is present, ampicillin is recommended, and gentamicin is added with a loading dose of 1.5 mg/kg administered intravenously, then 1 mg/kg administered every 8 hours. An alternative dosing of gentamicin is 5 mg/kg administered intravenously every 24 hours. See Unit 8, Prelabor Rupture of Membranes and Intra-amniotic Infection, in this book for additional recommendations regarding management of intra-amniotic infection.

- Whichever antibiotic is used, IV administration is preferred. Higher intra-amniotic concentrations are achieved with IV administration than with intramuscular administration.

C. Reduce maternal opioids

If used, opioid medication should be reduced in dosage and frequency. This is also to allow maternal and fetal metabolism of the medication and thereby reduce the risk of newborn respiratory depression.

D. Choose route of delivery

1. Vertex presentation

    The preterm fetus with a cephalic presentation may be delivered vaginally in the absence of any obstetric contraindication to vaginal delivery (eg, active genital herpes, prior classical cesarean delivery, placenta previa). The delivering practitioner should make every effort to achieve an atraumatic vaginal delivery. Obstetric interventions, such as planned cesarean delivery, "prophylactic" forceps delivery, or routine episiotomy, have not been shown to improve neonatal outcomes for preterm cephalic fetuses and should be reserved for specific indications, such as abnormal fetal heart rate patterns. Vacuum-assisted delivery is contraindicated in fetuses less than 35 weeks of gestation.

2. Non-vertex presentation

    Preterm fetuses at a viable gestational age (generally considered >23 to 24 weeks) that are in breech presentation typically have better short-term outcomes when delivered via cesarean than vaginal delivery. This is, in part, related to the rare but serious complication of head entrapment in an incompletely dilated cervix after delivery of the fetal trunk. As advancements in neonatal care continue to be made, the gestational age of potential viability will continue to be adjusted downward. Some centers report survival rates in excess of 50% for babies born at 22 weeks of gestation. Owing to the small number of babies born between 22 and 24 weeks of gestation and the lack of controlled studies to assess the effects of delivery route on survival and other outcomes, it is difficult to make a recommendation regarding the balance of risks and benefits of the route of delivery to the woman and the neonate. Current consensus opinion is that a cesarean delivery for a fetal indication (eg, breech presentation) is not recommended before $23^{0/7}$ weeks of gestation, may be considered between $23^{0/7}$ and $24^{6/7}$ weeks of gestation, and is recommended at or after $25^{0/7}$ weeks of gestation. In certain circumstances, the delivering practitioner may determine that a vaginal delivery is the best route for a particular non-vertex fetus. This may be due to extreme prematurity with anticipated low likelihood of survival, coexisting major fetal anomalies, serious maternal illness (increasing the risk of maternal complications of surgery), or, simply, rapid labor. Any time a vaginal breech delivery is anticipated, an essential element is the presence of an obstetrician skilled in breech delivery.

E. Be prepared for neonatal resuscitation

 Be prepared to resuscitate the preterm newborn.

Gentle handling is especially important for small preterm babies because tiny babies have particularly fragile skin, lungs, and cerebral blood vessels.

Consider the following information (review material in Book 1: Maternal and Fetal Evaluation and Immediate Newborn Care and Book 3: Neonatal Care):
- Provide resuscitation.
- Observe the baby for signs of respiratory distress. Use continuous positive airway pressure or intubate the baby early if respiratory distress develops.
- Postnatal surfactant administration acts with antenatal corticosteroids to reduce respiratory distress syndrome and mortality in extremely preterm newborns.
- Small preterm babies can become hypothermic *very* quickly. A warm delivery environment and the use of a plastic covering or chemical warming mattresses facilitates thermal support for the newborn. The delivery room temperature should be maintained at 22.7°C to 23.8°C [73.0°F–75.0°F]).
- Check the baby's blood pressure and hematocrit value.
- Screen the baby for hypoglycemia. Start IV fluids or feedings early.
- Consider performing cultures and starting antibiotics if the baby is sick or if maternal risk factors for infection are present.

Self-test C

Now answer these questions to test yourself on the information in the last section.

C1. True False Treatment with antenatal corticosteroids should be considered for all pregnant women with fetuses between 23 and 34 weeks of gestation when there is a strong possibility of preterm delivery.

C2. True False Preterm fetuses in breech presentation have higher short-term survival rates with cesarean delivery than with vaginal delivery.

C3. True False Early, aggressive intervention may allow preterm labor to be stopped and the pregnancy to continue for days or weeks.

C4. In which of the following situations might the use of antenatal corticosteroids be appropriate?

Yes	No	
___	___	A healthy woman in labor at 30 weeks of gestation with intact membranes and 4-cm cervical dilation, 60% effacement, and receiving tocolytic medication
___	___	A woman in labor, after prelabor rupture of membranes at 30 weeks of gestation, without evidence of intra-amniotic infection or other pregnancy complications, and receiving tocolytic medication
___	___	A woman in labor at 37 weeks of gestation, with ruptured membranes and foul-smelling amniotic fluid, being treated with intravenous antibiotics
___	___	A healthy woman in labor at 28 weeks of gestation, with ruptured membranes, 8-cm cervical dilation, and 100% effacement
___	___	A healthy woman in labor, with intact membranes at 33 weeks of gestation, being treated with intravenous magnesium sulfate

C5. When preterm delivery is unavoidable, which of the following measures are appropriate?

Yes	No	
___	___	Consider maternal-fetal transfer to a regional perinatal center for delivery.
___	___	Rush the woman immediately to a regional perinatal center for delivery.
___	___	Discontinue tocolytics as soon as the decision to allow labor to proceed is made.
___	___	Perform cesarean delivery for all fetuses with an estimated weight less than 1,500 g (<3 lb 5 oz).
___	___	Provide anesthesia for pelvic relaxation during delivery.
___	___	Notify pediatric staff.

C6. Indicate whether the side effects and signs of toxicity listed here are associated with magnesium sulfate, β-mimetic medication, or both.

Side Effect	Magnesium Sulfate	β-Mimetic Medications
Pulmonary edema	___	___
Rapid heart rate	___	___
Chest pain with cardiac ischemia	___	___
Hyperglycemia (high blood glucose level)	___	___
Loss of deep tendon reflexes	___	___
Hypokalemia (low serum potassium level)	___	___
Respiratory depression	___	___

Check your answers with the list that follows the Recommended Routines. Correct any incorrect answers and review the appropriate section in the unit.

PRETERM LABOR

Recommended Routines

All the routines listed below are based on the principles of perinatal care presented in the unit you have just finished. They are recommended as part of routine perinatal care.

Read each routine carefully and decide whether it is standard operating procedure in your hospital. Check the appropriate blank next to each routine.

Procedure Standard in My Hospital	Needs Discussion by Our Staff	Recommended Routine
_____	_____	1. Develop a system that allows outpatient evaluation, in an obstetric care area, of women with questionable preterm labor until it is determined that discharge home or hospitalization for continued treatment of preterm labor (or delivery) is appropriate.
_____	_____	2. Establish a protocol for prompt evaluation of preterm labor and, if appropriate, prompt intervention to stop labor.
_____	_____	3. Develop a system for appropriate consultation and referral of women at risk for preterm delivery.
_____	_____	4. Establish a system to ensure all pregnant women with fetuses between $23^{0/7}$ and $36^{6/7}$ weeks of gestation are evaluated for treatment with corticosteroids, if preterm delivery becomes a strong possibility.
_____	_____	5. Establish a system to notify nursery personnel whenever a preterm delivery is expected.

Self-test Answers

These are the answers to the Self-test questions. Please check them with the answers you gave and review the information in the unit wherever necessary.

Self-test A

A1. Preterm labor is defined as labor occurring before *37* weeks *0* days of gestation.

A2. Prematurity accounts for approximately *75*% of neonatal deaths that are not caused by congenital malformations.

A3. Approximately *10*% of babies born in the United States are born preterm.

A4. False *Reason:* Preterm labor often occurs in women who have no recognized risk factors.

A5. True

A6. True

A7. Any of the following symptoms:
- Abdominal cramping
- Change in vaginal discharge or onset of watery or mucoid discharge
- Low backache (intermittent or constant)
- Pelvic pressure
- Sense of heaviness in the vagina

A8.
Yes	No	
X	___	Intra-amniotic infection
X	___	Severe anemia
X	___	Gonorrhea
X	___	Maternal age of 18 years or younger
X	___	Cocaine use
X	___	Cervical insufficiency
X	___	Absence of prenatal care
X	___	Preterm prelabor rupture of membranes

A9. Any 3 of the following conditions:
- Previous preterm delivery
- Multifetal gestation
- Preterm prelabor rupture of membranes
- Infection, especially with chlamydia, gonorrhea, syphilis, or bacterial vaginosis

Self-test B

B1. If a woman is known to have cervical insufficiency, cerclage should be performed at *12 to 14* weeks of gestation.

B2. Any 3 of the following cervical changes:
- Effacement
- Dilation
- Softening
- Anterior position
- "Ballooning" of the lower uterine segment

B3. False *Reason:* Tocolysis is contraindicated in some situations.

B4. True

B5. True

PCEP BOOK 2: MATERNAL AND FETAL CARE

B6. **False** *Reason:* Even when cervical dilation is at least 4 cm, tocolysis might delay birth long enough for the fetus to benefit from corticosteroids administered to the mother. While maximum benefits are gained when steroids are started more than 24 hours before delivery, administration for less than 24 hours is also of value to a preterm fetus, especially one of 34 weeks' gestational age or younger. Tocolysis is appropriate unless imminent delivery is expected.

B7. True

B8. True

B9. Preterm labor is defined as persistent contractions (despite hydration and sedation) with cervical dilation of at least 2 cm or effacement of at least 80% before the start of the 38th week of gestation or cervical changes that occur during the observation period.

B10.

Yes	No	
X	___	Urinalysis
X	___	Discussion of treatment options and risks and benefits with the woman and her family.
X	___	Consideration of maternal-fetal referral for delivery at a regional perinatal center.
___	X	Internal monitoring of fetal heart rate and uterine activity (Even if the membranes are ruptured, use only external monitoring, unless the decision is made to allow labor to proceed. If labor is allowed, avoid internal monitoring when there is evidence of amniotic infection.)
X	___	Physical examination
X	___	Sterile speculum examination
X	___	Vaginal/rectal cultures

Self-test C

C1. True

C2. True

C3. True

C4.

Yes	No	
X	___	A healthy woman in labor at 30 weeks of gestation with intact membranes and 4-cm cervical dilation, 60% effacement, and receiving tocolytic medication
X	___	A woman in labor, after prelabor rupture of membranes at 30 weeks of gestation, without evidence of intra-amniotic infection or other pregnancy complications, and receiving tocolytic medication
___	X	A woman in labor at 37 weeks of gestation, with ruptured membranes and foul-smelling amniotic fluid, being treated with intravenous antibiotics
X	___	A healthy woman in labor at 28 weeks of gestation, with ruptured membranes, 8-cm cervical dilation, and 100% effacement
X	___	A healthy woman in labor, with intact membranes at 33 weeks of gestation, being treated with intravenous magnesium sulfate

C5.	Yes	No	
	X	___	Consider maternal-fetal transfer to a regional perinatal center for delivery.
	___	X	Rush the woman immediately to a regional center for delivery. (Transfer should not be conducted if there is a risk of delivery en route or if maternal or fetal condition is unstable. Treatment, as appropriate, should be provided before and during transport. Prompt, efficient transport may be indicated, but speed should never replace attention to patient stability and therapy. If transfer is appropriate, transport early.)
	X	___	Discontinue tocolytics as soon as the decision to allow labor to proceed is made. (If it is appropriate to transfer the woman to a regional perinatal center for delivery, tocolysis would be continued during the transport process.)
	___	X	Perform cesarean delivery for all fetuses with estimated weight less than 1,500 g (<3 lb 5 oz). (Cesarean delivery benefits small fetuses in breech presentation [except for the tiniest babies] but holds no advantage over vaginal delivery for small fetuses in vertex presentation.)
	X	___	Provide anesthesia for pelvic relaxation during delivery.
	X	___	Notify pediatric staff.

C6.	Side Effect	Magnesium Sulfate	β-Mimetic Medications
	Pulmonary edema	X	X
	Rapid heart rate	___	X
	Chest pain with cardiac ischemia	___	X
	Hyperglycemia (high blood glucose level)	___	X
	Loss of deep tendon reflexes	X	___
	Hypokalemia (low serum potassium level)	___	X
	Respiratory depression	X	___

Unit 9 Posttest

After completion of each unit there is a free online posttest available at www.cmevillage.com to test your understanding. Navigate to the PCEP pages on www.cmevillage.com and register to take the free posttests.

Once registered on the website and after completing all the unit posttests, pay the book exam fee ($15) and pass the test at 80% or greater to earn continuing education credits. Only start the PCEP book exam if you have time to complete it. If you take the book exam and are not connected to a printer, either print your certificate to a .pdf file and save it to print later or come back to www.cmevillage.com at any time and print a copy of your educational transcript.

Credits are only available by book, not by individual unit within the books. Available credits for completion of each book exam are as follows: Book 1: 14.5 credits; Book 2: 16 credits; Book 3: 17 credits; Book 4: 9 credits.

For more details, navigate to the PCEP webpages at www.cmevillage.com.

Unit 10: Inducing and Augmenting Labor

Objectives 316

1. What is induction and what is augmentation of labor? 319
2. When is induction of labor performed? 319
3. When should induction of labor *not* be performed? 320
4. What should be done before induction of labor is undertaken? 321
5. How can you tell if an induction of labor is likely to succeed? 321
6. What do you do if the Bishop score is low? 322
7. What do you do if the Bishop score is midrange? 327
8. What do you do if the Bishop score is high? 327
9. When should augmentation of labor be considered? 330
10. When may augmentation of labor *not* be appropriate? 330
11. How should you administer oxytocin? 331
12. What complications may occur with oxytocin infusion? 335
13. How long should you continue an oxytocin infusion? 336

Table

    Table 10.1. Bishop Scoring System 322

Recommended Routines 339

Objectives

In this unit you will learn

A. When induction of labor is performed, and when it is contraindicated

B. How to judge if an induction of labor is likely to be successful

C. When and how to use cervical ripening to facilitate induction of labor

D. When augmentation of labor is used, and when it should not be used

E. How oxytocin should be administered

F. How to determine when a normal contraction pattern has been achieved

G. What complications can occur with oxytocin administration

H. How to recognize and respond to complications of oxytocin administration

I. How long oxytocin should be given, and when it should be stopped

Unit 10 Pretest

Before reading the unit, please answer the following questions. Select the *one best* answer to each question (unless otherwise instructed). Record your answers on the test and check them with the answers at the end of the book.

1. **True   False**   According to the Bishop scoring system (use the following table), labor induction is unlikely to be successful in a woman whose cervix is of medium consistency, 20% effaced, midline position, and 2 cm dilated, with the fetus in vertex presentation at −3 station, unless she undergoes cervical ripening.

Bishop scoring system

	0	1	2	3
Dilation of cervix	Closed	1–2 cm	3–4 cm	5 cm
Effacement of cervix	0%–30%	40%–50%	60%–70%	80%
Station of presenting part	−3	−2	−1, 0	+1, +2
Consistency of cervix	Firm	Medium	Soft	
Position of cervix	Posterior	Midline	Anterior	

2. **True   False**   Oxytocin dosage should be expressed in milliunits (mU) per minute delivered intravenously.

3. **True   False**   Although induction of labor is done to produce the artificial onset of labor, the contraction pattern achieved should resemble one that occurs with the spontaneous onset of labor.

4. **True   False**   For most patients, isotonic solutions are preferable to hypertonic solutions, when oxytocin is administered intravenously.

5. **True   False**   Six or more contractions within 10 minutes represents normal labor.

6. Induction of labor is usually appropriate in all of the following situations, except when
   A. A woman has severe preeclampsia.
   B. Herpes lesions are on the vulva.
   C. There is prelabor rupture of membranes at 36 weeks of gestation and the pregnant woman is afebrile.
   D. A fetus is post-term.

7. Possible complications of oxytocin infusion include all of the following, except
   A. Uterine rupture
   B. Fetal heart rate abnormalities
   C. Tachysystole
   D. Chorioamnionitis

(continued)

317

Unit 10 Pretest (*continued*)

8. Which of the following conditions should be ruled out before oxytocin is administered for induction of labor?
    A. Post-term gestation
    B. Abnormal fetal presentation
    C. Prelabor rupture of membranes
    D. Maternal preeclampsia

9. Which of the following actions should you take first when uterine tachysystole occurs?
    A. Administer a tocolytic drug to the woman to relax the uterus.
    B. Turn the woman on her left side and give oxygen by mask.
    C. Stop the oxytocin infusion.
    D. Perform a cesarean delivery.

10. When oxytocin is administered for the induction of labor, the rate of infusion should be gradually but steadily increased until
    A. Delivery occurs.
    B. Baseline uterine tone increases to 20 mm Hg and higher.
    C. Regular contractions, lasting 90 seconds or longer, become established.
    D. A contraction pattern that resembles normal labor is established.

11. Which of the following risks is associated with prostaglandin cervical ripening medications?
    A. Neonatal sepsis
    B. Cervical bleeding
    C. Uterine tachysystole
    D. Maternal tachycardia

12. **True** False Maternal hyponatremia may be accompanied by mental confusion and seizures.

13. **True** False It is reasonable to administer oxytocin augmentation of labor for 18 to 20 hours if it is needed to achieve a normal contraction pattern.

14. True **False** Labor induction with oxytocin infusion should proceed simultaneously with local application of a prostaglandin preparation to ripen the cervix.

1. What is induction and what is augmentation of labor?

Induction of labor is the artificial initiation of labor before it begins spontaneously, including initiation of labor after spontaneous rupture of membranes without contractions. Induction may be accomplished with the intravenous (IV) administration of oxytocin, administration of vaginal or oral prostaglandin (PG), artificial rupture of membranes, membrane stripping, mechanical dilation (Foley catheter, cervical ripening balloon, or laminaria), and nipple stimulation.

Augmentation of labor is the further stimulation of labor that has already begun spontaneously but is not progressing normally. Labor augmentation should be considered when the natural labor process is not progressing as it should. The risks of augmentation should be weighed against those of a cesarean delivery, which is the only alternative to augmentation in the management of abnormally progressing labor.

2. When is induction of labor performed?

Labor may be induced for many reasons. Multiple factors must be taken into consideration when deciding to induce labor, to undertake a cesarean delivery, or *not* to intervene in a high-risk pregnancy.

Labor is generally induced when

- A gestational age is reached when the fetus is at increased risk of stillbirth or complications from remaining undelivered

or

- A medical or obstetric complication threatens the health of the mother or fetus and the situation can be expected to improve if the fetus is delivered

or

- Electively, after $39^{0/7}$ weeks of gestation (the approach should be individualized and made with the patient after considering the risks, benefits, and alternatives)

and

- Vaginal delivery is preferable to cesarean delivery.

Medical and obstetric complications that potentially threaten the health of the mother or fetus include, but are not limited to
- Placental abruption
- Prelabor rupture of membranes, when delivery is indicated (see Unit 8, Prelabor Rupture of Membranes and Intra-amniotic Infection, in this book).
- Intra-amniotic infection, regardless of gestational age.
- Hypertensive disorders of pregnancy, when appropriate (see Unit 1, Hypertension in Pregnancy, in this book).
- Maternal medical illness with evidence of declining maternal or fetal health (unless fetal or maternal condition is such that cesarean delivery is deemed safer than labor and vaginal delivery). Conditions include but are not limited to diabetes mellitus, renal disease, cardiovascular disease, chronic pulmonary disease, and antiphospholipid syndrome.
- Fetal compromise, as demonstrated by tests of fetal growth or well-being.
- Fetus at late term or post-term gestation (when dates are *certain,* begin considering induction at $41^{0/7}$ weeks of gestation and undertake by $42^{0/7}$ weeks).
- Fetal death.

- Women at 39 or more weeks of gestation with a history of rapid labor(s) and geographic difficulties in reaching a hospital.
- Other (numerous uncommon indications for labor induction also exist; consult with maternal-fetal medicine specialists about individual circumstances).
- Labor may be induced electively if the pregnancy is well dated, with a gestational age greater than 39 weeks, and with maternal consent. A favorable cervix is recommended but is not essential. Recent data suggest that in low-risk nulliparous women, elective induction of labor may reduce the risk of a cesarean delivery when compared to awaiting spontaneous labor.

Every induction of labor should have specific indications recorded in the woman's chart.

3. When should induction of labor *not* be performed?

The following conditions are *contraindications* to the induction of labor. Some exceptions may be reasonable, however, such as prolapsed umbilical cord with a deceased fetus.

- Category III fetal heart rate pattern.
- Placenta previa.
- Vasa previa (uncommon, difficult to diagnose condition in which the umbilical vessels cover the cervical os). It may be possible to palpate the vessels or see them during a sterile speculum examination or with ultrasonography. If found, cesarean delivery is indicated.
- Umbilical cord that is prolapsed or in front of the fetal presenting part. (The latter situation is known as *funic presentation*.)
- Active genital herpes lesions.
- Prior classical (vertical) cesarean incision.
- Previous myomectomy entering the endometrial cavity.
- Fetopelvic disproportion, if known to be present prior to labor. (This is uncommon. An example is if a fetus is known to have clinically significant hydrocephalus.)
- Contracted maternal pelvis or bony abnormalities that encroach on the birth canal.
- Invasive cervical carcinoma.
- Abnormal fetal presentations (face, brow, compound, transverse lie, breech).

Like any medical procedure, induction of labor is not without risks. However, the risks are small enough in appropriate patients that it can be undertaken either for appropriate medical indications or electively for pregnant women whose fetal gestational age is $39^{0/7}$ weeks or more.

4. What should be done before induction of labor is undertaken?

A. Obtain informed consent
Explain to the woman and her family the reasons for an induction, how it will be done, and the accompanying risks. Discuss the possible need for repeat induction attempts or cesarean delivery.

B. Assess fetal maturity, unless maternal or fetal condition necessitates delivery
A gestational age of at least $39^{0/7}$ weeks should be established before undertaking an induction without a medical indication. Criteria that should be fulfilled are given in Book 1: Maternal and Fetal Evaluation and Immediate Newborn Care, Unit 2, Fetal Age, Growth, and Maturity.

C. Assess cervix, pelvis, fetal size, and presentation
Before an induction begins, the woman and fetus should be assessed to rule out the presence of contraindications to induction.

D. Prepare equipment and personnel to provide continuous electronic monitoring and possible surgical intervention
This is recommended because of the increased risk for uterine tachysystole when oxytocin is administered. Oxytocin should be administered and monitored by nursing personnel who are knowledgeable and skilled in oxytocin administration. A guideline for the administration of oxytocin in a standardized manner should be developed by a multidisciplinary group. A physician who is capable of performing a cesarean delivery, along with corresponding personnel and support services, should be readily available.

5. How can you tell if an induction of labor is likely to succeed?

A. Examine the woman
Natural preparation for the onset of labor is a gradual process, controlled by a multitude of incompletely understood interactions of biochemical, biophysical, and hormonal systems. Softening and thinning (effacement) of the cervix occurs—a process termed *ripening*. The lower uterine segment thins as it is drawn toward the increasingly active myometrium of the fundus. This pulls the cervix from its normal position of pointing posteriorly to an anterior position. In the anterior position, the cervix can more readily be palpated by the examiner's finger and seen during a speculum examination.

The closer to labor the patient is when examined, the more the
- Cervix will be pulled anteriorly
- Cervix will be effaced and softened
- Internal cervical os will be dilated
- Uterine contractions will be felt by the patient and examiner
- Uterine muscle (myometrium) will be more sensitive to oxytocin administered intravenously

B. Calculate a Bishop score (Table 10.1)
The Bishop score indicates the likelihood that an induction attempt will be successful. In general, a score of 8 and higher indicates that induction of labor will be successful, whereas a score of 6 or lower is considered unfavorable, and cervical ripening will be necessary.

Table 10.1. Bishop Scoring System

	0	1	2	3	Score
Dilation of the cervix	Closed	1–2 cm	3–4 cm	5–6 cm	_____
Effacement of the cervix	0%–30%	40%–50%	60%–70%	80%	_____
Station of the presenting part[a]	−3	−2	−1, 0	+1, +2	_____
Consistency of the cervix	Firm	Medium	Soft		_____
Position of the cervix	Posterior	Midline	Anterior		_____
				Total score =	_____

[a] By using a −3 to +3 scale (not a −5 to +5 scale).

Derived from Bishop EH. Pelvic scoring for elective induction. *Obstet Gynecol.* 1964;24(2):266–268.

Response to oxytocin is influenced by the degree of cervical dilation, the gestational age of the fetus, the number of previous deliveries, and individual uterine sensitivity. *Uterine response to oxytocin is unpredictable and varies widely among women.*

The Bishop score should be used as a guide to indicate which women are more likely to respond to oxytocin induction and when administration of PGs for cervical ripening is more likely to be helpful.

Example: Findings of a cervix 1 cm dilated (1), 50% effaced (1), medium consistency (1), posterior position (0), and fetal station of −3 (0) would receive a total score of 3.

6. What do you do if the Bishop score is low?

A. Consider cervical ripening

In women who have an indication for delivery and no contraindications to induction, a Bishop score of 6 or lower indicates that cervical ripening should be considered. Preparation of the cervix with medication or mechanical dilation increases the likelihood of successful induction of labor. These techniques or medications should be used only when induction of labor is indicated.

All cervical ripening techniques produce uterine contractions. Uterine contractions produced by a cervical ripening agent may, in some cases, go on to produce labor. In addition, PG preparations may make the uterus more sensitive to oxytocin.

There are several common methods used to promote cervical ripening.
1. Stripping of the membranes (also known as *sweeping of the membranes*)
   Manual separation of the membranes from the decidua (transformed endometrium during pregnancy)
2. Mechanical techniques
   Dilation of the cervix accomplished by inserting an osmotic dilator into the cervical canal, which swells as a result of absorbing fluid, or by inserting a Foley catheter or a cervical ripening balloon through the cervical canal, inflating the balloon, and leaving it inflated within the lower uterine segment
3. Prostaglandins
   Topical application of one of several PG preparations

B. Contraindications and risks of cervical ripening techniques

 All techniques for cervical ripening carry risks. Their risks and indications should be explained to the woman and recorded in her chart.

1. Stripping (sweeping) of the membranes
   a. Contraindications
      - Cervical infection
      - Active genital herpes
      - Group B streptococcal colonization (relative contraindication; may increase the risk of intra-amniotic infection)
      - Recent unexplained vaginal bleeding
      - Placenta previa
   b. Risks
      - Infection
      - Prelabor rupture of membranes due to accidental amniotomy
      - Bleeding from an unidentified placenta previa
2. Mechanical techniques
   a. Contraindications
      - Cervical infection
      - Ruptured membranes
      - Active genital herpes
      - Recent unexplained vaginal bleeding
   b. Risks
      - Infection
      - Prelabor rupture of membranes
      - Bleeding from an unidentified placenta previa
3. Prostaglandins
   a. Contraindications
      - Previous cesarean or other uterine surgery (increased risk of uterine rupture)
      - Presence of excessive uterine activity
      - Known hypersensitivity to PGs
      - Recent unexplained vaginal bleeding
   b. Relative contraindications
      - Ruptured membranes
      - Unexplained vaginal bleeding during the current pregnancy
      - History of difficult labor or traumatic delivery
      - Grand multiparity
      - Multifetal gestation or suspected fetal macrosomia
   c. Risks
      The onset of excessive force or frequency of uterine contractions is the primary risk of using PG ripening agents.

d. Excessive uterine stimulation may result in *tachysystole*—more than 5 contractions in 10 minutes, averaged over a 30-minute period.

Tachysystole may reduce blood flow to the intervillous space within the placenta. At times, this may lead to fetal heart rate changes. Although rare, excessive uterine activity may also result in uterine rupture.

Tachysystole can occur with use of any prostaglandin preparation to ripen the cervix or oxytocin to induce or augment labor.

C. Cervical ripening techniques
   1. Stripping of the membranes
   Membranes are "stripped" or "swept" by inserting a gloved finger through the internal os and then sweeping the finger, in a circular motion, along the lower uterine segment. This separates the membranes from their attachment to the decidua, which, in turn, causes the release of PGs.

   The release of PGs has a direct influence on cervical ripening and causes the uterus to contract. Uterine contractions also promote the cervical changes that are associated with cervical ripening.

   2. Mechanical techniques
   - Osmotic dilators used for mechanical dilation of the cervix include natural seaweed (*Laminaria japonica*) tents and several types of synthetic osmotic dilators. One to 4 dilators are inserted into the cervix during a sterile speculum examination. Generally, osmotic dilators are inserted on an outpatient basis.
   - Insertion of a Foley catheter into the cervical canal, followed by inflation of the 30- to 40-mL balloon of the catheter, has also been used safely as a mechanical dilator. There are cervical dilation balloons currently available that are specifically designed for this use. This is usually done as an inpatient procedure, although use of such balloons in outpatients has been found to be a safe option.

   Mechanical and biochemical methods of cervical ripening have been shown to be effective in ripening the cervix.

   3. Prostaglandins
   Two forms of PG used for cervical ripening are PGE_2 and PGE_1.
      a. Dinoprostone vaginal insert (Cervidil)
      Each vaginal insert contains 10 mg of dinoprostone (PGE_2) in a sustained-release preparation (it has a slower rate of release than dinoprostone gel).
      - Store the inserts in a refrigerator. Warming before use is not necessary.
      - Avoid the use of a lubricant during the insertion. If the insert becomes coated, the release of dinoprostone may be hindered.
      - Place the insert manually into the vagina, with the end containing the drug capsule placed across the posterior fornix and the woven tail left outside the vagina, for easy removal later.
      - Leave the insert in place until the onset of labor or for 12 hours, whichever comes first. The U.S. Food and Drug Administration (FDA) labeling for dinoprostone indicates a single use only. At least one prospective study has

been conducted to explore the use of a second sequential insert if cervical ripening has not occurred after the first; however, the data on the effectiveness of this approach are limited.
- Oxytocin can be initiated 30 minutes after the PG insert is removed.

b. Dinoprostone cervical gel (Prepidil)
This gel comes in prefilled syringes, which contain 0.5 mg of dinoprostone (PGE_2).
- Store the syringes in a refrigerator. Allow the gel to reach room temperature before use, but do *not* use an external heat source, such as a water bath or microwave, to warm the gel.
- Administration of dinoprostone gel may be repeated 2 or 3 times, at 6- to 12-hour intervals, but should not exceed 1.5 mg of dinoprostone in 24 hours.
- Use a speculum for visualization while the gel is inserted into the cervical canal, by using a shielded catheter supplied by the manufacturer. A disk (shield) surrounds the catheter, which blocks the opening of the cervix to minimize the backflow of gel into the vagina. The shield size used depends on the degree of cervical effacement. (See the manufacturer's directions.)
- Select the length of catheter according to the length of the cervix. The tip of the catheter should protrude only a short distance beyond the shield into the cervical canal because the gel should be inserted *below* the internal os and away from the membranes. (Use with ruptured membranes is not recommended.) If the cervix is long, use the catheter with the tip 2 cm beyond the shield; if the cervix is short, use the catheter with the 1-cm tip.
- Oxytocin administration may be initiated 6 to 12 hours after the last dose of dinoprostone gel.

c. Misoprostol tablets (Cytotec)
Each tablet contains 100 mcg of misoprostol (an analog of PGE_1). This drug inhibits gastric acid secretion and is licensed for that purpose. It is not approved by the FDA for use during pregnancy, but off-label use for cervical ripening and labor induction has been recognized by the American College of Obstetricians and Gynecologists as "safe and effective when used appropriately" (ACOG Practice Bulletin No. 107: induction of labor. *Obstet Gynecol*. 2009;114[2 Pt 1]:386–397. Reaffirmed 2019).
- Each 100-mcg tablet of misoprostol needs to be divided into 25-mcg quarters. *Scoring and division of each tablet needs to be done with meticulous care and accuracy by skilled personnel.*
- Dosage is a 25-mcg segment placed in the vagina every 4 to 6 hours or a 50-mcg segment placed every 6 hours, for a maximum of 4 doses (total dosage is 100–200 mcg over 16–24 hours). Dosing misoprostol every 6 hours may have a lower rate of uterine tachysystole. The 50-mcg dose may be associated with a higher rate of fetal heart rate decelerations and uterine tachysystole. Misoprostol can also be administered buccally or orally, and dosing parameters may differ.
- Misoprostol has been shown to be as effective as dinoprostone in producing cervical ripening. In addition, misoprostol more often goes on to produce labor, without the need for oxytocin infusion. Misoprostol carries a higher risk for adverse maternal and fetal responses with doses higher than 25 mcg or when given more frequently than every 3 to 6 hours.

d. Contraindications
PGs should *not* be used in women with a prior cesarean delivery or major uterine surgery. The safety of PG use in women with multifetal gestation or fetal macrosomia is unknown.

D. Monitoring prostaglandin medications

Hospitalization is recommended for women undergoing cervical ripening attempt(s) with any of the PG medications. After placement of the ripening agent, a woman should rest on her side (sometimes the Trendelenburg position is used with dinoprostone gel) for 30 minutes after application. During this time, monitor her vital signs frequently.

If contractions that are too frequent or too strong develop, their onset most often occurs in the first 4 hours after application of a PG medication but may not be seen for as long as 9 or 10 hours after application.

When using Cervidil, uterine activity and fetal heart rate should be monitored continuously
- For at least 30 minutes before application
- Throughout the period of cervical ripening
- For at least 30 minutes after removal of the vaginal insert

When using Prepidil or Cytotec, uterine activity and fetal heart rate should be monitored continuously for at least 2 hours after the last dose of a cervical ripening agent and should be continued if regular uterine contractions persist.

1. If excessive contractions develop
   a. If the dinoprostone vaginal insert is being used, it may be removed. This may help to reduce excessive contractions.

   Note: The dinoprostone insert is the only PG cervical ripening agent that can be removed after administration. Misoprostol tablets dissolve and cannot be removed. Dinoprostone gel also cannot be removed, even by irrigation of the vagina. Vaginal irrigation has not been shown to be effective in treating excessive uterine activity.

   b. Use in utero resuscitative measures.
   Respond to excessive uterine activity or a change in the fetal heart rate pattern by providing such measures as turning the woman on her side and giving oxygen by mask. In most cases, a category II fetal heart rate pattern will resolve as uterine tachysystole subsides. If it does not, manage as you would for any other episode of suspected fetal compromise.

   c. Consider administering a tocolytic medication.
   If the abnormal pattern does not quickly subside, consider giving terbutaline, 0.25 mg, subcutaneously.

2. If labor does not begin
   Dinoprostone and misoprostol may initiate labor, as well as produce cervical ripening. Oxytocin may not be needed. If labor does not begin, allow a rest period before beginning induction of labor.

   The rest period should be *at least*
   - 30 minutes after removing a dinoprostone vaginal insert
   - 6 to 12 hours after the last dose of dinoprostone gel
   - 4 to 6 hours after the last dose of misoprostol

In addition to increasing the likelihood of successful induction of labor, cervical ripening with PGs has been associated with a reduction in the incidence of prolonged labor and the amount of oxytocin needed.

If labor has not begun by the end of the rest period, oxytocin infusion may then be started. Start with a low dose. The effects of PG on the myometrium generally increase the uterine sensitivity to oxytocin.

Do not administer oxytocin too soon after the use of any prostaglandin preparation. If labor has not started, wait the full *rest period before beginning induction of labor with oxytocin.*

7. What do you do if the Bishop score is midrange?

If the Bishop score is 6 to 8, the need for delivery is high, and there are no contraindications to labor induction, consider cervical ripening before attempting to induce labor. Cervical ripening will increase the likelihood of successful induction and/or decrease the need for oxytocin.

If the cervix becomes ripe, proceed to oxytocin induction or amniotomy (described later) to induce labor.

If the cervix does not become ripe, oxytocin induction may still be successful. It should be considered before moving to cesarean delivery.

8. What do you do if the Bishop score is high?

If the Bishop score is at least 8, particularly if the woman is multipara, labor induction by artificial rupture of membranes (amniotomy) may be successful, without requiring oxytocin infusion.

  A. Amniotomy technique

    A sterile plastic hook, specifically designed for this purpose, is inserted through the cervix and used to rupture the membranes. Continuous fetal heart rate monitoring should be used before, during, and immediately after the procedure.

    Be sure the fetal head is well-applied to the cervix and the umbilical cord cannot be palpated. The head should not be moved during the procedure.

Once the membranes have ruptured, delivery must occur. Only rupture the membranes in a patient for whom a firm commitment to move to delivery has been made.

  Note: When there is an urgent need for induction, amniotomy may be done together with oxytocin infusion, even if the Bishop score is low and cervical dilation is minimal, in an effort to speed the onset of labor and reduce the time to delivery. Performing amniotomy with a low Bishop score increases the risk for intra-amniotic infection.

B. Amniotomy contraindications and risks
   1. Contraindications
      - Non-vertex presentation
      - Head not well-applied to the cervix
      - Umbilical cord is presenting part (funic presentation)
      - Vasa previa or placenta previa
      - Active genital herpes
      - Unwillingness to discontinue induction or perform cesarean delivery if induction attempt fails
   2. Relative contraindications
      - Group B streptococci colonization. May be acceptable after administration of prophylactic antibiotics.
      - Maternal HIV infection. Delaying amniotomy can reduce the risk of vertical transmission.
   3. Risks
      - Prolapsed or compressed umbilical cord
      - Infection
      - Umbilical cord compression
      - Bleeding from an unidentified placenta previa or vasa previa

Self-test A

Now answer these questions to test yourself on the information in the last section.

A1. All of the following conditions are contraindications to labor induction, except
   - **A.** Placenta previa
   - **B.** Previous cesarean delivery with a classical incision
   - **C.** Active herpes infection
   - **D.** Post-term pregnancy

A2. Why is a Bishop score calculated?

A3. A Bishop score of 7 indicates

A4. What may be done to improve the likelihood of successful labor induction in a woman with a low Bishop score?

A5. Using Table 10.1, calculate a Bishop score for a woman whose cervix is
   - **A.** Closed, soft, posterior position, and 50% effaced, with the fetus at −2 station

   - **B.** 3-cm dilated, soft, anterior position, and 70% effaced, with the fetus at 0 station

A6. Give at least 2 situations for which labor induction may be appropriate.

A7. Give at least 2 contraindications to stripping of the membranes.

A8. The main risk associated with cervical ripening is

A9. **True   False**   There is no limit on the number of attempts that may be made to ripen a cervix in preparation for oxytocin induction of labor.

A10. **True   False**   Oxytocin induction of labor may be started as soon as treatment with a prostaglandin cervical ripening agent has been inserted.

Check your answers with the list that follows the Recommended Routines. Correct any incorrect answers and review the appropriate section in the unit.

9. When should augmentation of labor be considered?

Labor augmentation with oxytocin may be indicated in the following situations:
- Hypotonic uterine dysfunction
- Secondary arrest of labor

See Unit 11, Abnormal Labor Progress and Difficult Deliveries, in this book, for further information about these conditions.

Note: In women who require augmentation of labor, artificial rupture of membranes has a variable effect on the progression of labor.

10. When may augmentation of labor *not* be appropriate?

A. When a normal contraction pattern is present

Uterine contractions with the following characteristics are considered normal:
- *Frequency:* 2 to 3 minutes apart (3–5 contractions within 10 minutes)
- *Duration:* 45 to 70 seconds each
- *Strength (intensity)*
    — "Strong" at palpation (difficult to indent the uterine wall with your fingers at the peak of a contraction)
    or
    — Peak pressure of 50 mm Hg or more (measured with an internal pressure monitor)

If labor progress has failed despite normal contractions, other reasons for lack of progress should be investigated.

Normal contractions cannot be improved with oxytocin.

B. When fetopelvic disproportion is present

This occurs when the size or the position of the fetus and the size or shape of a woman's pelvis do not allow passage of the fetus. This may be due to
- A contracted maternal pelvis
- Abnormal fetal presentation or abnormal position of the fetal head
- Fetal malformation or abnormal condition (eg, hydrocephalus, fetal hydrops)
- Fetal macrosomia (a large fetus, estimated weight >4,000 g [>8 lb 13 oz])

Oxytocin should not be administered when fetal malposition, fetal malpresentation, or fetopelvic disproportion are known to be present.

C. When contraindications or cautions exist for oxytocin

Use of oxytocin to stimulate labor that began spontaneously is *contraindicated* with
- Prior classical (vertical) cesarean incision
- Prior myomectomy or other full-thickness uterine surgery
- Transverse fetal lie
- Active genital herpes

These conditions require cesarean delivery.

Oxytocin should be *used with caution* in the following situations:
- Abnormal uterine distention (multifetal gestation, hydramnios)
- The presenting part of the fetus positioned above the pelvic inlet (more likely to be present with a contracted pelvis or abnormal fetal presentation)
- Abnormal fetal presentations (face, brow, compound, breech)
- Grand multiparity (5 or more previous deliveries)
- Previous low-transverse cesarean delivery

The use of oxytocin is associated with an up to twofold increase in the risk of uterine rupture. The risk of uterine rupture appears to be related to the dose of oxytocin, although an upper limit of oxytocin dosing during trial of labor after cesarean delivery has not been established.

D. When hypertonic uterine inertia is present
Oxytocin is not useful in the management of this uncommon disorder. See Unit 11, Abnormal Labor Progress and Difficult Deliveries, in this book, for additional information.

E. When there is fetal intolerance to uterine contractions
Although quick delivery is indicated when a category II or III fetal heart rate pattern does not respond to the usual interventions (turning patient, increasing IV fluids, giving oxygen) and vaginal delivery is remote, stimulating even sluggish contractions with oxytocin is likely to make fetal condition worse. Strong, frequent contractions may not allow sufficient relaxation time between contractions for adequate placental perfusion. If placental blood flow is restricted, fetal oxygenation will be diminished, thus increasing the risk of fetal compromise.

Oxytocin is contraindicated whenever evidence of fetal intolerance to labor is present.

11. How should you administer oxytocin?

A. Prepare for use of oxytocin
While oxytocin is used frequently and can be safely administered, even in high-risk situations, risks do accompany the use of this drug. Those risks may be associated with the underlying maternal or fetal condition that indicates the need for oxytocin or with complications directly associated with the medication. Regardless of how low risk a situation seems, adequate preparations should be taken *every* time oxytocin is given.

Oxytocin is a high-risk medication. Indications for its use should be documented for each patient.

B. Use a standard guideline for dosage and rate advancement
There are many acceptable guidelines for the use of oxytocin. Use of *one* standard guideline, however, will help avoid confusion and errors that may accompany oxytocin administration. Specifically, the number of unintended neonatal intensive care unit admissions, Apgar scores below 7 at 5 minutes, and primary cesarean delivery rates have been shown to decrease when using a standardized approach to oxytocin administration. Whichever guideline your hospital uses, it is recommended it be the same for all patients.

Use only IV administration of oxytocin for labor induction or augmentation. Buccal, nasal, or intramuscular administration of oxytocin should not be used to induce or augment labor. Rate of uptake of the drug with these administration routes cannot be controlled or modified, and uterine tachysystole is more common.

Things you should keep in mind when using oxytocin include
1. Individualize dosage
   Follow the standard guideline for oxytocin administration adopted by your institution and increase until the desired pattern of uterine contractions has been established.
2. Recognize the risk of uterine tachysystole
   Excessive uterine stimulation can have adverse consequences for a woman and her fetus. The risk of excessive stimulation is influenced by
   - The dose of oxytocin (milliunits per minute rate of infusion)
   - The frequency of increasing the infusion rate
   - Sensitivity of the myometrium

   The faster the rate of infusion and the more frequently the rate is increased, the higher the risk of overstimulating the uterus.
3. Use isotonic solutions
   Oxytocin has antidiuretic effects, which promote fluid retention. For most women who receive oxytocin, use lactated Ringer injection for oxytocin dilution and routine maintenance IV fluids.
4. Use a standard dilution
   Medication errors can be minimized by having only one concentration of oxytocin solution available on the labor and delivery unit. A pharmacy- or manufacturer-prepared solution of 30 units of oxytocin in 500 mL of lactated Ringer injection or physiological (normal) saline solution results in a concentration in which a pump setting of 1 mL/h delivers an infusion rate of 1 mU/min, and this 1:1 ratio is preserved with infusion rate increases. For example, with this oxytocin concentration, a 2-mL/h infusion rate results in 2 mU/min being delivered.
5. Select an appropriate route of administration
   - When used during the intrapartum period, oxytocin should be diluted before administration and delivered intravenously via an infusion pump.
   - IV administration of undiluted oxytocin can cause maternal hypotension and cardiac arrhythmia.
   - Undiluted oxytocin should not be administered by any route for induction or augmentation of labor.

6. Control the rate of IV infusion
   - Oxytocin should be provided in premixed preparations, and then the IV tubing should be flushed with the mixture.
   - Connect the oxytocin solution with a side port, at a point near the patient, of the main IV infusion line.
   - Use an IV pump to control the rate of infusion.
7. Control the rate of dosage increase

   The initial effect of a given dose (milliunits per minute) of oxytocin may occur within a few minutes. The maximum effect of a specific dose, however, may not be fully achieved for 30 to 45 minutes.

   Likewise, the initial effect of stopping an oxytocin infusion may be observed within a few minutes. Some effects, however, may last for 30 to 45 minutes after an oxytocin infusion is stopped or the rate is reduced.

   Reported initial infusion rates range from 1 to 6 mU/min (1–6 mL/h) with interval increases ranging also from 1 to 6 mU/min. The usual interval to increase the infusion rate ranges from 30 to 60 minutes. Regular increases are performed until the desired contraction pattern of 5 contractions in each 10-minute period is achieved. Each institution should have a single standard administration guideline for all patients.
8. Recognize limits of effectiveness

   If a patient has not established a satisfactory labor pattern after sufficient oxytocin administration, the plan of care should be reevaluated with the patient.

Self-test B

Now answer these questions to test yourself on the information in the last section.

B1. Which type of intravenous fluids should be delivered when oxytocin is administered?
_____

B2. True False In an emergency, an initial dose of oxytocin may be given by intravenous push, followed by a continuous infusion of dilute oxytocin.

B3. True False The more frequently the rate of oxytocin is increased, the more likely uterine tachysystole will occur.

B4. Thirty units of oxytocin in 500 mL of normal saline was prepared by your hospital pharmacy. What initial intravenous pump setting should be set to deliver 1 mU/min?
_____

How should the rate be changed to deliver 1.5 mU/min?
_____

B5. Normal labor has contractions with the following characteristics:

Frequency: _____

Duration: _____

Strength: _____

B6. Name at least 3 situations in which labor augmentation is not appropriate.
_____
_____
_____

B7. List at least 3 things you should keep in mind when administering oxytocin.
_____
_____
_____

B8. Given a normal maternal pelvis and term gestation, all of the following conditions are contraindications or relative contraindications to labor augmentation, except
   A. Hypotonic uterine dysfunction
   B. Face presentation
   C. Hydramnios
   D. Twins

B9. True False Fetal compromise is diagnosed when a laboring multiparous woman is at 8-cm cervical dilation and the fetus is at 0 station. To speed delivery, you should start an oxytocin infusion at 2 mU/min.

B10. True False Membranes should be ruptured so internal uterine pressure monitoring can be used whenever oxytocin is infused.

Check your answers with the list that follows the Recommended Routines. Correct any incorrect answers and review the appropriate section in the unit.

12. What complications may occur with oxytocin infusion?

A. Excessive uterine stimulation
  1. Cause
     Uterine tachysystole may develop because of PG medications used for cervical ripening or infusion of oxytocin for labor induction or augmentation.

     During oxytocin infusion, excessive uterine stimulation may occur because
     - A larger dose is given than is needed because the dose is too high or is increased too frequently. Most adverse responses to oxytocin infusion are dose related.
     or
     - The myometrium becomes more sensitive to a previously satisfactory dosage of oxytocin.

     Sometimes, after a normal labor pattern has been achieved and a stable infusion of oxytocin has been used for an hour or more, uterine tachysystole may develop unexpectedly. The myometrium becomes more receptive to oxytocin because more receptors, and corresponding muscle fibers, respond simultaneously to oxytocin. As a result, the same dosage of oxytocin may cause an increase in the number or strength of contractions. Many women will maintain active labor without the aid of oxytocin once active labor has been established, so it is reasonable to decrease the rate of infusion when this occurs.
  2. Risks
     a. Maternal risks
        - Lacerations of the cervix, vagina, or perineum (results from rapid propulsion of the fetus through the birth canal)
        - Uterine rupture (results from excessive strength of contractions; rare, particularly in the absence of a uterine scar)
     b. Fetal and neonatal risks
        The forces that accompany rapid transit through the birth canal or reduced placental perfusion can result in
        - Restricted placental blood flow
        - Fetal hypoxia
        - Birth trauma
        - Bruising
        - Intracranial bleeding (rare, more likely in preterm babies)
        - Need for resuscitation at birth
  3. Treatment
     If uterine tachysystole develops, labor may progress so rapidly that delivery will occur before the situation can be corrected. If recognized early, however, promptly stopping or reducing the oxytocin infusion may help. Immediate management depends on the fetal heart rate pattern.
     a. Normal fetal heart rate pattern
        Reduce the rate of the oxytocin infusion, usually by half.
     b. Abnormal fetal heart rate pattern
        - *Stop* the oxytocin infusion.
        - Consider administration of a tocolytic agent if excessive uterine activity and fetal heart rate pattern do not quickly resolve after other interventions (for example, terbutaline [0.25 mg, administered subcutaneously])

- Provide other measures of in utero resuscitation: Turn the woman onto her side or from one side to the other, provide an IV fluid bolus, and give oxygen by non-rebreather mask.

If contraction frequency decreases, uterine tonus returns to normal, and the concerning fetal heart rate pattern disappears, oxytocin may be restarted at a slower rate. In general, the infusion is restarted at half the rate that was being used when the excessive uterine stimulation developed, and the interval between rate increases is lengthened.

B. Water intoxication

As noted previously, oxytocin has an antidiuretic effect and should be mixed only in isotonic solutions. Although uncommon, if oxytocin is administered in IV fluids that contain glucose but no sodium, with prolonged administration of large doses, the antidiuretic effect of oxytocin may lead to retention of fluid without retention of sodium. The severe form of hyponatremia (low serum sodium level) is water intoxication.

Clinical signs of water intoxication begin with decreased urinary output and headache and may progress rapidly to mental confusion and seizures. These signs resemble the onset of eclampsia. The 2 signs can be differentiated by blood pressure (increased in eclampsia) and serum sodium level (low with water intoxication, within reference range in eclampsia).

Water intoxication should be avoided by
- Using only normal saline or a balanced salt solution for IV fluids
- Monitoring intake and output

If water intoxication occurs, severely restrict the volume of fluid given to the patient. Overly rapid correction of hyponatremia may lead to permanent neurological damage. Consult with regional perinatal center specialists.

13. How long should you continue an oxytocin infusion?

When oxytocin is used to induce or augment labor, the goal is to mimic the pattern of normal labor as closely as possible. Labor is normally *progressive,* with contractions becoming stronger and more frequent and lasting longer, as cervical dilation and fetal descent progress.

Oxytocin primarily stimulates the frequency of uterine contractions. Usually, but *not* always, contraction strength and duration increase with increased contraction frequency. Uterine contractions that have the characteristics of normal labor represent an appropriate and adequate response to oxytocin.

A. Induction of labor
1. Establishment of labor
   Throughout the course of the induction, the urgency of need for delivery should be periodically reassessed. If labor has not been established and maternal or fetal condition warrants delivery, cesarean delivery may be indicated. If the indication for delivery is less urgent, consider the option of discontinuing the oxytocin and allowing the woman to rest overnight. An attempt at induction may be repeated once or twice on successive days. If labor has not been established after 2 or 3 induction attempts, consider
   - Sending the patient home, if the mother and fetus are stable and the need for delivery is not urgent (eg, elective induction)
   - Rupturing the membranes (if you are prepared for cesarean delivery if labor does not ensue)
   - Performing a cesarean delivery

2. Management after labor is established
    - When contractions occur more frequently than every 2 minutes (from the start of one to the start of the next), their effectiveness in producing cervical effacement and dilation is likely to diminish. As soon as contractions are occurring every 2 to 3 minutes, maintain the oxytocin infusion at that rate, increasing it further if the contraction frequency decreases.
    - Generally, as labor progresses, less oxytocin is needed. The goal is to use the minimum effective dose of oxytocin to maintain a normal contraction pattern. After at least 6 cm cervical dilation has been reached and uterine activity is normal, consider reducing the rate of oxytocin infusion by approximately 10% to 25%.
    - If labor progress continues satisfactorily after 30 to 60 minutes of infusion at a lower rate, reduce the rate of oxytocin infusion again. The aim is to continue this "stair-step" system of decreasing the oxytocin until the infusion is stopped entirely, with labor continuing on its own.
    - Observe the uterine response carefully to be sure it does not decline. In some cases, reduction in the rate of oxytocin infusion will be accompanied by reduced labor quality. In this situation, the rate of oxytocin should be increased to the previous effective dosage.

B. Augmentation of labor

Augmentation of labor with an oxytocin infusion or artificial rupture of membranes may be used to increase the frequency or strength of contractions after the onset of spontaneous labor or contractions after spontaneous rupture of membranes. Adequate uterine response may be seen promptly, or the response may be delayed for 2 to 4 hours. Most women promptly resume normal labor progress if there are no other problems.

If a normal labor pattern is not achieved after 4 to 6 hours of oxytocin infusion, reassess the woman's condition and be sure there is no other cause for failure to progress, such as fetopelvic disproportion or fetal malposition.

Augmentation should be considered unsuccessful if
- A normal contraction pattern cannot be achieved after 6 or more hours of oxytocin infusion. Consider the use of an intrauterine pressure catheter to quantitatively assess contraction strength.

or

- Progress is not made after 4 hours of oxytocin infusion with a normal labor pattern and documentation of adequate uterine contraction with intrauterine pressure catheter, or 6 hours of oxytocin infusion with a normal labor pattern and no documentation of adequate uterine contractions.

If no other cause exists for failure to respond adequately to oxytocin augmentation, consider
- A period of rest and hydration

or

- Cesarean delivery

Self-test C

Now answer these questions to test yourself on the information in the last section.

C1. When contractions occur more often than every 2 minutes, their effectiveness in producing cervical dilation and effacement usually _____.

C2. Oxytocin primarily increases the _____ of contractions.

C3. True False When used for labor induction, the rate of oxytocin infusion should be increased every 15 minutes until 8-cm cervical dilation is achieved.

C4. True False When labor is being augmented, if there is no progress beyond 6 cm and there are 4 hours or more of adequate contractions or 6 hours or more of inadequate contractions, you should consider a cesarean delivery.

C5. Risks of excessive uterine stimulation include

Yes	No	
___	___	Uterine rupture
___	___	Birth trauma
___	___	Vaginal lacerations
___	___	Postpartum endometritis
___	___	Neonatal hypoglycemia
___	___	Intracranial bleeding in the newborn
___	___	Perineal tears
___	___	Fetal asphyxia

C6. What should you do if uterine tachysystole occurs when oxytocin is being infused? _____

C7. True False When oxytocin is used to induce labor, the urgency of the need for delivery should be reassessed periodically.

C8. True False In a patient undergoing oxytocin induction of labor, the dose that first brings about normal labor is the dose that should be maintained until delivery.

C9. True False Contraction strength and duration always increase when oxytocin is used to increase contraction frequency.

C10. True False Water intoxication is likely to occur if only balanced salt intravenous solutions are used with an oxytocin infusion.

C11. True False Whenever an oxytocin infusion is used, intake and output should be monitored.

Check your answers with the list that follows the Recommended Routines. Correct any incorrect answers and review the appropriate section in the unit.

INDUCING AND AUGMENTING LABOR

Recommended Routines

All the routines listed below are based on the principles of perinatal care presented in the unit you have just finished. They are recommended as part of routine perinatal care.

Read each routine carefully and decide whether it is standard operating procedure in your hospital. Check the appropriate blank next to each routine.

Procedure Standard in My Hospital	Needs Discussion by Our Staff	Recommended Routine
_____	_____	1. Establish a protocol for patient care and monitoring when prostaglandins are used for cervical ripening.
_____	_____	2. Establish a system to identify and record the reasons for use of oxytocin and the evaluation done to rule out contraindications, whenever labor is induced or augmented.
_____	_____	3. Establish protocols for the use of oxytocin that include • Uniform dilution of oxytocin for intravenous administration • A standard interval for the rate of intravenous oxytocin infusion change (increase and decrease) • Administration of oxytocin only by the intravenous route for labor induction or augmentation
_____	_____	4. Establish a flow sheet for the administration of oxytocin that shows the dosage rate of oxytocin (milliunits per minute), and every change in the rate, with the corresponding • Time • Maternal vital signs • Fetal heart rate and pattern • Contraction frequency, duration, and strength • Uterine tonus
_____	_____	5. Establish guidelines for staffing and personnel availability whenever oxytocin is given, including • Nurse to patient ratio • Attending physician or certified nurse midwife • Surgical and anesthesia staff • Continuous electronic fetal heart rate and uterine contraction monitoring
_____	_____	6. Establish guidelines for the response to uterine tachysystole.
_____	_____	7. Develop a system whereby an emergency cesarean delivery can be started within 30 minutes of the decision to operate, at any time of the day or night.

Self-test Answers

These are the answers to the Self-test questions. Please check them with the answers you gave and review the information in the unit wherever necessary.

Self-test A

A1. D. Post-term pregnancy

A2. A Bishop score is calculated to indicate the likelihood that an attempt at induction of labor will be successful and when cervical ripening is likely to be most helpful.

A3. A Bishop score of 7 indicates *it is likely that an induction of labor will be successful.*

A4. Any of the following actions may be done:
  - Cervical ripening with a prostaglandin preparation
  - Stripping of the membranes
  - Mechanical dilators

A5. A. Closed *(0)*, soft *(2)*, posterior position *(0)*, and 50% effaced *(1)*, with the fetus at −2 station *(1)*; *total score: 4*

  B. 3-cm dilated *(2)*, soft *(2)*, anterior position *(2)*, and 70% effaced *(2)*, with the fetus at 0 station *(2)*; *total score: 10*

A6. Any 2 of the following situations:
  - Prelabor rupture of membranes, when delivery is indicated
  - Chorioamnionitis
  - Complicated gestational hypertension or preeclampsia
  - Maternal medical illness with evidence of declining maternal or fetal health
  - Fetal jeopardy as demonstrated by tests of fetal growth or well-being
  - Placental abruption (grade 1 with no fetal compromise or grade 3 with fetal death and a stable woman)
  - Fetus approaching post-term gestation (when dates are certain, consider induction at 41 weeks of gestation; undertake induction at 42 weeks)
  - Fetal death
  - Woman at 39 or more weeks of gestation, with a history of rapid labor(s) and geographic difficulties in reaching a hospital
  - Other, various, uncommon individual indications

A7. Any 2 of the following contraindications:
  - Cervical infection
  - Active genital herpes infection
  - Recent unexplained vaginal bleeding

A8. The main risk associated with cervical ripening is *uterine tachysystole*.

A9. False *Reason:* Repeated use of a dinoprostone vaginal insert is not recommended. Dinoprostone gel may be repeated 2 or 3 times (with 6–8 hours of rest between applications), but the total dose should not exceed 1.5 mg in 24 hours.

A10. False *Reason:* A period of rest should follow the use of any of the prostaglandin cervical ripening agents.

Self-test B

B1. Isotonic solutions—physiological (normal) saline solution or other fluid that contains sodium

B2. False   *Reason:* Intravenous push of undiluted oxytocin can cause maternal hypotension and cardiac arrhythmia.

B3. True

B4. Initial intravenous rate = 1.0 mL/h; rate to deliver 1.5 mU/min = intravenous rate of 1.5 mL/h

B5. Frequency: every 2 to 3 minutes (3–5 contractions in 10 minutes)
Duration: 45 to 70 seconds
Strength: strong at palpation (or 50 mm Hg measured with an internal monitor)

B6. Any 3 of the following situations:
- When labor is normal
- When fetopelvic disproportion is present
- Generally, for any of the situations when labor induction is not recommended
- When hypertonic uterine inertia is present
- When there is fetal intolerance to labor

B7. Any 3 of the following things:
- Individualize the dosage.
- Recognize the risk of uterine tachysystole.
- Use a standard dilution.
- Use isotonic solutions.
- Select an appropriate route of administration.
- Control the rate of intravenous infusion.
- Calculate the intravenous rate for milliunits per minute dosage.
- Control the rate of dosage increase.
- Recognize the limits of effectiveness.

B8. A. Hypotonic uterine dysfunction

B9. False   *Reason:* Oxytocin will increase the frequency, and usually the strength and duration, of contractions. Any or all of these effects may limit placental blood flow and thereby worsen the fetal response. Oxytocin should not be used when there is evidence of fetal compromise.

B10. False   *Reason:* Prolonged rupture of membranes increases the risk of infection for the woman and the newborn. Artificial rupture of membranes should not be done unless you are willing and prepared to perform a cesarean delivery if the induction attempt fails. Intrauterine pressure monitoring should only be used when indicated. It is not required for all patients who receive oxytocin.

Self-test C

C1. When contractions occur more often than every 2 minutes, their effectiveness in producing cervical dilation and effacement usually *decreases or diminishes*.

C2. Oxytocin primarily increases the *frequency* of contractions.

C3. False *Reason:* The dose should be increased by 1 to 2 mU/min every 30 to 60 minutes until a regular contraction pattern (contractions every 2–3 minutes) is achieved and sustained.

C4. True

C5.

Yes	No	
X	___	Uterine rupture
X	___	Birth trauma
X	___	Vaginal lacerations
___	X	Postpartum endometritis
___	X	Neonatal hypoglycemia
X	___	Intracranial bleeding in the newborn
X	___	Perineal tears
X	___	Fetal asphyxia

C6. Immediately reduce the rate of oxytocin infusion, usually by half. Maternal hydration, administration of oxygen, and lateral positioning may also be useful.

C7. True

C8. False *Reason:* Generally, less and less oxytocin is needed once labor becomes established. After 6-cm cervical dilation is achieved, you should begin to reduce the amount of oxytocin infused. In most cases, but not all, the oxytocin can be reduced in increments until it is stopped completely, with labor progressing on its own. Occasionally, labor quality declines and oxytocin needs to be continued until delivery occurs. You should observe uterine response closely and use the minimum amount of oxytocin to maintain a normal labor pattern.

C9. False *Reason:* Oxytocin works primarily by increasing contraction frequency. Contraction strength and duration usually, but not always, increase with increased contraction frequency.

C10. False *Reason:* Only normal saline solution or balanced salt solutions should be used with oxytocin infusion to avoid the possibility of water intoxication.

C11. True

Unit 10 Posttest

After completion of each unit there is a free online posttest available at www.cmevillage.com to test your understanding. Navigate to the PCEP pages on www.cmevillage.com and register to take the free posttests.

Once registered on the website and after completing all the unit posttests, pay the book exam fee ($15) and pass the test at 80% or greater to earn continuing education credits. Only start the PCEP book exam if you have time to complete it. If you take the book exam and are not connected to a printer, either print your certificate to a .pdf file and save it to print later or come back to www.cmevillage.com at any time and print a copy of your educational transcript.

Credits are only available by book, not by individual unit within the books. Available credits for completion of each book exam are as follows: Book 1: 14.5 credits; Book 2: 16 credits; Book 3: 17 credits; Book 4: 9 credits.

For more details, navigate to the PCEP webpages at www.cmevillage.com.

Unit 11: Abnormal Labor Progress and Difficult Deliveries

Objectives 347

1. How is labor diagnosed? 351
2. What is the normal progress of labor? 351
3. What constitutes abnormal labor? 354
4. What are the risks of abnormal labor? 354
5. When should you suspect abnormal labor? 357
6. What are the causes of abnormal labor? 359
7. How should you investigate abnormal progress during labor? 360
8. How is abnormal labor treated? 366
9. What are operative vaginal deliveries? 377
10. When are operative vaginal deliveries performed, and what can you do to make them safe? 379
11. What are the maternal risks of prolonged labor or difficult delivery? 383
12. What are the fetal and neonatal risks of prolonged labor? 383
13. How do you recognize and treat rapid labor? 384
14. How should you handle emergent, or potentially emergent, conditions during labor? 387
15. How should you manage an abnormal third stage of labor? 394

Tables and Figures

- Table 11.1. Characteristics of Latent and Active Labor 351
- Table 11.2. Characteristics of Normal Spontaneous Labor 355
- Table 11.3. Causes of Delay in Labor Progress 360
- Table 11.4. Characteristics of Uterine Dysfunction 361
- Table 11.5. Suggested Response to Delay of Labor Progress 374
- Figure 11.1. Labor Curves: Normal Progress, First Stage of Labor 358
- Figure 11.2. Labor Curves: Normal and Abnormal Progress for a Nullipara Woman During the First Stage of Labor 358
- Figure 11.3. Positioning of the Fetus During Labor 362
- Figure 11.4. Clinical Pelvimetry: Measurement of Diagonal Conjugate 363
- Figure 11.5. Face Presentation With the Mentum (Chin) Posterior 368

Figure 11.6. Spontaneous Rotation of Face Presentation During Descent 368

Figure 11.7. Application of Forceps Blades for an Outlet Delivery 377

Figure 11.8. Thigh Flexion for Treatment of Shoulder Dystocia 391

Figure 11.9. Shoulder Rotation for Treatment of Shoulder Dystocia 392

Figure 11.10. Delivery of the Posterior Arm 393

Recommended Routines **397**

UNIT 11: ABNORMAL LABOR PROGRESS AND DIFFICULT DELIVERIES

Objectives

In this unit you will learn

A. How to differentiate latent from active labor

B. What maternal, fetal, and neonatal risks accompany abnormal labor

C. How to recognize normal and abnormal labor progress

D. When and how to investigate abnormal labor progress

E. How to treat the causes of abnormal labor

F. When forceps or a vacuum extractor is used and how to ensure safe application

G. How to respond to emergent, or potentially emergent, fetal conditions, including

- Meconium-stained amniotic fluid
- Fetal heart rate abnormalities
- Complications of maternal analgesia or anesthesia
- Prolapsed umbilical cord
- Shoulder dystocia

H. How to identify and manage an abnormal third stage of labor

Unit 11 Pretest

Before reading the unit, please answer the following questions. Select the *one best* answer to each question (unless otherwise instructed). Record your answers on the test and check them against the answers at the end of the book.

1. Shoulder dystocia occurs more commonly in all of the following conditions, except
    A. Fetal macrosomia
    B. Late term gestation
    C. Maternal diabetes
    D. Vaginal birth after cesarean delivery

2. You see the sudden onset of severe variable decelerations on a fetal heart rate tracing. Of the following actions, what is the *first* thing you should do?
    A. Check for umbilical cord prolapse.
    B. Check the woman's blood pressure.
    C. Prepare to administer a tocolytic medication.
    D. Prepare for emergency cesarean delivery.

3. **True / False** — With meconium-stained amniotic fluid, the baby's mouth and nose should be suctioned after delivery of the head, but before delivery of the shoulders.

4. **True / False** — Narcotics given to a laboring woman may cause minimal or absent fetal heart rate variability.

5. **True / False** — Face presentation puts a baby at risk for spinal cord injury.

6. **True / False** — The fetal head should be engaged before a forceps delivery is attempted.

7. **True / False** — Once normal fetal size, presentation, and position and adequate pelvic size have been determined, oxytocin augmentation is the treatment of choice for hypertonic uterine dysfunction.

8. **True / False** — When cord prolapse occurs, one appropriate way to elevate the presenting part off of the cord is to fill the woman's bladder with 500 mL of sterile saline and have her assume the knee-chest position.

9. **True / False** — Contraction quality is poor, but baseline tonus is usually increased with hypotonic uterine dysfunction.

10. Which of the following conditions should *always* be present before forceps or vacuum extraction delivery is attempted?

Yes	No	
___	___	Estimated fetal weight of 4,000 g (8 lb 13 oz) or more
___	___	Adequate maternal anesthesia
___	___	Complete cervical dilation
___	___	Evaluation of fetal size, presentation, and position
___	___	Oxytocin augmentation of labor

UNIT 11: ABNORMAL LABOR PROGRESS AND DIFFICULT DELIVERIES

11. In which of the following situations is oxytocin augmentation of labor likely to be useful (assuming normal fetal size, presentation, and position and normal pelvic size are present)?

Yes	No	
___	___	Arrested second stage with normal contraction pattern
___	___	Hypotonic uterine dysfunction during the active phase
___	___	Hypertonic uterine dysfunction during the latent phase
___	___	Maternal fatigue with weak pushing efforts but normal labor pattern

12. Maternal risks of rapid labor include all of the following complications, except
  A. Postpartum hemorrhage
  B. Postpartum endometritis
  C. Lacerations of the birth canal
  D. Uterine atony

13. Which of the following interventions are appropriate when rapid cervical dilation is occurring and rapid delivery is anticipated?

Yes	No	
___	___	Begin broad-spectrum antibiotics.
___	___	Investigate for placental abruption.
___	___	Check cervical dilation frequently.
___	___	Prepare for delivery.
___	___	Anticipate the need for neonatal resuscitation.
___	___	Place the woman in reverse Trendelenburg position.
___	___	Administer large doses of narcotic analgesia to the laboring woman.

14. Which of the following are associated with vaginal breech delivery?

Yes	No	
___	___	Placental abruption
___	___	Birth trauma
___	___	Growth-restricted fetus
___	___	Prolapsed umbilical cord

15. True False If there is excessive bleeding during the third stage of labor, oxytocin should be administered to cause the uterus to contract and expel the placenta.

16. True False The second stage of labor normally lasts 6 hours or longer.

17. True False Oxytocin infusion may be appropriate treatment for second-stage arrest of labor.

18. True False If delivery of the placenta does not occur within 30 minutes of delivery of the baby, but there is no evidence of vaginal bleeding, it is best to wait for spontaneous delivery of the placenta.

(continued)

Unit 11 Pretest (*continued*)

19. True False Ultrasonographic estimation of fetal weight is less accurate when the fetal head is deep in the woman's pelvis.

20. True False The hallmark of active labor is contractions with progressive cervical dilation.

21. True False Goiter and tumors of the fetal neck are associated with an increased likelihood of a fetus being in face or brow presentation.

22. True False The most common cause of prolonged labor is breech presentation.

23. True False A woman is exhausted and can no longer push effectively. The fetus is vertex, right occiput posterior, at +3 station. Manual rotation of the head and low forceps delivery is one appropriate approach to this situation.

24. True False Artificially rupturing the membranes to stimulate labor in a woman with a prolonged latent phase will require a cesarean delivery if labor does not progress.

25. True False When fetal gestational age is 34 weeks or less and an operative vaginal delivery is indicated, a vacuum extractor is preferred to forceps.

26. Which of the following conditions is *most* likely to be a cause of a prolonged latent phase?
    A. Fetal malformation
    B. Uterine fibroids
    C. Excessive maternal sedation
    D. Grand multiparity

27. Which of the following conditions is the *best* indication of active labor?
    A. Regular contractions
    B. Rupture of membranes
    C. Painful contractions
    D. Cervical dilation

28. Once labor becomes established, clues to abnormal progress include all of the following situations, except
    A. The cervix becomes edematous.
    B. The fetal presenting part remains unengaged.
    C. Contractions occur every minute.
    D. Cervical dilation averages 1.5 cm/h.

29. Evaluation of a prolonged active phase reveals fetal hydrocephalus. The fetus is vertex, with a reassuring fetal heart rate pattern. Which of the following actions are appropriate to take?

Yes	No	
___	___	Begin oxytocin augmentation.
___	___	Drain the hydrocephalus with a needle and monitor labor for fetal descent.
___	___	Advise the parent or parents that hydrocephalus is a fatal malformation.
___	___	Perform cesarean delivery.

UNIT 11: ABNORMAL LABOR PROGRESS AND DIFFICULT DELIVERIES

1. How is labor diagnosed?

During the last few weeks of pregnancy, there is a gradual increase in uterine activity that leads to the onset of labor. Pregnant women observe that the irregular contractions they have been experiencing begin to increase in regularity and intensity. The contractions can gradually become more painful. Obstetric caregivers document the onset of active labor by identifying progressive cervical dilation, which is almost always accompanied by painful and palpable uterine contractions. A woman whose cervix is dilated 6 cm or more on arrival at a hospital can be assumed to be in labor.

Women with less than 6 cm of cervical dilation may or may not be in active labor. A woman in latent labor may be experiencing painful contractions with little or no cervical dilation. A period of observation is needed. The general characteristics of false labor and true labor are listed in Table 11.1.

Table 11.1. Characteristics of Latent and Active Labor	
False Labor	**True Labor**
Uterine Contractions	
• Usually irregular but can become regular • Duration varies • Strength varies • Wane or cease over time	• Increasingly regular • Increasing duration • Increasing strength • Persistent
Cervical Dilation	
• No change	• Cervical change present

If contractions continue, but the cervix has not begun to change progressively after observation and monitoring for 1 to 2 hours, the woman remains in the latent phase of labor. If contractions cease, labor has not yet begun. Women in latent labor may not need to be observed continuously in a health care setting. Unless there are specific risk factors or other contraindications, these women may be discharged, with instructions for changes that should prompt them to return to the hospital.

Diagnosing and monitoring labor involves performing vaginal examinations on the woman. Her consent or permission to perform these examinations should be obtained before each examination.

2. What is the normal progress of labor?

A. Time of onset
   The exact time at which labor begins is often difficult to determine. Establishing the time of labor onset is important only when it is needed to determine that labor is prolonged. In many cases, the time of hospital admission is used as the time of onset of labor. However, this may not be accurate if a woman began having regular uterine contractions hours before arrival at the hospital.

B. Contraction pattern
   Normal contraction frequency, duration, and strength are described in Unit 10, Inducing and Augmenting Labor, in this book.

C. Stages of labor

Normal labor usually progresses in a predictable pattern. Uterine contractions become more frequent, last longer, are accompanied by more discomfort, and are associated with identifiable changes in the maternal cervix and fetal station.

1. First stage of labor

   The first stage of labor is divided into 2 phases that span the time from the onset of labor until the cervix is completely dilated.

   a. Latent phase

   The latent phase begins with the onset of regular contractions and ends when the cervix begins to dilate at a more rapid rate. Most of the work of uterine contractions during the latent phase goes to softening and effacing the cervix. The length of the latent phase varies widely among women. The transition from the latent phase to the active phase occurs at approximately 6 cm of cervical dilation.

   Hospital admission often occurs during the latter part of the latent phase. It is important for health professionals to understand that progression of cervical dilation from 4 cm to 6 cm may take 6 hours or more in women having a normal labor.

   b. Active phase

   This begins when the cervix starts to dilate more rapidly and ends with complete dilation of the cervix. Most of the work of uterine contractions during the active phase goes to cervical dilation. During the active phase, each centimeter of cervical dilation may occur over 30 to 90 minutes in women progressing normally.

   Fetal descent is usually minimal during the first stage of labor, often just 1 to 2 cm. Most women will not feel the urge to push until the cervix is fully dilated and the second stage of labor has been reached. Some women will have an urge to push earlier, late in the first stage. Strong pushing efforts prior to full cervical dilation should be avoided, as they can lead to cervical edema and subsequent laceration, as well as maternal exhaustion.

    The critical feature of progress in the first stage of labor is cervical dilation.

2. Second stage of labor

   This stage begins with complete dilation of the cervix and ends with delivery of the baby.

   a. Descent

   Cervical dilation is said to be *complete, full,* or *10 cm* when no cervix around the presenting fetal part can be felt by the examiner's finger. With the resistance of the cervix gone, fetal descent is more rapid because maternal pelvic structures are less resistant to pressure applied to the presenting part. With the continued pressure of uterine contractions, plus the added force of maternal pushing efforts, the presenting part descends deeper into the woman's pelvis.

   b. Rotation

   The fetal head normally enters the true pelvis in a flexed attitude, with the chin close to the chest. The posterior fontanel and sagittal suture are the landmarks most easily felt during vaginal examination.

The occipitofrontal diameter of the fetal head (from the forehead to the back of the skull) is greater than the biparietal (transverse) diameter. Because the maternal pelvis is usually wider transversely at the inlet, the head enters the pelvis with the sagittal suture oriented transversely and the posterior fontanel oriented toward the left or right side of the pregnant woman's pelvis (occiput transverse position).

The pelvis becomes narrower below the inlet and is narrowest between the ischial spines. At that point, the largest diameter of the pelvis is from the symphysis to the sacrum (anterior to posterior). This creates a twisting funnel through which the fetus must pass. As fetal station approaches the level of the ischial spines, the downward pressure on the fetus forces the longer part of the head to rotate to the largest diameter of the maternal pelvis. Thus, the head rotates 90° to *occiput anterior* or *occiput posterior*. The sagittal suture is now oriented anteroposterior rather than transverse. This process of the fetal head turning, as labor progresses, to accommodate the size and shape of the maternal pelvis is referred to as *internal rotation*.

As long as contractions remain strong and the woman pushes well, rotation and descent will progress if the size of the pelvis and the fetus and the position of the fetal presenting part allow it.

The second stage of labor can be separated into passive and active phases. During the passive phase, uterine activity leads to passive descent of the fetal head. The active phase is also known as the *expulsive phase,* and it involves pushing and bearing down from the patient.

Guidelines exist that define the acceptable duration of the second stage of labor, but it is reasonable and acceptable to exceed those guidelines if the probability of a vaginal delivery is high and clinical judgement establishes that adequate progress is being made and fetal monitoring remains reassuring. There is no consistent relationship between any specific duration of the second stage of labor and maternal and/or neonatal adverse outcomes. However, there does appear to be consensus that the passive phase is not implicated in adverse outcomes, other than its contribution to the overall duration of the second stage of labor. A period of passive second stage may provide maternal benefit, but this is not corroborated in the literature.

 The critical feature of progress in the second stage of labor is descent of the fetal presenting part.

3. Third stage of labor
   This stage begins after the birth of the baby and ends when the placenta is delivered. Delivery of the placenta usually occurs 5 to 10 minutes after delivery of the baby. If it does not occur spontaneously within 30 minutes, manual removal of the placenta is most often needed.
4. Fourth stage of labor
   The fourth stage is not a classic stage of labor but is used to identify the period that begins after delivery of the placenta and ends 1 hour later.

   During this time, the uterus contracts normally to prevent excessive postpartum bleeding. It is the time when postpartum hemorrhage occurs most often and is therefore the time after delivery when careful observation and monitoring of the maternal condition is especially important.

3. What constitutes abnormal labor?

Labor is abnormal if it progresses either more slowly or more rapidly than normal. Abnormally slow labor is more common than abnormally rapid labor, but in both cases, abnormal labor progress is associated with risks for a woman and her fetus. *Slow labor* can be

- *Protracted* (slow rate of progress)
- *Prolonged* (long time for progress to occur)
- *Arrested* (progress stops)

Rapid labor is also abnormal and is defined as completion of labor and vaginal birth within 3 hours of the first contraction.

   A. First stage/cervical dilation

      Dilation is protracted when cervical dilation is slower than the normal rate, prolonged if dilation does not progress within a specified period, or arrested if dilation stops entirely.

   B. Second stage/fetal descent
- For nulliparous women, allow up to 4 hours for the second stage or 3 hours of pushing prior to diagnosing arrest of labor.
- For multiparous women, allow up to 3 hours for the second stage or 2 hours of pushing prior to diagnosing arrest of labor.

      For most women, the second stage of labor lasts less than 2 hours. Longer durations of the second stage may be acceptable, as long as progress (fetal descent) is being made and the woman and the fetus remain stable, with a normal fetal heart rate pattern.

      Table 11.2 lists the characteristics of labor, including the normal rate of progress and the length of each stage and phase.

4. What are the risks of abnormal labor?

All labor carries risks of morbidity and mortality for the woman and the fetus. When labor progresses normally, risks are minimal. When labor progress is delayed or extremely rapid, the risks increase.

Intervention into the physiological process of labor, however, also carries risks. The risks that accompany medical intervention must be weighed against the risks that accompany continued observation of suspected abnormal labor. The goal of medical intervention in the process of labor should be to reduce the risks to the woman and the fetus.

When labor progress is abnormal—particularly when it is abnormally slow—there may be more than one cause. When more than one cause is present, the effect of each abnormality is magnified, and the likelihood of successful vaginal delivery is significantly reduced.

Table 11.2. Characteristics of Normal Spontaneous Labor				
Period	**Defining Events**	**Cervical Dilation**	**Duration (Nullipara)**	**Duration (Multipara)**
First stage	Onset of labor until complete cervical dilation. Cervical dilation and effacement and fetal descent occur.	0–10 cm		
Latent phase	Onset of contractions until beginning of the active phase. Progress may occur at very slow rates.	0–6 cm	Up to 20 h[a]	Up to 14 h[a]
Active phase	Onset of predictable rate of cervical dilation	6–10 cm	Up to 8 h Up to 10 h with an epidural 0.5–1.0 cm/h	Up to 6 h Up to 8 h with an epidural 1.0–1.5 cm/h
Second stage	Complete dilation of the cervix until delivery of the baby		Up to 5 h 1-cm descent per hour	Up to 5 h 2-cm descent per hour
			If descent is continuing to occur and mother and baby are stable, it is not necessary to place a time limit on the duration of the second stage.	
Third stage	Delivery of the baby until delivery of the placenta		Up to 30 min	Up to 30 min
Fourth stage	First hour after delivery of the placenta		Not a traditional stage of labor but represents the period during which postpartum hemorrhage is most likely to occur.	

[a] The duration of latent labor may be longer when labor is being induced.

Self-test A

Now answer these questions to test yourself on the information in the last section.

A1. True   False   The contractions of false labor do not persist or cause progressive cervical dilation.

A2. True   False   If a woman enters a hospital with contractions and cervical dilation of 6 cm or more, she can be assumed to be in true labor.

A3. An active phase of labor with cervical dilation progressing at a rate of 0.8 cm/h would be called a(n) _____ active phase.

A4. An active phase that lasted longer than 6 hours would be called a(n) _____ active phase.

A5. When the cervix is completely dilated, but fetal station does not change during a 2-hour period, it is called _____.

A6. Describe the stages of labor.

The first stage of labor starts with the onset of labor and continues until _____.

The second stage of labor starts with _____ and continues until _____.

The third stage of labor starts after _____ and ends with _____.

The "fourth stage" of labor starts after _____ and ends _____. It is the time when the risk of postpartum hemorrhage is the _____.

A7. Normal cervical dilation during the **active phase** of labor in a nullipara woman is _____ cm/h and in a multipara woman is _____ cm/h.

A8. Normal duration of the **active phase** of labor in a nullipara woman is _____ hours or less and in a multigravida woman is _____ hours or less.

A9. Usual duration of the **second** stage of labor in a nullipara woman is _____ hours or less and in a multigravida woman is _____ hours or less.

A10. The critical feature of progress in the first stage of labor is _____ and in the second stage of labor is _____.

Check your answers with the list that follows the Recommended Routines. Correct any incorrect answers and review the appropriate section in the unit.

5. When should you suspect abnormal labor?

A. Clinical clues

If prolonged labor occurred in one pregnancy, it is likely to recur in subsequent pregnancies. There is also an increased risk for rapid labor to recur. Although the risk for recurrence of abnormal labor is increased, labor in a subsequent pregnancy may also progress normally.

Once labor begins, signs of abnormal labor progress may be found long before a diagnosis can be established. Recognizing the clues enables you to anticipate that labor may not progress well, identify a problem early, and prepare for treatment that may be needed.

The following 7 factors may indicate that labor will not progress normally.
- *Poor application of the fetal head to the cervix:* suggests fetopelvic disproportion (FPD)
- *Deflexed fetal head:* indicates FPD may be present
- *Unengaged fetal head:* indicates FPD may be present
- *Low-intensity contractions:* indicates hypotonic uterine dysfunction may be present
- *Continuous contractions, seemingly without uterine relaxation:* indicates hypertonic dysfunction
- *Edema of the cervix:* indicates FPD, with the fetal head compressing the cervix against the pelvic bones, thus limiting lymphatic return in the lower portion of the cervix
- *Pushing uncontrollably before complete dilation:* indicates occiput posterior, with the occiput pushing the rectum against the sacrum, thus giving the woman the sensation of an urge to push

B. Labor progress curve

The labor of any woman may be plotted on a graph (a "partogram") that shows a normal labor pattern (nullipara and multipara women are plotted separately, on their respective normal curves). If the resulting curve deviates significantly from the general, normal pattern, further investigation into the progress of labor is recommended.

Normal labor patterns are shown in Figure 11.1. For most women, labor begins before the time of hospital admission; therefore, much of the latent phase may not be included in the graph.

Figure 11.2 shows another normal labor curve for a nullipara woman, plus plots for 3 abnormal labors. This graph shows hospital admission earlier in the course of labor than is shown in Figure 11.1. Therefore, more of the latent phase is seen.

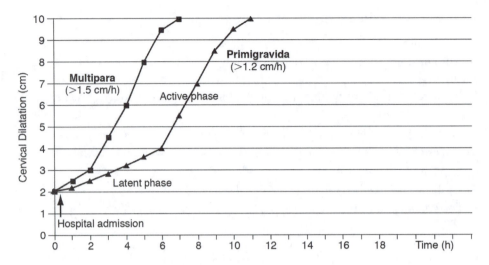

Figure 11.1. Labor Curves: Normal Progress, First Stage of Labor

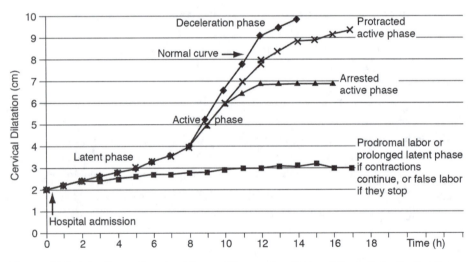

Figure 11.2. Labor Curves: Normal and Abnormal Progress for a Nullipara Woman During the First Stage of Labor

6. What are the causes of abnormal labor?

A significant proportion of abnormal labor progress can be attributed to a problem, or a combination of problems, with

- Maternal pelvic size or shape (passage)
- Fetal size, position, or presentation (passenger)
- Contraction strength and effectiveness (power)

Keep the 3 P's in mind.
- *Passage*
- *Passenger*
- *Power*

Some factors can cause delay in labor progress at more than one point in labor. In addition, it is common for a combination of factors to be responsible for abnormal progress. For example, slightly large fetal size and a mild degree of pelvic contraction may, together, result in arrest of fetal descent. It is not always possible to determine which factor, or combination of factors, is the cause of abnormal labor.

A fourth P, for *psyche*, has been proposed as an important factor in assessing labor progress. A woman's state of mind and how she perceives her accomplishments in labor may be influenced by

- The woman's level of fear
- Her understanding of the labor process
- Her confidence in her ability to cope with labor and parenthood
- The support she receives from her family and others
- The response she receives from health professionals
- The labor environment

For women who feel overwhelmed by labor, the psychological stress added to the physical stress may interfere with normal labor progress.

Despite normal pelvic size, normal fetal position and size, and normal uterine contractions, labor will not progress normally in some women.

Possible causes of delayed labor progress are listed in Table 11.3, along with the period of labor in which they are likely to occur. Psychological influences, although important, are difficult to isolate or quantify and are not listed.

Table 11.3. Causes of Delay in Labor Progress

Period	Uterine Dysfunction (Power)	Fetopelvic Disproportion (Passage)	Fetal Position (Passenger)	Other Causes
Stage 1: Cervical Dilation				
Prolonged *latent phase*	Hypotonic (uncommon) or hypertonic (uncommon)	Uncommon	Uncommon	False labor; induced labor
Prolonged or arrested *active phase*	Hypotonic (common) or hypertonic (uncommon)	Common	Uncommon	Uterine overdistension: check for hydramnios, twins
Prolonged *deceleration phase*	Hypotonic (common) or hypertonic (rare)	Common	Common[a]	Occiput posterior
Stage 2: Fetal Descent				
Prolonged or arrested *descent*	Hypotonic (uncommon) or hypertonic (rare)	Common	Common[a]	Inadequate pushing; excessive sedation or anesthesia; fetal malposition or malformation (rare)

[a] Fetopelvic disproportion (smaller pelvis or larger fetus) is the cause in about one-half of the patients who develop delay in labor progress at this point. Fetal malformations or tumors also may obstruct passage through the birth canal (hydrocephalus is the malformation most often associated with fetopelvic disproportion).

Note: Uterine dysfunction delays cervical dilation. Fetopelvic disproportion and abnormal fetal positions primarily interfere with descent of the presenting part. Uterine dysfunction and fetopelvic disproportion may be present at the same time.

7. How should you investigate abnormal progress during labor?

 Investigate all causes. More than one cause of abnormal labor may be present.

A. Power: assess uterine contractions
   Power relates to uterine contractions and, in the second stage, to maternal pushing efforts.
   - Has labor definitely begun? If not, see Section 1, How is labor diagnosed? for the management of early labor.
   - If labor is in the *latent phase,* was the labor *induced*? If so, this phase may take longer than when labor has a spontaneous onset, and some portion occurs before hospital admission.
   - Is *contraction quality* normal?
     — *If yes*, investigate other causes of abnormal labor.
     — *If no*, determine whether hypotonic or hypertonic uterine dysfunction is present (Table 11.4) and treat accordingly.
     — *If uncertain* and membranes are *already* ruptured and there are no contraindications to internal monitoring, consider inserting an intrauterine pressure catheter to allow more precise evaluation of uterine function.

UNIT 11: ABNORMAL LABOR PROGRESS AND DIFFICULT DELIVERIES

Table 11.4. Characteristics of Uterine Dysfunction		
Characteristic	**Hypotonic (Common)**	**Hypertonic (Rare)**
Contractions	Poor quality, low intensity, irregular	Irregular; may be nearly continuous with little relaxation; difficult to time onset and end; quality of contractions often does not match with patient's perception of pain.
Baseline tonus	Normal	Usually increased
Pain	Minimal	Continuous, usually felt in the back; often out of proportion to contraction strength
Fetal heart rate abnormalities	Rare	Frequently coincident
Oxytocin	Usually helpful in achieving normal labor	Usually not useful

 Do not rupture the membranes artificially unless you are committed to delivery at this time. You must be prepared to perform a cesarean delivery if labor does not progress after rupturing the membranes.

- If *hypotonic contractions* are present, is the uterus overdistended? Check for twins or polyhydramnios.
- Is the fetus in vertex presentation with the *occiput posterior*? Occiput posterior may be associated with a prolonged deceleration phase late in the first stage or delay in descent during the second stage of labor.
- If labor is in the *second stage*:
  — Is *epidural or spinal anesthesia* (may slow the second stage) being used?
  — Is there *excessive maternal sedation*?
  — Is maternal *pushing ineffective*?

B. Passenger: determine the size and position of the fetus
When there is significant delay in the progress of labor, reevaluate the size, presentation, and position of the fetus. Look for findings that might have been overlooked in earlier examination(s) and for things that might have changed.

Fetal lie refers to the orientation of the fetal long axis to the woman's spine, by using the spinal columns as reference points. A longitudinal lie is present when the spines of the woman and fetus are parallel to each other; both vertex and breech presentation are longitudinal lies. Transverse lie is present when the fetal spine is perpendicular to the maternal spine and the fetal spine or abdomen and small parts are the presenting part.

Presentation refers to the part of the fetus that leads into the pelvis. The general term for a fetus whose head is presenting above the pelvis is *cephalic presentation*. Vertex presentation refers to the crown of the head presenting with the fetal neck flexed. The fetal face or brow may also be the presenting part if the fetal neck is extended. Buttocks first is called a *breech presentation* but also may be labeled more specifically as *frank, complete, footling,* or *double footling,* depending on the exact presentation (see Section 8, How is abnormal labor treated?).

PCEP BOOK 2: MATERNAL AND FETAL CARE

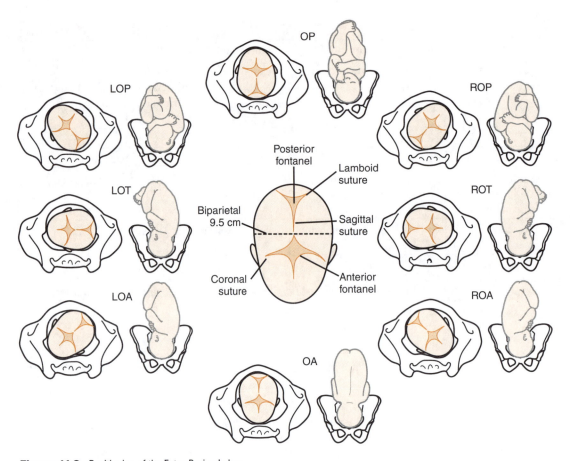

Figure 11.3. Positioning of the Fetus During Labor
LOA, left occiput anterior; LOP, left occiput posterior; LOT, left occiput transverse; OA, occiput anterior; OP, occiput posterior; ROA, right occiput anterior; ROP, right occiput posterior; ROT, right occiput transverse.

Position refers to the relationship of the fetal presenting part to the maternal pelvis. For example, a normal vertex presentation may be left occiput anterior, right occiput anterior, or right or left occiput posterior (Figure 11.3).

1. Clinical evaluation
   a. Palpate the maternal abdomen
      - Recheck Leopold maneuvers to determine fetal lie and presentation.
      - Reassess the size of the fetus.
   b. Perform digital vaginal examination
      This helps identify the presenting part and its position and determine fetal station. Be especially careful if an abnormal presentation is suspected.

 While vertex presentation, with the occiput being the leading part, is the most common presentation by far, the fetal genitalia, hand, face, foot, or umbilical cord can also be the presenting part.

2. Ultrasonography (US) examination
   US is useful in determining
   - Fetal lie, presentation, and position
   - Estimation of fetal weight, with the following limitations:
     — When the head is deep in the pelvis, the fetal biparietal diameter cannot be measured accurately, thus reducing the accuracy of fetal weight estimates.
     — Oligohydramnios reduces the accuracy of fetal weight estimation.
     — The accuracy of fetal weight estimation decreases as fetal weight increases. The range of error of US estimates of fetal weight is up to 20%. Therefore, the potential range of error with an estimated fetal weight of 3,000 g is ±600 g, where the range of error for a 4,000-g estimated fetal weight is ±800 g.
   - Presence of fetal malformation that may obstruct labor progress (eg, hydrocephalus) or lethal anomaly that might contraindicate a cesarean delivery (eg, anencephaly)
   - Location of the placenta

C. Passage: determine the maternal pelvic size
   1. Clinical evaluation
      Pelvic abnormalities can contribute to delay of labor progress. Clinical estimation of the size of the pelvis will help determine if any gross abnormalities in the shape of the midpelvis or pelvic outlet are present. The diagonal conjugate provides an estimate of the anteroposterior dimension of the pelvis (Figure 11.4). Although the transverse diameter may be narrow with a normal anteroposterior size, this is uncommon. In most cases, if the diagonal conjugate is normal, the transverse diameter of the pelvis is normal too.

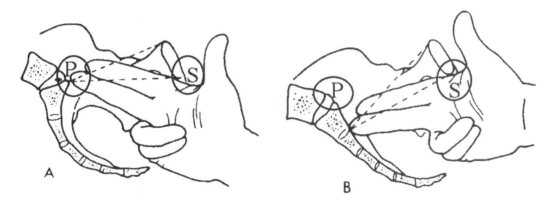

Figure 11.4. Clinical Pelvimetry: Measurement of Diagonal Conjugate. A, The distance between the tip of the middle finger on the sacral promontory (P) and the point where the hand meets the symphysis pubis (S) is the diagonal conjugate. B, Often, the middle finger cannot reach the sacral promontory (P). When this happens, the diagonal conjugate can be assumed to be 12.5 cm or more.

 If there is any suspicion of a placenta previa, do not perform a digital pelvic examination until ultrasonography findings have ruled it out.

a. Obtain the diagonal conjugate measurement
- Insert your index and middle finger into the vagina.
- Hold these 2 fingers together and trace the anterior surface of the sacrum until your middle finger reaches the sacral promontory (the most prominent portion of the upper sacrum).
- Keep your middle finger firmly in place on the sacral promontory and pivot your hand upward until the web of your thumb reaches the symphysis pubis.
- Mark the point on the lateral surface of your hand, where it touches the symphysis.
- Withdraw your hand and measure the distance between the mark and the tip of your middle finger.

b. Interpret the diagonal conjugate measurement
- *Diagonal conjugate less than 11.5 cm:* When the diagonal conjugate is less than 11.5 cm, the obstetric conjugate (the distance between the sacral promontory and the *inside* edge of the symphysis pubis, which represents the space available to the fetus) will average less than 10 cm. The biparietal diameter of a term fetus is often 9.5 to 10.0 cm. An average-sized, term fetus may manifest cephalopelvic disproportion when the diagonal conjugate is less than 11.5 cm.
- *Diagonal conjugate larger than 11.5 cm:* A pelvic inlet of this size is adequate for the birth of most fetuses. A diagonal conjugate close to 11.5 cm, however, may not be adequate for a very large fetus.

D. Summarize your findings

Make a summary of your findings after *systematically* evaluating
- The quality of the uterine contractions
- The size, presentation, and position of the fetus
- The general size of the pelvis
- Other factors that may be considered
  — Placental location (particularly if there is a reason to suspect placenta previa)
  — Presence/absence of major fetal malformation (particularly if there is a reason to suspect fetal hydrocephalus)
  — Uterine overdistension (multifetal gestation, polyhydramnios)
  — The level of maternal sedation or anesthesia
  — The effectiveness of maternal pushing (if in the second stage); maternal exhaustion
  — The ability of a woman to cope with labor
  — Fetal status

Identify the probable cause(s) of the delayed progress of labor and document these in the patient's medical record.

Self-test B

Now answer these questions to test yourself on the information in the last section.

B1. Which of the following conditions are associated with *prolonged first stage* of labor?

Yes	No	
___	___	Fetopelvic disproportion
___	___	Large fetus
___	___	Post-term pregnancy
___	___	Polyhydramnios
___	___	Low-intensity uterine contractions
___	___	Malpositioned fetus
___	___	Woman addicted to cocaine

B2. Which of the following conditions are associated with *prolonged second stage* of labor?

Yes	No	
___	___	Fetopelvic disproportion
___	___	Inadequate pushing
___	___	Fetal malposition
___	___	Hypotonic uterine dysfunction

B3. This graph shows a _____ of labor.

B4. True   False   With thorough investigation, a clear cause or causes of abnormal labor can always be determined.

B5. True   False   Hypertonic uterine dysfunction is uncommon, but hypotonic uterine dysfunction is common.

B6. True   False   Fetopelvic disproportion may be caused by a small pelvis, a large fetus, or a combination of both factors.

B7. Name at least 4 early clues to abnormal labor.

_____
_____
_____
_____

> **B8.** Match the following characteristics with the corresponding type of uterine dysfunction:
>
> ____ Minimal pain   **a.** Hypotonic
>
> ____ Usually responds well to oxytocin treatment   **b.** Hypertonic
>
> ____ Increased baseline tonus
>
> ____ Fetal distress is more common
>
> ____ Normal baseline tonus
>
> ____ Nearly continuous contractions
>
> **B9.** All causes of abnormal labor relate to p_____, p_____, or p_____, and sometimes p_____.
>
> **Check your answers with the list that follows the Recommended Routines. Correct any incorrect answers and review the appropriate section in the unit.**

8. How is abnormal labor treated?

Treatment of a particular cause of abnormal labor may vary, depending on the point in labor when the problem arises. In addition, more than one factor may be responsible for delayed labor progress. When more than one cause for abnormal labor is identified, cesarean delivery may be indicated by the combination of factors, even when no individual factor alone would warrant cesarean delivery.

Evidence of a category II or III fetal heart rate tracing at any point during labor requires immediate reevaluation of labor and delivery management and may necessitate intervention in the interest of the fetus, regardless of labor progress.

A. Uterine dysfunction
   1. Hypertonic uterine dysfunction
      This rare type of uterine dysfunction occurs when the uterus does not relax fully between contractions or contracts in an uncoordinated pattern. If it develops, it almost always does so during the latent phase of labor. Hypertonic uterine dysfunction is separate from uterine hypertonus, which may follow excessive oxytocin administration.

      If oxytocin is being used to induce or augment labor and hypertonic uterine dysfunction develops, the oxytocin should be stopped and labor progress should be observed for up to 1 hour. At that time, respond to whatever pattern is present after the period of observation. Many times, after discontinuing oxytocin in such a situation, a normal labor pattern will develop.

      Another potential cause of hypertonic dysfunction is placental abruption. Be sure an abruption has been ruled out before proceeding with the care outlined in the following text:
      a. Provide therapeutic rest. Either
         • Provide analgesic medication to allow the patient to rest or sleep
         or

- Provide lumbar epidural anesthesia (intrathecal narcotics may be used instead of epidural anesthesia) and intravenous (IV) fluid hydration. Maintain adequate maternal hydration to avoid hypotension.

  Most women with a prolonged latent phase due to hypertonic uterine dysfunction, who are treated with therapeutic rest, will progress into the active phase and continue with normal labor progress.

  b. Consider cesarean delivery

  If normal labor does not follow the rest period, low-dose oxytocin augmentation may be attempted. There is an increased risk, however, that hypertonic uterine dysfunction will recur. In that case, cesarean delivery may be associated with less risk of fetal compromise and newborn respiratory and/or neurological depression than continued augmentation of labor, particularly if cervical dilation is minimal and a vaginal delivery is predicted to be a number of hours away.

2. Hypotonic uterine dysfunction

   After labor has been established, as documented by uterine contractions with progressive cervical dilation, hypotonic uterine dysfunction may develop. This occurs when contractions become ineffective because they become less frequent, of lower intensity, or of shorter duration.

   a. Begin oxytocin augmentation (see Unit 10, Inducing and Augmenting Labor, in this book). When the pelvis is normal and the fetus is of normal size, presentation, and position, oxytocin augmentation is successful in correcting abnormal labor progress in about 80% of women with hypotonic uterine dysfunction.

   b. Be prepared to perform cesarean delivery if oxytocin augmentation does not cause progress to resume.

3. Secondary arrest of labor

   Progress during labor may simply stop. If contractions are normal but progress has not occurred for 2 hours or longer, investigate other causes of abnormal labor and consider cesarean delivery.

   a. If contractions have diminished, consider oxytocin augmentation of labor.

   b. Be prepared to perform cesarean delivery if oxytocin augmentation does not cause progress to resume.

 Whenever abnormal labor develops, consider the possibility that fetal malpresentation, fetal malposition, or fetopelvic disproportion is present.

B. Fetal presentation or position

An abnormal presentation detected during pregnancy may have corrected itself by the time labor begins. Many times, however, malpresentation is not recognized until it is revealed through investigation of abnormal labor progress.

If malpresentation is found, evaluate maternal pelvic size (if not already done) and placental location. A contracted pelvis and a low-lying placenta may be associated with abnormal presentation.

Management depends on the specific abnormal presentation or position.
1. Brow or face presentation

    When the fetal neck is extended, the fetal head usually cannot pass through the pelvis (Figure 11.5). Sometimes, with a large pelvis and good labor, the head may convert into a flexed attitude with the pressure from uterine contractions. The result will be a vertex presentation, which can be expected to deliver vaginally.

    a. Management
    - *Avoid* internal fetal heart rate monitoring. Accurate placement of a fetal scalp electrode is more difficult, and inaccurate placement may result in damage to the fetal face or eye.

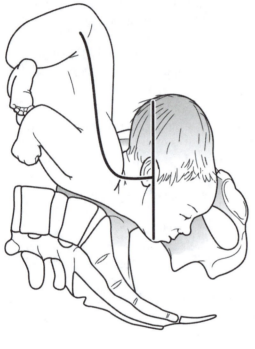

Figure 11.5. Face Presentation With the Mentum (Chin) Posterior. With face presentation, vaginal delivery cannot be accomplished safely, unless the fetus's chin rotates to anterior positioning with descent (Figure 11.6).

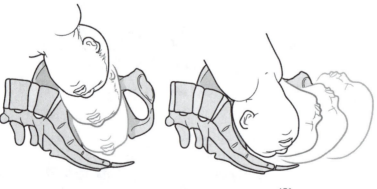

Figure 11.6. Spontaneous Rotation of Face Presentation During Descent. Spontaneous rotation from right mentum posterior to mentum anterior during descent allows vaginal delivery, with the chin coming directly under the symphysis pubis. Rotation is shown in 45° increments.

UNIT 11: ABNORMAL LABOR PROGRESS AND DIFFICULT DELIVERIES

- Brow and face presentations prior to labor may flex into normal vertex presentation during early labor. Some will not, and some brow presentations will change to face presentations.
- Fetal neck teratomas and goiters are associated with an increased risk of face and brow presentation.
- If the chin (mentum) is posterior (with face presentation) and does not rotate spontaneously to anterior positioning with descent, vaginal delivery is contraindicated because of the risk of spinal cord trauma to the abnormally extended fetal neck and the risks associated with forceps rotation.
- If a brow presentation does not flex to become vertex, or if a face presentation does not rotate to become mentum anterior within 2 hours of the onset of the second stage, a cesarean delivery is usually necessary.
- If a cesarean delivery is necessary, special attention should be given to gentle delivery of the deflexed head; this will help avoid fetal spinal cord injury.

b. Neonatal risks
- If the baby has a nuchal teratoma or goiter, emergency care at delivery, particularly endotracheal intubation, may be needed.
- Severe facial and laryngeal edema may occur with face presentation. Endotracheal intubation may be needed to maintain an open airway.
- The baby should be assessed for spinal cord injury.
- Severe facial bruising may occur. Check the baby's bilirubin levels.

2. Compound presentation
This occurs when an extremity presents alongside the presenting part. For example, a fetus in vertex position may have a hand in front of or beside the head.

a. Management
- Do not attempt to replace the extremity into the uterus because trauma to the woman or fetus, or prolapse of the umbilical cord, may occur.
- If a compound presentation is present early in labor with a fetus in vertex presentation, most babies can be delivered vaginally. As labor progresses, the hand will usually retract into the uterus.
- If a compound presentation occurs with a fetus in non-vertex position or is associated with delay of labor progress, cesarean delivery is recommended.

b. Neonatal risks
- These depend on presentation (eg, vertex, breech), route of delivery, and other risk factors, if any.
- Bruising or trauma to the presenting extremity may occur. Examine carefully. If bruising is severe, check the baby's bilirubin levels. A fracture can occur but is rare.

3. Transverse lie
This occurs when the body of the fetus lies horizontally in the uterus, across the birth canal entrance. It is associated with contracted pelvis, placenta previa, uterine fibroids, abnormal uterine shape, high parity (several previous deliveries), and certain congenital malformations in the fetus—particularly hydrocephalus.

a. Management
- In most cases, transverse lie detected earlier in pregnancy will have changed spontaneously to vertex, or sometimes to breech, presentation by the time labor starts.

- If transverse lie persists, the fetus appears normal, and placenta previa is not present, consider external cephalic version (turning the fetus) at 36 weeks of gestation or later.
- If transverse lie is first detected early in labor, a *gentle* attempt at external version may be successful. After the active phase has begun, external version is not recommended.
- If transverse lie cannot *easily* be changed to vertex, a cesarean delivery is needed for safe delivery. If the fetus is in a back-down transverse lie, a vertical incision (classical cesarean) is performed because the larger incision allows an easier delivery of the fetus than a low transverse incision.
- After delivery, check for maternal fibroids, uterine duplication, or other abnormal shape of the uterine cavity.

b. Neonatal risks
- If the uterine cavity is abnormally shaped, restriction of normal fetal movement may lead to joint contractures or clubbed feet. Assess the newborn for these positional deformities.

4. Breech presentation

Breech presentation is classified as follows:
- Frank breech: buttocks presenting, hips flexed, knees extended
- Complete breech: buttocks presenting, hips flexed, knees flexed
- Footling breech: one or both feet presenting, hips incompletely flexed, knees incompletely flexed

The risk of asphyxia, umbilical cord prolapse, and birth trauma are increased with vaginal breech delivery. Fetal head entrapment may also occur after the body is delivered. Because the circumference of the fetal body is generally smaller than the circumference of the fetal head—particularly in preterm fetuses—the cervix can entrap the aftercoming head, especially if the cervix is not completely dilated. Preterm fetuses, especially those weighing less than 2,500 g (<5 lb 8 oz), are at highest risk for fetal head entrapment, which can be fatal.

Contemporary research has documented an increase in perinatal morbidity and mortality in planned vaginal breech delivery. Many obstetricians have not been trained in the skills of vaginal breech delivery. Cesarean delivery is the most commonly recommended route of delivery for all viable fetuses remaining in breech presentation at the onset of labor.

a. Vaginal versus cesarean delivery decision factors
- Regardless of presentation earlier in pregnancy, nearly all fetuses turn spontaneously to cephalic presentation by 36 weeks. If a fetus remains in breech presentation at 36 weeks, the woman should be presented with options that include external cephalic version and planned cesarean delivery. Approximately 50% to 65% of attempted external cephalic versions result in a fetus in cephalic presentation. These women may then await the onset of labor or undergo induction of labor after 39 weeks. After counseling, a woman may also decline external cephalic version and request a planned cesarean delivery.

- Vaginal breech delivery is controversial. If a woman has arrived at the hospital with a viable fetus in breech presentation and delivery is imminently occurring, a vaginal breech delivery may be considered if the following criteria are met. Otherwise, efforts should be made to perform a cesarean delivery.
    — Fetal gestational age of 35 weeks or older
    — Frank or complete breech
    — Adequate maternal pelvic size
    — Flexed fetal head (as documented with radiography or US)
    — Normal fetal heart rate pattern
    — Normal progress of spontaneous labor
    — Availability of continuous fetal monitoring
    — Availability of a physician experienced and skilled in vaginal breech delivery
    — Capability (staff and equipment) for rapid cesarean delivery
    — Prior vaginal delivery
- Recommend a cesarean delivery if *any* of the following conditions exist:
    — Fetal gestational age of 34 weeks or earlier
    — Footling breech
    — Contracted pelvis according to clinical pelvimetry
    — Hyperextended fetal head (significantly increases the likelihood of traumatic delivery and injury to the fetus's neck and spinal cord)
    — Abnormal fetal heart rate pattern
    — Abnormal progress of spontaneous labor
    — Lack of availability of a physician experienced and skilled in vaginal breech delivery
    — Absence of anesthesia personnel and facilities for immediate cesarean delivery throughout labor
    — Patient declines to undergo attempted external cephalic version.

b. Management
- Avoid the artificial rupture of membranes because there is an increased risk of umbilical cord prolapse with breech presentation.
- If membranes rupture spontaneously, examine the woman to be sure cord prolapse has not occurred.
- If internal fetal heart rate monitoring is needed, place the electrode carefully to avoid damage to the fetal genitalia or anus.

If vaginal delivery is undertaken
- Allow spontaneous delivery to the umbilicus, and then use *gentle* assistance to deliver the arms and head.
- Generally, one person is needed to support the baby's legs and thorax, while the second person delivers the head.

c. Neonatal risks
Anticipate the need for resuscitation and evaluation.

5. Occiput posterior
While this is one of the normal positions for a vertex presentation, it is much less common than occiput anterior and is often associated with hypotonic uterine dysfunction and non-flexed attitudes of the fetal head (the head is in either a neutral or extended position).

a. Management
- If labor is progressing normally, continue to observe labor progress. The fetus may rotate to occiput anterior or remain occiput posterior, but vaginal delivery may occur in either case.
- If hypotonic uterine dysfunction is present, but there is no evidence of FPD, a trial of oxytocin augmentation is warranted.
- If oxytocin is used, follow the guidelines in Unit 10, Inducing and Augmenting Labor, in this book, starting with a low dose (1–2 mU/min) and increasing until an effective uterine contraction pattern is achieved. If progress is not made after an appropriate period of augmentation, cesarean delivery may be necessary.
- If the fetal head has reached the pelvic floor but spontaneous delivery has not occurred, management options include manual rotation, low or outlet forceps in occiput posterior position, or vacuum extraction in occiput posterior position. Rotational forceps may be considered, but only by an experienced practitioner. The vacuum extractor should never be used to actively rotate the fetal vertex; spontaneous rotation may occur with descent during traction. If attempts at operative vaginal delivery are unsuccessful, deliver by cesarean section.
- Serious lacerations of the birth canal, including fourth-degree perineal tears (laceration extends into the woman's rectum), may result from spontaneous delivery of the fetus.

In occiput posterior position or from operative vaginal delivery (See Section 9, What are operative vaginal deliveries?), maternal positioning to encourage the rotation of the fetal head may be attempted if there are no contraindications.

b. Neonatal risks
These depend on the course of labor, type of delivery (spontaneous or operative vaginal deliveries) and other risk factors, if any.

C. Congenital malformation

Investigation of delayed progress in labor sometimes demonstrates a fetal malformation or condition (eg, hydrocephalus, hydrops) that obstructs descent. These situations often require cesarean delivery.

Not all fetal malformations necessitate cesarean delivery. A lethal malformation that does not obstruct fetal descent, such as anencephaly, does not require cesarean delivery. In these situations, cesarean delivery has no benefit to the fetus but exposes the woman to the risks of surgery and anesthesia.

The management of other malformations (eg, meningomyelocele, encephalocele, gastroschisis, omphalocele) should be discussed with specialists at a regional perinatal center. In some cases, the route of delivery may affect neonatal outcome. In addition, even the smoothest neonatal transport may be more traumatic for a baby than maternal-fetal transfer would be. Delivery at a hospital that can provide full evaluation and surgical treatment of the baby also allows the mother to be with her baby. Referral of a woman for delivery at a regional perinatal center is recommended if a fetal malformation is identified before labor or during *early* labor.

When a congenital malformation is identified, maternal-fetal referral for delivery at a regional perinatal center is usually preferable to neonatal transport.

D. Fetopelvic disproportion

Incompatibility in size between the fetus and pelvis, whether it is because of a small maternal pelvis, large fetal size, or fetal anomaly, is also sometimes called *cephalopelvic disproportion.*

Clinical pelvimetry, estimation of fetal size, and determination of fetal position are used together to decide if FPD is present.
- Does the pelvis seem small enough to cause or contribute to the delay in labor?
- Does the fetus seem large enough to cause or contribute to the delay in labor?
- Is an abnormal presentation or fetal malformation present? If so, is it responsible for the delay in labor?

If FPD is found, it is managed with cesarean delivery.

E. Anesthesia

Slowing of the active phase of the second stage of labor may occur with epidural or spinal anesthesia, but only because a woman might be unable to feel the appropriate location in which to direct her maternal effort during pushing. More coaching may be needed, particularly in a nulliparous woman, to overcome the lack of sensation. The epidural infusion may also be decreased to improve sensation of the pelvic floor.

F. Ineffective pushing

Complete cervical dilation does not immediately bring the urge to push in all women. The decision to transition from the passive phase into the active phase of the second stage of labor should be individualized to the patient and the current clinical scenario. Maternal positioning to enhance fetal descent should be promoted. Provided that fetal descent continues, waiting for a woman to feel ready to push may lengthen the second stage but may also reduce the need for operative delivery.

Some women may need to avoid pushing (in the case of certain maternal cardiac, pulmonary, or cerebrovascular diseases). Other than these uncommon situations, management options include the following:

1. Consider that medication may be responsible for ineffective pushing
   Consider allowing epidural or spinal analgesia or narcotic analgesia to wear off.
2. Consider providing a period of rest
   Sometimes a woman becomes exhausted or is unable to push effectively after a long, difficult labor and a lengthy second stage with the need for active pushing over an extended period. If the woman is well, the fetal heart rate pattern is category I, and the arrest of descent is because of the inability of the woman to push any more, consider a period of rest, ensuring adequate pain relief and maternal comfort during rest. Many times, a woman will be able to push more effectively after a period of rest. The duration needed for recuperative rest varies. Use maternal position changes to promote fetal descent during this period, if possible.
3. Consider a trial of forceps or vacuum extraction delivery
   Be prepared for cesarean delivery if the trial does not proceed *easily*. Operative deliveries are presented later in this unit.
4. Consider delivering the baby by cesarean delivery.

G. Summarize your plan

Earlier, you summarized your findings on the probable cause(s) of delay in labor progress for a patient. Now you should expand that summary to include an outline of your management plan. Discuss this plan with the woman and her family.

If your initial plan does not proceed as expected, you will need to review your findings, reconsider your plan, and outline a revised plan. Keep the woman and her family informed regarding the expected and actual course of events. Discuss any revisions in your management plan with them.

At each junction in therapy, you should *systematically* review your findings and revise your plan as the situation changes. It is important that you approach the management of abnormal labor in a systematic way, as well as document your findings, your actions, and the maternal and fetal response to each step as care is given.

Management of abnormal labor is summarized in Table 11.5. Review the steps for each period of labor.

Table 11.5. Suggested Response to Delay of Labor Progress[a]	
Consider the P's: *passage, passenger, power.* Investigate each as a possible cause of abnormal labor (more than one may contribute to a delay). Consider the woman's *psyche,* too. Depending on your findings, provide treatment for the cause(s) or proceed directly to cesarean delivery.	
Period of Labor	**Actions to Take[b]**
First Stage (Cervical Dilation)	
Prolonged	1. Allow excessive sedation to wear off. Alternatively, if a woman is not overly sedated, providing analgesia or sedation to produce therapeutic rest (sleep) may be beneficial.
	2. If, after therapeutic rest, contractions persist but fail to produce adequate progress, investigate whether there is fetopelvic disproportion, malposition, or malpresentation. Deliver by cesarean if • Fetopelvic disproportion is found. or • Fetal indications are present.
	3. If the maternal pelvis is considered adequate and there are no fetal contraindications, consider oxytocin[c] augmentation. The goal is to achieve at least 4 hours of a normal contraction pattern.
Prolonged or arrested active phase	1. If due to hypotonic uterine dysfunction, consider oxytocin[c] augmentation to achieve at least 4 hours of a normal contraction pattern.
	2. Deliver by cesarean if • Fetopelvic disproportion is found. or • Fetal indications are present. or • An oxytocin trial fails to produce labor progress after at least 4 hours of normal contractions.

(continued)

Table 11.5. Suggested Response to Delay of Labor Progress[a] (*continued*)	
Period of Labor	**Actions to Take[b]**
Second Stage (Fetal Descent)	
Prolonged or arrested	1. If contractions have been normal, maternal pushing has been strong for 2 hours but without progress, and the fetus is at +1 station or higher, deliver by cesarean.
	2. If due to hypotonic uterine dysfunction, consider oxytocin[c] augmentation to achieve 1 hour of a normal contraction pattern.
	3. Consider allowing narcotic sedation or epidural/spinal anesthesia to wear off.
	4. If maternal exhaustion prevents effective pushing, consider hydration and sedation or conduction anesthesia. (Two hours of rest is usually adequate.)
	5. Consider a trial of forceps or vacuum extraction if the vertex position is at +2 station or below.
	6. Deliver by cesarean if • Fetopelvic disproportion is found. or • Fetal indications are present. or • An oxytocin trial fails to produce labor progress after 2 hours of normal contractions. or • A trial of forceps or vacuum extraction does not proceed *easily*.

[a] *Fetal well-being is assumed.* Evidence of fetal distress at any point requires immediate reevaluation, and possible revision, of a management plan.

[b] Whenever abnormal labor develops, consider the possibility that fetal malpresentation, fetal malposition, or fetopelvic disproportion is present.

[c] See Unit 10, Inducing and Augmenting Labor, in this book, for information about oxytocin use.

PCEP BOOK 2: MATERNAL AND FETAL CARE

Self-test C

Now answer these questions to test yourself on the information in the last section.

C1. True False Breech presentation is associated with increased risk for umbilical cord prolapse.

C2. True False Often, more than one factor contributes to abnormal progress of labor.

C3. True False Although occiput posterior is a normal vertex presentation, it is associated with hypotonic uterine dysfunction and an increased likelihood of birth canal lacerations.

C4. True False Hypertonic uterine dysfunction is treated with therapeutic rest.

C5. True False Maternal exhaustion and inadequate pushing may be an indication for cesarean delivery.

C6. True False Maternal exhaustion and inadequate pushing may be an indication for forceps or vacuum extraction delivery.

C7. True False Maternal exhaustion and ineffective pushing may be an indication for a period of rest with pain relief and hydration.

C8. True False Evaluation of abnormal labor should be followed by a summary, written in the patient's chart, of the suspected cause(s) and the subsequent management plan.

C9. True False Face presentation, with the chin posterior, is an indication for cesarean delivery.

C10. Compound presentation occurs when _____.

C11. Hypertonic uterine dysfunction occurs when _____.

C12. Which of the following actions is *not* indicated when abnormal fetal position is detected early in labor?
   A. Prepare for immediate cesarean delivery.
   B. Evaluate the size of the maternal pelvis.
   C. Evaluate the fetus for congenital malformations.
   D. Determine the location of the placenta.

C13. Cesarean delivery is performed more frequently for breech presentation than for vertex presentation because
   A. The cervix may not allow passage of the head after delivery of the body.
   B. The risk of asphyxia and birth trauma are higher with vaginal breech delivery.
   C. Fewer physicians are skilled in breech delivery than in cesarean delivery.
   D. All of the above

C14. Before oxytocin augmentation of labor is started, _____ and _____ should be ruled out.

C15. In which of the following situations may oxytocin augmentation of labor be appropriate?

Yes	No	
___	___	Hypertonic uterine dysfunction during the active phase
___	___	Secondary arrest of labor
___	___	Hypotonic uterine dysfunction during the deceleration phase
___	___	Hypotonic uterine dysfunction during the active phase

C16. True False If external version cannot *easily* convert a transverse lie to a vertex lie, a cesarean delivery is needed for safe delivery.

C17. True False A 30-year-old woman who easily delivered 3 healthy term babies and is now pregnant at 39 weeks of gestation with the fetus in breech position represents a high-risk pregnancy.

Check your answers with the list that follows the Recommended Routines. Correct any incorrect answers and review the appropriate section in the unit.

9. What are operative vaginal deliveries?

Operative vaginal delivery refers to one that is assisted by the use of obstetric forceps or a vacuum extractor.

 Training, skill, and experience are essential *for safe forceps or vacuum extractor delivery.*

A. Forceps
There are many types of obstetric forceps, some of which have specific uses. Each branch of a pair of forceps is applied to the fetal head separately and then locked together before traction is applied. Safe forceps delivery requires proper application of the forceps, followed by rotation and traction maneuvers that change progressively according to fetal station and descent. Traction and rotation should be *gentle* and coordinated with uterine contractions and maternal pushing.

Figure 11.7 shows the proper application of obstetric forceps to the fetal head for an outlet forceps delivery. The technique shown is with the fetus in vertex, occiput anterior presentation, and crowning. Techniques are different for other fetal presentations and for low or mid-forceps application.

B. Vacuum extractor
A soft or rigid plastic suction cup (metal cups are no longer commonly used) is applied to the leading edge of the fetal skull, in the midline over the sagittal suture, and between but not overriding the fontanels. The specific placement is dependent on the device being used, and appropriate training of the obstetrician should be assured. Correct placement is generally straightforward when the fetal position is occiput anterior but can be much more difficult with other vertex positions. Care should be taken to avoid trapping maternal tissue (vaginal or cervical) under the cup edges. Once the cup is applied, do not attempt to twist or rotate it in an effort to rotate the fetal head because lacerations of the fetal scalp may result.

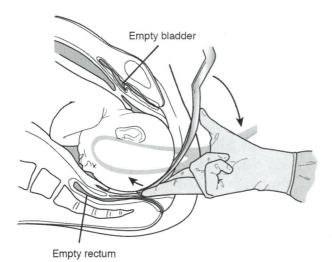

Figure 11.7. Application of Forceps Blades for an Outlet Delivery. After the left blade (Simpson forceps are shown) is in place, the right blade is applied. The 2 blades are then interlocked at the handles, and *gentle* traction is applied. Correct positioning of both blades is essential.

Traction should be coordinated with uterine contractions and simultaneous maternal pushing. Rotation will occur naturally as the descending head follows its normal course through the birth canal. Descent of the fetal head should occur with each uterine contraction and application of traction. Vacuum-assisted deliveries should be limited to 3 contractions during the descent phase, 3 contractions during the outlet extraction phase, 2 to 3 "pop offs," and a total time of 15 to 30 minutes. Close monitoring of the procedure and maternal and fetal tolerance is essential.

C. Types of forceps or vacuum extractor deliveries (Source: ACOG Practice Bulletin No. 219. Operative vaginal birth. *Obstet Gynecol*. 2020;135(4):e149-e159)

The following definitions use the system that describes station as the level of the leading point of the skull in centimeters, by using a scale of −5 to +5, with 0 being the level of the maternal ischial spines.

1. Outlet forceps or vacuum extraction
   This procedure has the same risk of perinatal morbidity and mortality as spontaneous delivery. It is defined by the following:
   - Fetal scalp is visible without manually separating the labia.
   - Fetal skull has reached the pelvic floor.
   - Sagittal suture is in the anteroposterior diameter of the pelvis or in the right or left occiput anterior or posterior position (ie, no more than 45° from vertical).
   - Rotation does not exceed 45° from the vertical midline.

2. Low forceps or vacuum extraction
   The leading point of the fetal skull is at +2 station or lower but not on the pelvic floor.
   Use of forceps is divided into 2 categories.
   - *Rotation of 45° or less:* Left or right occiput anterior rotated to occiput anterior or left or right occiput posterior rotated to occiput posterior.
   - *Rotation more than 45°:* Rotation and delivery with forceps requires much skill and experience, is more likely to be unsuccessful, and is associated with increased neonatal morbidity. A vacuum extractor is not used in this situation. See Section 10, When are operative vaginal deliveries performed, and what can you do to make them safe?

3. Mid-forceps or mid-pelvic vacuum extraction
   The fetal head is engaged in the pelvis, but the leading part of the fetal skull is above +2 station. It is associated with a higher likelihood of maternal or fetal morbidity and is more likely to be unsuccessful but, in skilled hands, may still be of lower morbidity than a cesarean delivery.

4. High forceps or vacuum extraction
   The fetal head is unengaged. It is associated with an unacceptable degree of risk to the woman and the fetus and is not performed in modern obstetrics.

 There is never *an indication for the use of high forceps or high vacuum extraction.*

10. When are operative vaginal deliveries performed, and what can you do to make them safe?

The potentially serious risks associated with the use of obstetric forceps or vacuum extractors can be minimized with adequate preparation, clear indications for use, and recognition that cesarean delivery is preferable to a traumatic assisted vaginal delivery. When the instruments cannot be applied smoothly, or when rotation or traction does not produce the desired results with minimum effort, the attempt should be stopped, and a cesarean delivery should be performed.

A. Meet basic requirements
Before forceps or vacuum extractor delivery is considered, the following conditions need to be ensured.
1. Maternal informed consent for the procedure
2. Physician trained, experienced, and skilled in the use of forceps or vacuum extractor
3. Adequate anesthesia given to the woman
Anesthesia personnel should be continuously available if mid-forceps or mid-pelvis vacuum extraction is attempted.
4. Capability to perform cesarean delivery immediately if an attempt at forceps or vacuum extractor delivery does not proceed easily
5. Fully dilated cervix
6. Engaged fetal head
7. Empty maternal bladder
8. Thorough assessment of fetal presentation and position, fetal size, gestational age, and maternal pelvic size
Do this to be certain vaginal delivery is possible and for accurate application of forceps or a vacuum extractor.
9. Safe fetal age, size, position, and presentation
   a. Forceps or vacuum extractor delivery is not advisable in the following situations:
   - There is a suspected or known fetal coagulation defect.
   - There is a known or suspected demineralizing fetal skeletal condition (eg, osteogenesis imperfecta).
   - Any non-vertex presentation occurs, including face or brow presentation.
   - Position of the presenting part cannot be identified.
   b. Vacuum extraction also should be avoided when
   - Gestational age is 34 weeks or less (risk of intracranial hemorrhage is increased in preterm fetuses).
   - Rotation is required to effect delivery.

Forceps or vacuum extractors should never be applied unless there is complete cervical dilation and the fetal head is engaged.

B. Use only when indicated
1. Evidence of category II or III fetal heart rate tracing
If the need for rapid delivery develops at a time when the fetal head is deep in the maternal pelvis, low forceps (or even mid-forceps/mid-pelvis vacuum extraction) may be faster and safer than an emergency cesarean delivery. Preparations for cesarean

delivery should continue while forceps or vacuum extractor delivery is attempted, in case the trial does not proceed easily and must be abandoned.
2. Arrested descent during the second stage
Slow rate of fetal descent is acceptable, as long as the woman and the fetus show no signs of distress. When there is *no* fetal descent for 2 hours, with a normal labor pattern, arrest of descent is diagnosed. Depending on the fetal station, perform a cesarean delivery, a forceps delivery, or a vacuum extraction.
3. Ineffective voluntary pushing
In certain situations, a woman should not push (due to cardiac, pulmonary, or cerebrovascular disease). In other cases, a woman may not be able to push effectively because of exhaustion or excessive sedation or anesthesia (see sections 8E and 8F).

C. Select the appropriate technique
1. Vacuum extraction
Use of a vacuum extractor is appropriate whenever the use of forceps also would be considered, as long as the gestational age is more than 34 weeks. A vacuum extraction may be safer than forceps when the fetal head is rotated 45° or more from the midline. This situation can be a difficult forceps delivery, but with vacuum extraction, the head may rotate naturally when traction is applied to the vacuum extractor. Increase suction gradually within the cup. Control suction to stay within the recommended limit. Follow manufacturers' recommendations for the specific cup used in your hospital.
2. Low or outlet forceps or vacuum extraction
Use of these techniques is appropriate whenever an operative vaginal delivery is indicated.
- Abnormal fetal heart rate patterns or maternal compromise are best treated with a prompt vaginal delivery.
- Delayed or arrested second stage of labor occurs without FPD, malpresentation, or malformation.
- Maternal pushing is ineffective.
3. Mid-forceps or mid-pelvis vacuum extraction
This technique has limited uses. When the fetal head is higher in the pelvis, operative vaginal delivery becomes more difficult, and the risk of complications rises. Mid-forceps or mid-pelvis vacuum extraction may, however, be appropriate when
- There is arrest of descent above +2 station but below 0 station, in the apparent absence of FPD. (This situation most often develops when there is ineffective maternal pushing.)
- Abnormal fetal heart rate patterns or maternal compromise dictate delivery sooner than it can be expected to occur spontaneously, and the obstetrician concludes that a mid-forceps or mid-pelvic vacuum extraction can be accomplished more expeditiously than a cesarean delivery.

When application of the vacuum extractor or forceps is easy and subsequent rotation or traction occurs with minimal force, delivery is usually successful without trauma to the fetus or the woman. When the application, rotation, or traction does not proceed smoothly, it is usually better to abandon the attempt and perform a cesarean delivery.

Every attempt at delivery with mid-forceps or mid-pelvis vacuum extraction should be considered a trial.

If the attempt does not proceed easily, you should be willing and prepared to abandon it and promptly perform a cesarean delivery.

D. Prepare adequately

Each of the following items should be ensured before operative vaginal delivery is attempted.
1. Prepare the woman
   - Confirm maternal consent
   - Empty the woman's bladder
   - The woman's buttocks should overhang the bed or table slightly
   - The woman's legs should be supported in stirrups but not restrained (due to possible shoulder dystocia)
2. Provide anesthesia
   - Outlet and low forceps or vacuum extraction deliveries can usually be performed with pudendal nerve block or local infiltration or with epidural or spinal anesthesia.
   - Mid-forceps or mid-pelvis vacuum extraction deliveries require major conduction (spinal or epidural) anesthesia or, occasionally, inhalation anesthesia, with anesthesia personnel in attendance during the procedure.
3. Organize personnel and equipment

   An operative vaginal delivery should be treated like any other surgical procedure, with indications, maneuvers to bring about application of the forceps or vacuum extractor and delivery, and post-delivery condition of the woman and the newborn recorded in the medical record.

Whenever a mid-forceps or mid-pelvis vacuum extraction is undertaken, it is preferable to use an operating room and a table where an unsuccessful attempt can be followed promptly by a cesarean delivery.

Cesarean setup, with surgical and anesthesia staff present during the mid-forceps or mid-pelvis vacuum extraction trial, is recommended.

4. Anticipate care for the newborn (See also Section 12, What are the fetal and neonatal risks of prolonged labor?)
   - Risk for birth trauma, including fractures and intracranial bleeding, is increased
   - Need for resuscitation may be increased

Self-test D

Now answer these questions to test yourself on the information in the last section.

D1. True False The *only* reason to use low forceps is to speed delivery when there is evidence of fetal compromise.

D2. True False Mid-forceps or mid-pelvis vacuum extraction delivery is higher risk than low forceps or low vacuum extraction delivery.

D3. True False Outlet forceps is an unnecessary procedure that is associated with a high risk of fetal morbidity.

D4. True False When a vacuum extractor is used, traction on the fetal head should be coordinated with uterine contractions and maternal pushing.

D5. True False When low forceps is used, rotation of the fetal head more than 45° requires considerable skill and is associated with an increased risk of trauma to the fetus.

D6. When a vacuum extractor is used, all of the following statements are correct, except
   A. The vacuum cup should be centered over the anterior fontanel.
   B. Delivery should occur within 15 minutes after the cup is applied.
   C. Descent of the fetal head should occur with each contraction and simultaneous application of traction with the vacuum extractor.
   D. In certain situations, vacuum extraction may be safer than forceps.

D7. Every mid-forceps or mid-pelvis vacuum extractor delivery attempt should be considered a _____. If the procedure does not proceed _____, you should be willing and prepared to perform a cesarean delivery promptly.

D8. Forceps or vacuum extractor should *never* be applied unless
   1. _____ and
   2. _____.

D9. Match the procedures in the left column with the best choice from the right.
   _____ Low forceps   a. Contraindicated before 35 weeks of gestation.
   _____ Mid-forceps   b. Fetal head is below +2 station.
   _____ Vacuum extraction   c. Use is seldom indicated.

Check your answers with the list that follows the Recommended Routines. Correct any incorrect answers and review the appropriate section in the unit.

UNIT 11: ABNORMAL LABOR PROGRESS AND DIFFICULT DELIVERIES

11. What are the maternal risks of prolonged labor or difficult delivery?

Maternal and fetal risks may not end with birth of the baby. You should anticipate possible complications and continue to monitor the woman and newborn after delivery.

A. Prolonged labor

Prolonged labor carries an increased risk of intra-amniotic infection. Minimize the number of digital examinations and monitor the woman for signs of infection, including postpartum endometritis after delivery has occurred.

Review the indications for intrapartum antibiotics. (See Unit 3, Infectious Diseases in Pregnancy, in this book for specific guidance on group B streptococcus.)

B. Prolonged labor or difficult delivery
  1. Lacerations of the birth canal
     Lacerations of the cervix, vagina, or perineum, with tears that may extend into the rectum or parametrium (area around the cervix and lower uterus), may occur. After delivery, visually inspect the birth canal.
  2. Postpartum hemorrhage
     Women are at increased risk for postpartum hemorrhage because of uterine atony with any of the following circumstances of abnormal labor.
     - Prolonged labor
     - Prolonged second stage of labor
     - Intra-amniotic infection
     - Prolonged use of oxytocin
     - Increased risk of genital tract lacerations is associated with forceps or vacuum extractor use.
  3. Maternal exhaustion
     This may interfere with a woman's ability to interact with and care for her newborn.
  4. Macrosomic fetus
     Large fetuses are associated with prolonged labor. Delivery of a macrosomic fetus carries additional risks (see Book 1: Maternal and Fetal Evaluation and Immediate Newborn Care, Unit 6, Gestational Age and Size and Associated Risk Factors; Book 2, Unit 5, Obstetric Risk Factors: Prior or Current Pregnancy; and Book 2, Unit 7, Gestational Diabetes).

C. Cesarean delivery

If required, cesarean delivery carries the risks associated with any surgery and use of anesthesia.

12. What are the fetal and neonatal risks of prolonged labor?

A. Risks associated with prolonged labor

By itself, lengthy labor usually does not cause fetal harm, but it may increase the risk of neonatal infection.
  - Review the baby's risk for infection; consider conducting blood cultures.
  - Observe and monitor the baby for signs of infection.
  - Begin antibiotics, if appropriate, based on risk factors or clinical condition (see Book 3: Neonatal Care, Unit 8, Infections).

B. Risks associated with medical management and/or interventions for prolonged labor
1. Oxytocin augmentation or induction
   Medical stimulation of labor may increase the risk of abnormal fetal heart rate patterns, especially if uterine tachysystole occurs.
2. Operative deliveries
   Mid-pelvis vacuum extraction or mid-forceps deliveries are sometimes associated with shoulder dystocia, but neither is a cause of shoulder dystocia. Failure of fetal descent may lead to the need for use of the instruments, and abnormal progress of labor in the second stage is associated with an increased risk of shoulder dystocia.
   a. Vacuum extraction
      Any of the following side effects may occur as a result of a vacuum extractor applied to the fetal scalp:
      - Caput succedaneum
      - Cephalohematoma
      - Subgaleal hemorrhage (rare)
      - Scalp avulsion or bleeding (rare)
      - Intracranial bleeding (rare, but higher if gestational age is <34 weeks)
   b. Forceps delivery
      Any of the following side effects may occur with a forceps delivery:
      - Cephalohematoma
      - Facial bruises or abrasions
      - Subgaleal hemorrhage (rare)
      - Facial nerve palsy (rare)
      - Skull fracture (rare)
      - Intracranial bleeding (rare)
3. Maternal medication
   Narcotics given to the woman close to delivery may cause neonatal respiratory depression.

13. How do you recognize and treat rapid labor?

A. Risk factors and recognition
   Rapid labor cannot be predicted, although it is more often associated with high parity (several previous births) and oxytocin infusion during labor. If rapid labor occurred in one pregnancy, it is more likely to happen in a woman's subsequent pregnancies, but it does not always recur. The onset of rapid labor also may be triggered by placental abruption.

   Rapid or tumultuous labor may produce strong contractions with very little relaxation time between them, accompanied by rapid cervical dilation and rapid fetal descent. Because of the extremely forceful and frequent uterine contractions, fast labors are often accompanied by abnormal fetal heart rate patterns and newborn respiratory and/or neurological depression. The rapid, forceful passage of the baby through the birth canal may also result in maternal trauma.
   1. Maternal
      - *During labor:* Patients often report severe, nearly constant pain. Cervical dilation progresses at a rate of 3 to 4 cm/h or faster. Uterine rupture can occur from the strong and frequent contractions, but it is rare.

- *Postpartum*
  - Hemorrhage due to uterine atony
  - Lacerations of the birth canal or perineum
  - Disseminated intravascular coagulation, if placental abruption was the cause of the rapid labor
2. Fetal
   - Frequent strong contractions may compromise placental blood flow, reduce oxygen exchange, and lead to fetal compromise.
   - Rapid fetal descent and delivery may lead to birth trauma.
3. Neonatal
   - Anticipate the possible need for neonatal resuscitation and, if needed, monitor for post-resuscitation complications.
   - Consider whether computed tomography is needed to evaluate the baby for subarachnoid, subdural, or intraventricular hemorrhage.
   - Assess the baby for birth trauma, including bruising or fractures of the skull, humerus, or clavicles.

B. Treatment

If labor seems to be progressing rapidly
1. Discontinue oxytocin infusion immediately if it is being used.
2. Monitor the fetus continuously.
3. Provide in utero resuscitative measures if abnormal fetal heart rate patterns develop.
4. Check cervical dilation regularly.
5. Consider the use of terbutaline.
   If there is evidence of fetal compromise, a 0.25-mg dose of terbutaline may be given subcutaneously to relax the uterus and decrease the frequency of uterine contractions as part of intrauterine resuscitation or during preparation for emergency vaginal or cesarean delivery.
6. Consider possibility of placental abruption
   Placental abruption may irritate the uterus and cause tumultuous labor. Refer to evaluation and management of abruption in Unit 2, Obstetric Hemorrhage, in this book.
7. Prepare for delivery
   There is often little that can be done to slow rapid labor. Anticipate the possible complications the woman and the newborn may have, and be prepared to treat them.

Self-test E

Now answer these questions to test yourself on the information in the last section.

E1. With rapid labor, abnormal fetal heart rate patterns may develop due to _____.

E2. Which of the following risks are increased with *rapid* labor?

Yes	No	
___	___	Facial nerve palsy
___	___	Maternal pulmonary edema
___	___	Fetal intracranial hemorrhage
___	___	Fetal distress
___	___	Broken clavicle
___	___	Uterine rupture
___	___	Perineal tears

E3. Which of the following risks are increased with *prolonged* labor?

Yes	No	
___	___	Postpartum hemorrhage
___	___	Postpartum endometritis
___	___	Birth canal lacerations
___	___	Neonatal infection
___	___	Placental abruption
___	___	Disseminated intravascular coagulation
___	___	Maternal hypertension

E4. Which of the following risks are increased with *forceps or vacuum extractor* deliveries?

Yes	No	
___	___	Fetal intracranial hemorrhage
___	___	Cephalohematoma
___	___	Birth canal lacerations
___	___	Neonatal infection
___	___	Facial nerve palsy
___	___	Postpartum hemorrhage

E5. Which of the following actions should be taken when rapid labor is identified?

Immediately	Within Several Minutes	Not Indicated	
___	___	___	Check the maternal blood pressure.
___	___	___	Stop oxytocin, if it is being infused.
___	___	___	Check the cervical dilation.
___	___	___	Check the fetal station.
___	___	___	Perform emergency cesarean delivery.
___	___	___	Check the fetal heart rate pattern.

Check your answers with the list that follows the Recommended Routines. Correct any incorrect answers and review the appropriate section in the unit.

14. How should you handle emergent, or potentially emergent, conditions during labor?

A. Obstetric hemorrhage (See Unit 2, Obstetric Hemorrhage, in this book.)

B. Meconium-stained amniotic fluid
   1. Risk for meconium aspiration
      - May occur in normal pregnancies and labors
      - Is more common with breech presentation and in post-term pregnancies
      - May be associated with a hypoxic event, which may cause relaxation of the rectal sphincter and release of meconium

      Regardless of the reason meconium came to be in the amniotic fluid, its presence places the baby at risk for meconium aspiration. Severe neonatal respiratory distress may result.
   2. Warning sign for previous possible fetal stress
      If meconium-stained fluid is seen when the membranes rupture, begin fetal heart rate and uterine contraction monitoring, if not already initiated. Anticipate the need for neonatal resuscitation.
   3. Management at delivery
      At delivery, management should not be altered because of meconium staining of the amniotic fluid. Suctioning of the mouth and nares before delivery of the shoulders is not recommended. If the baby is vigorous at birth, the mouth and nose may be bulb-suctioned during delayed cord clamping, while the baby is placed skin-to-skin with the mother. If the baby is not vigorous, the baby should be passed to the pediatrics team or other personnel in attendance, who are trained in the Neonatal Resuscitation Program. Endotracheal intubation is not automatically performed solely because of the presence of meconium. However, clearing meconium from a baby's nose and mouth is still a good practice, as long as it does not delay handing the newborn to the pediatrics team for further management. See Book 1: Maternal and Fetal Evaluation and Immediate Newborn Care, Unit 5, Resuscitating the Newborn, for additional, *essential* information about delivery room management. For non-vigorous babies, endotracheal suctioning is indicated to suction the trachea directly and help prevent meconium aspiration syndrome.

C. Fetal heart rate abnormalities (See Book 1: Maternal and Fetal Evaluation and Immediate Newborn Care, Unit 3, Fetal Well-being.)
   1. Whenever there is a category II fetal heart rate pattern, perform in utero resuscitative measures.
      - Turn off oxytocin, if in use.
      - Position the woman on her side (or put her in knee-chest position).
      - Consider giving 100% oxygen by non-rebreather mask.
      - Increase the rate of IV fluid infusion.
      - Check the maternal blood pressure.
      - Perform a vaginal examination to assess labor progress.

      Use other measures, according to individual situation.
      - Elevate the fetal head off the prolapsed cord, if present.
      - Consider administering tocolytic drugs to relax the uterus.
      - Ask the woman to stop pushing.

2. Prepare for emergency delivery and neonatal resuscitation
If a persistent category II (>60 minutes when vaginal delivery is remote and intrauterine resuscitation has not corrected the pattern, especially when recurrent decelerations are present) or category III fetal heart rate pattern exists, proceed with delivery via emergency cesarean or assisted vaginal delivery, as appropriate for cervical dilation and fetal station. Be prepared for resuscitation of the newborn.

D. Maternal analgesia or anesthesia
   1. Medications, dosage, and timing of administration
   Systemic opioids generally provide relief during labor by reducing anxiety and producing mild sedation, rather than analgesia. Use the least amount of analgesic needed to make the woman comfortable. Recommended medications include
   - Butorphanol tartrate, 1 to 2 mg, administered intramuscularly or intravenously, every 4 to 6 hours
   - Fentanyl, 50 to 100 mcg, administered intravenously, every 30 to 60 minutes
   - Nalbuphine, 10 to 20 mg, administered intravenously, intramuscularly, or subcutaneously, every 2 to 4 hours, up to a maximum of 160 mg

   For all of these medications, dosage and frequency of administration should be determined according to each woman's individual response to them. Analgesia delivered with small, patient-controlled IV boluses is often used.

   Opioids given to a laboring woman can cause neonatal respiratory and/or neurological depression, particularly if multiple doses are given over time or if large doses are given close to delivery. Avoid using long-acting opioids or administering large doses of opioids if delivery is anticipated to occur within 2 to 3 hours, and be prepared for neonatal resuscitation, including the administration of naloxone hydrochloride, if labor progresses more rapidly than expected. Short-acting, rapidly metabolized opioids such as fentanyl may be preferred.

   2. Consider the possibility of maternal substance use
   Excessive need for narcotic analgesia may indicate a substance use disorder.

   3. Effects on the fetus and newborn
   Small amounts of opioids administered to a laboring woman usually do not negatively affect a healthy fetus, unless multiple doses are given over a long labor. They do, however, cause diminished fetal heart rate variability.

   Epidural, spinal, or general anesthesia generally do not, by themselves, adversely affect the fetus. However, if regional anesthesia causes maternal hypotension (low blood pressure), the fetus may be compromised by poor blood flow to the placenta. General anesthesia will result in some degree of fetal anesthesia with possible need for resuscitation or assisted ventilation, until the effects of the anesthetic have resolved.

   If the baby demonstrates respiratory or neurological depression at birth
   - Assist with ventilation, as necessary; give oxygen, as appropriate.
   - *After* the baby is stable and well oxygenated, consider the use of naloxone hydrochloride to reverse the effects of narcotics given to the mother. Naloxone hydrochloride is *not* a resuscitation drug and should be used only after the baby is adequately ventilated. (See Book 1: Maternal and Fetal Evaluation and Immediate Newborn Care, Unit 5, Resuscitating the Newborn.)

- Be cautious about the use of naloxone hydrochloride if maternal opioid use disorder is suspected. In this situation, naloxone hydrochloride administration may precipitate acute withdrawal reaction in the baby.

If maternal opioid use disorder is suspected, the administration of naloxone hydrochloride may cause an acute withdrawal reaction in the baby.

E. Prolapsed umbilical cord
   1. Risk factors
   Prolapse of the umbilical cord cannot be predicted, but certain conditions increase the risk of occurrence. The possibility of cord prolapse should be considered or investigated if any of the following risk factors are present:
   - Cord presentation
   - Preterm labor
   - Spontaneous prelabor rupture of membranes
   - Artificial rupture of membranes before the presenting part is engaged
   - Non-vertex presentation
   - Polyhydramnios
   - Multifetal gestation
   2. Diagnosis
      - Variable fetal heart rate decelerations are associated with cord compression, which can occur when the cord is compressed between a fetal part and the uterine wall. The sudden onset of deep, variable fetal heart rate declarations is often the first sign of cord prolapse.
      - Prolapse may be visible or hidden. A prolapsed cord may be felt in the vagina or may be palpable, through intact membranes, in front of the presenting part (cord presentation).
   3. Management

Umbilical cord prolapse is a fetal emergency. Fetal asphyxia can occur. Prompt intervention is essential to preserve or restore fetal health.

- If the diagnosis is clear, continue external fetal monitoring and perform emergency cesarean delivery as soon as possible.
- If fetal heart rate monitoring indicates fetal compromise, elevate the fetal presenting part off of the prolapsed cord until a cesarean delivery can be performed.
- The following maneuvers may lift the presenting part off of the cord without compressing the cord in the vagina:
  — Insert a gloved hand into the woman's vagina and hold the presenting part off of the cord.
  — Insert a Foley catheter into the woman's bladder, fill it with 400 to 500 mL of sterile saline, and put the patient in knee-chest position. (This maneuver is less commonly performed, as it takes several minutes longer.)

4. Neonatal care
   Be prepared for prompt and aggressive resuscitation. If resuscitation is needed, monitor for possible post-resuscitation complications.

F. Shoulder dystocia (impaction of the fetal shoulders after delivery of the head)
   1. Risk factors
      Risk increases as fetal weight increases but does not always occur, even with the largest babies, and is possible with all but the smallest fetuses. Large fetal size therefore increases the risk but is not predictive of the occurrence of shoulder dystocia.

      Women who gave birth to one macrosomic baby are more likely to have macrosomic babies in subsequent pregnancies. Women with abnormal glucose tolerance or diabetes mellitus are also more likely to have large babies. Many large babies, however, are born to women with no known risk factors. Neither estimated fetal weight nor labor progress is an adequate predictor of shoulder dystocia. Pregnancy and labor may be uncomplicated until the shoulders become impacted after delivery of the head. Most shoulder dystocia deliveries occur in women without apparent risk factors.

       Shoulder dystocia is unpredictable. You should be prepared for the possibility of shoulder dystocia with every delivery.

   2. Diagnosis
      The baby's head delivers and promptly "snaps back" against the woman's perineum. The usual traction on the head does not produce delivery of the anterior shoulder. Avoid excess lateral traction on the head, which may lead to strain on the nerve fibers of the brachial plexus, which arise from spinal nerves C5 through T1 and supply the upper extremity. Injury to these nerves may result in temporary or permanent brachial plexus injury and loss of upper-extremity function. About half of brachial plexus injuries occur in the absence of shoulder dystocia, and most shoulder dystocias do not result in brachial plexus injury.

   3. Management
      When shoulder dystocia occurs, it suddenly poses immediate and grave danger to the fetus.

       Urgent and coordinated action is needed. If the shoulders remain trapped, severe damage or fetal death may result from asphyxia within minutes of delivery of the head.

      Summon additional help to the delivery room immediately, including nursing, anesthesiology, and a pediatrics team prepared for resuscitation.

      Systematically and quickly perform the following steps, until delivery is accomplished:
      a. Primary maneuvers
         - Hip flexion (McRoberts maneuver)
           With her legs out of stirrups, help the woman flex her hips by pulling her thighs onto her abdomen and chest, so her knees are near her breasts. Ask the woman to grasp tightly behind her knees to hold this position, or have assistants hold the legs in this position (Figure 11.8).

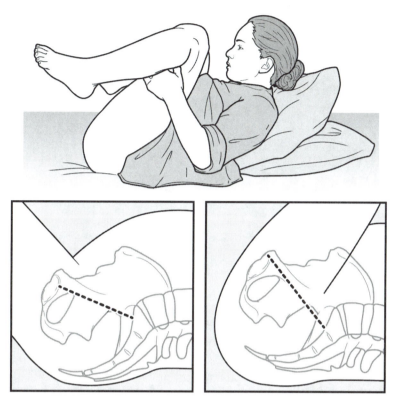

Figure 11.8. Thigh Flexion for Treatment of Shoulder Dystocia. Sharp flexion of the maternal hips increases the useful size of the pelvic outlet. Note the change in relationship of the pelvic bones with full hip flexion.

- Suprapubic pressure
  One person then applies pressure downward and laterally, just above the symphysis pubis (suprapubic pressure). Suprapubic pressure is applied from behind the fetal anterior shoulder to effect rotation anteriorly; the person applying suprapubic pressure should be positioned on the side of the mother the fetal spine is facing. This is done while another person exerts gentle downward traction on the baby's head (not shown).

Often, the McRoberts maneuver and suprapubic pressure promptly result in delivery of the anterior shoulder. If delivery does not occur, however, proceed quickly to secondary maneuvers.

b. Secondary maneuvers

Secondary maneuvers are those that require intravaginal manipulation of the baby's position to rotate the shoulders out of the vertical orientation. The order in which secondary maneuvers are applied is dictated by the orientation of the baby (right vs left occiput transverse), by the amount of space available within the vagina for manipulation, and—to some extent—if the operator is right-handed or left-handed.

- Woods screw maneuver
  To rotate the shoulders into an oblique orientation, pressure is applied by the operator anteriorly against the clavicle of the posterior shoulder to effect rotation. In some cases, it is necessary to rotate the posterior arm and shoulder 180°, so the posterior shoulder becomes the anterior shoulder (Figure 11.9).

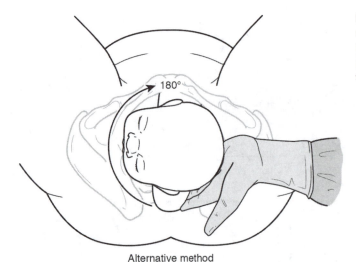

Figure 11.9. Shoulder Rotation for Treatment of Shoulder Dystocia. Compared with backward rotation, forward rotation of the posterior shoulder is more likely to compress the shoulder girdle (reducing its size).

- Rubin maneuver
  Alone, or in conjunction with the Woods maneuver, pressure is applied to the anterior or posterior scapula, again attempting to rotate the shoulders into an oblique orientation.

Simultaneously, a second person applies suprapubic pressure on the anterior shoulder (wedged against the symphysis pubis) by pressing on the lower maternal abdomen (not shown).

If shoulder rotation was not successful, proceed immediately to

c. Delivery of the posterior arm (Barnum maneuver)
Often, it is only the anterior shoulder that is affected. The posterior pelvis may have adequate space. Delivery of the posterior arm is almost always successful in freeing the shoulders but is more likely than the shoulder rotation maneuver (Figure 11.10) to be accompanied by fracture of the humerus or clavicle, primarily when the procedure is done incorrectly.

If the baby is still not delivered, proceed to

d. Cephalic replacement (Zavanelli maneuver)
Replace the fetal head into the pelvis before delivering the baby with cesarean delivery.
  - Gently rotate the head back to occiput anterior, flex the neck, and apply gentle upward pressure, after which the head will retract into the vagina.
  - Do *not* push the head inward. If it is going to retract, it will do so by itself, from the upward pull of the extended shoulders.
  - Perform an immediate cesarean delivery. Upward displacement of the fetal head by an assistant is likely necessary to elevate the head to the uterine incision.
  - Continue to monitor the fetal heart rate while awaiting cesarean delivery. If fetal bradycardia occurs, cord compression may be present and may be relieved by
    — Further elevation of the head by putting the woman in knee-chest position or

— Administration of tocolytic drugs to diminish uterine contractions
— Terbutaline, 0.25 mg, administered subcutaneously
or
— Magnesium sulfate, 4 to 6 g, administered intravenously, over 20 minutes
4. Postdelivery considerations
   a. Maternal
      Check for vaginal, cervical, perineal, or rectal lacerations.
   b. Neonatal
      • Be prepared for prompt and aggressive resuscitation. If needed, monitor the baby for possible post-resuscitation complications.
      • Obtain a radiograph if there is reason to suspect fracture of the humerus or clavicle.
      • Evaluate the baby for brachial plexus nerve injury (Erb palsy).

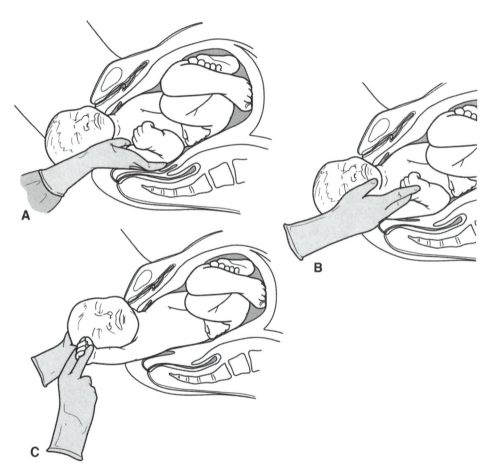

Figure 11.10. Delivery of the Posterior Arm. A, Insert your hand into the vagina, posterior to the baby; grasp the posterior arm from the shoulder to the elbow, and slide it across the baby's chest. B, Grasp the baby's hand. C, Bring the hand and arm forward, out of the vagina.

15. How should you manage an abnormal third stage of labor?

The third stage of labor lasts from delivery of the baby to delivery of the placenta, which is normally a period of less than 30 minutes. After delivery of the baby, the placenta usually separates from the uterine wall because of continued uterine contractions. Once separated, it descends into the cervix and is then expelled from the vagina by the pushing efforts of the woman.

When the placenta has not been delivered within 30 minutes after delivery of the baby, it should be removed manually. Clinical situations have 2 main categories: excessive bleeding and little or no bleeding.

Historically, oxytocin was not administered until after delivery of the placenta. Numerous studies have shown that the immediate administration of oxytocin after delivery of the baby, combined with controlled cord traction, results in less blood loss. This practice is known as "active management of the third stage of labor" and is addressed in greater detail in Unit 2, Obstetric Hemorrhage, in this book.

A. Excessive bleeding (see Unit 2, Obstetric Hemorrhage, in this book)
While there is normally a gush of blood from the vagina immediately after separation of the placenta from the uterine wall, continued uterine contractions stop excessive blood flow. If heavy bleeding persists, life-threatening hemorrhage can result. If the placenta separates but is not expelled from the uterus, the bulk of the placenta prevents the uterus from contracting enough to close off the bleeding arteries and veins.

Take the following steps to deliver the placenta:
1. Insert one hand into the vagina and explore the cervix.
   If the placenta can be felt, grasp it and pull it out. Puncturing the placenta with your fingers is appropriate if you need to do so to get a grip on it.
2. If the placenta cannot be felt in the cervix, continue upward into the uterus.
   Grasp the placenta and pull it out of the uterus.
3. Inspect the placenta carefully for missing pieces.
   If fragments are missing, explore the uterus again for the remaining pieces.
   If available, anesthesia should be given to the mother. If bleeding is profuse, however, there may not be time to wait for anesthesia personnel. In this case, IV sedation with narcotics or tranquilizers may be helpful.

B. Little or no bleeding
Examine the vagina and cervix for the placenta. If it is not there, *do not enter the uterus*. The placenta has not separated from the uterine wall and manually separating it may cause hemorrhage. General anesthesia will probably be required to relax the uterus enough to get your hand inside.
1. Make the following preparations before attempting to remove the placenta.
   a. Summon anesthesia personnel
   b. Send blood for crossmatching
      Ask that at least 2 units of blood be prepared.
   c. Start an IV line or increase the infusion rate of an existing IV line

UNIT 11: ABNORMAL LABOR PROGRESS AND DIFFICULT DELIVERIES

2. As soon as blood is available and the woman has been anesthetized
   a. Explore the uterus and find the placental edge.
      If a distinct placental edge can be felt, systematically loosen the adhered areas of the placenta. Once separated, grasp the placenta and pull it out of the uterus.
      - Place one hand on the woman's abdomen to hold the fundus in place.
      - Insert your other hand into the uterus. Using your fingertips held together, with the palm of your hand facing the inside of the uterus (and the back of your hand against the uterine wall), begin to work your fingers under the edge of the placenta.
      - Proceed until the placenta separates completely.
   b. If a distinct placental edge cannot be found, *stop*.
      Placenta accreta may be present. Placenta accreta occurs when the tissue of the placenta invades the uterine wall, making separation of the placenta impossible. Prior to any management, it is advisable to ensure that the patient has two large-bore IV access sites because massive hemorrhage may result, particularly if efforts to separate the placenta continue and uterine rupture occurs. Because the placenta has grown into the uterus and cannot be separated from it, an abdominal hysterectomy is almost always required to remove it.

Self-test F

Now answer these questions to test yourself on the information in the last section.

F1. Which of the following factors are associated with increased risk for umbilical cord prolapse?

Yes	No	
___	___	Maternal obesity
___	___	Premature rupture of membranes
___	___	Non-vertex presentation
___	___	Multifetal gestation
___	___	Preterm labor
___	___	Hydramnios
___	___	Growth-restricted fetus

F2. When an umbilical cord prolapses, what should you do in the time between diagnosis and emergency cesarean delivery?
_____
_____
_____

F3. True   False   Meconium in the amniotic fluid always indicates that an episode of fetal compromise has occurred.

F4. True   False   If a woman received large or frequent doses of narcotic medication during labor and the newborn demonstrates respiratory or neurological depression, naloxone hydrochloride should be given *immediately* in the delivery room.

F5. True   False   Only babies weighing 4,000 g (8 lb 13 oz) and more are at risk for shoulder dystocia.

F6. True   False   If maternal anesthesia causes hypotension, the fetus may be compromised because of poor blood flow to the placenta.

F7. True   False   If a woman is addicted to narcotics, drug withdrawal reaction in the baby may be brought on by administration of neonatal naloxone hydrochloride.

F8. True False There is an increased risk of umbilical cord prolapse with vaginal delivery of twins.

F9. True False Delivery of the placenta should occur spontaneously within 30 minutes of birth of the baby.

F10. Meconium in the amniotic fluid (check all that apply)

Yes	No	
____	____	May be a sign of fetal compromise
____	____	Occurs more frequently in post-term pregnancies
____	____	May lead to meconium aspiration
____	____	May be a normal finding

F11. Describe the McRoberts maneuver.
_____
_____
_____

F12. True False When umbilical cord prolapse occurs, the fetal heart rate pattern seen most often is sudden development of *late* decelerations.

F13. True False Severe neonatal respiratory distress may result from meconium aspiration.

F14. True False Unless shoulder dystocia is treated and the baby is delivered within minutes, death or severe asphyxia may occur.

F15. True False Placenta accreta is best managed by separation of the adherent areas of the placenta with your fingertips.

F16. Which of the following events can be predicted before they occur?
  A. Umbilical cord prolapse
  B. Rapid labor
  C. Shoulder dystocia
  D. All of the above
  E. None of the above

F17. Which of the following options are part of in utero resuscitative measures that should be taken whenever a non-reassuring fetal heart rate pattern develops?

Yes	No	
____	____	Turn off oxytocin infusion, if being used.
____	____	Check for a prolapsed umbilical cord.
____	____	Check the maternal blood pressure.
____	____	Give the woman 100% oxygen by mask.
____	____	Turn the woman onto her side.
____	____	Conduct a vaginal culture, and then begin broad-spectrum antibiotics.
____	____	Administer 50 mcg of fentanyl intravenously.

Check your answers with the list that follows the Recommended Routines. Correct any incorrect answers and review the appropriate section in the unit.

UNIT 11: ABNORMAL LABOR PROGRESS AND DIFFICULT DELIVERIES

ABNORMAL LABOR PROGRESS AND DIFFICULT DELIVERIES

Recommended Routines

All the routines listed below are based on the principles of perinatal care presented in the unit you have just finished. They are recommended as part of routine perinatal care.

Read each routine carefully and decide whether it is standard operating procedure in your hospital. Check the appropriate blank next to each routine.

Procedure Standard in My Hospital	Needs Discussion by Our Staff	Recommended Routine
_____	_____	1. Establish a protocol for the assessment of women in questionable labor, including documentation of • Cervical dilation • Fetal station • Fetal presentation • Contraction characteristics • Care provided • Response to therapy
_____	_____	2. Establish guidelines for the augmentation of labor (see also Unit 10, Inducing and Augmenting Labor, in this book), including documentation of • Factors that indicate the need for oxytocin • Evaluation to rule out contraindications to the use of oxytocin • Uniform dilution for oxytocin • Standard interval for the rate of infusion change
_____	_____	3. Establish guidelines for the use and application of forceps and a vacuum extractor. For mid-forceps or a mid-vacuum extractor, establish guidelines for personnel and readiness for immediate cesarean delivery if the trial fails.
_____	_____	4. Establish guidelines for response to rapid labor.
_____	_____	5. Establish guidelines for response to emergent or potentially emergent fetal situations, including • Meconium-stained amniotic fluid • Fetal heart rate abnormalities • Complications of maternal anesthesia or narcotic analgesia • Prolapsed umbilical cord • Shoulder dystocia
_____	_____	6. Develop a system whereby an emergency cesarean delivery can be started within a maximum of 30 minutes, at any time of the day or night.

Self-test Answers

These are the answers to the Self-test questions. Please check them with the answers you gave and review the information in the unit wherever necessary.

Self-test A

A1. True

A2. True

A3. An active phase of labor with cervical dilation progressing at a rate of 0.8 cm/h would be called a *protracted* active phase.

A4. An active phase that lasted longer than 6 hours would be called a *prolonged* active phase.

A5. When the cervix is completely dilated, but fetal station does not change during a 2-hour period, it is called *arrest of descent* or *arrested second stage*.

A6. The first stage of labor starts with the onset of labor and continues until *the cervix is fully dilated*.

The second stage of labor starts with *full cervical dilation* and continues until *delivery of the baby*.

The third stage of labor starts after *delivery of the baby* and ends with *delivery of the placenta*.

The "fourth stage" of labor starts after *delivery of the placenta* and ends *1 hour later*. It is the time when the risk of postpartum hemorrhage is the *greatest*.

A7. Normal cervical dilation during the **active phase** of labor in a nullipara woman is *0.5 to 1.0 cm/h* and in a multipara woman is *1.0 to 1.5 cm/h*.

A8. Normal duration of the **active phase** of labor in a nullipara woman is *8 to 10* hours or less and in a multigravida woman is *6 to 8* hours or less.

A9. Usual duration of the **second** stage of labor in a nullipara woman is *5* hours or less and in a multigravida woman is *5* hours or less. (Five hours is *acceptable*, as long as the woman and the fetus are well and labor progress [fetal descent] is being made.)

A10. The critical feature of progress in the first stage of labor is *cervical dilation* and in the second stage of labor is *fetal descent*.

Self-test B

B1.

Yes	No	
	X	Fetopelvic disproportion
X		Large fetus
	X	Post-term pregnancy
X		Polyhydramnios
X		Low-intensity uterine contractions
X		Malpositioned fetus
	X	Woman addicted to cocaine

B2.

Yes	No	
X		Fetopelvic disproportion
X		Inadequate pushing
X		Fetal malposition
X		Hypotonic uterine dysfunction

B3. This graph shows a *protracted* (cervical dilation has progressed at 1.2 cm/h—slow rate for a primigravida woman—and 1.5 cm/h—slow for a multipara woman) *and prolonged* (6 hours since 5-cm dilation, and 10 cm not yet reached) *active phase* of labor. (See Table 11.2.)

B4. False Reason: In about 10% of labors with abnormal progress, a clear cause is never found.

B5. True

B6. True

B7. Any 4 of the following early clues:
- Application of the fetal head to the cervix is poor
- Deflexed fetal head
- Unengaged fetal head
- Poor contractions
- Continuous contractions, seemingly without letting up
- Edema of the cervix
- Pushing uncontrollably before complete dilation

B8. <u>a</u> Minimal pain

<u>a</u> Usually responds well to oxytocin treatment

<u>b</u> Increased baseline tonus

<u>b</u> Fetal distress is more common

<u>a</u> Normal baseline tonus

<u>b</u> Nearly continuous contractions

B9. All causes of abnormal labor relate to *passage, passenger,* or *power,* and sometimes *psyche*.

Self-test C

C1. True

C2. True

C3. True

C4. True

C5. True

C6. True

C7. True

C8. True

C9. True

C10. Compound presentation occurs when *an extremity presents alongside the presenting part.*

C11. Hypertonic uterine dysfunction occurs when *the uterus does not relax between contractions or contracts in an uncoordinated way.*

C12. A. Prepare for immediate cesarean delivery.

C13. D. All of the above

C14. Before oxytocin augmentation of labor is started, *fetal malposition or malpresentation* and *fetopelvic disproportion* should be ruled out.

C15. Yes | No
___ | _X_ Hypertonic uterine dysfunction during the active phase
_X_ | ___ Secondary arrest of labor
_X_ | ___ Hypotonic uterine dysfunction during the deceleration phase
_X_ | ___ Hypotonic uterine dysfunction during the active phase

C16. True

C17. True

Self-test D

D1. False *Reason:* Use of low forceps is appropriate to speed delivery when there is evidence of fetal distress, for delayed or arrested second stage (no fetopelvic disproportion or malposition), or for ineffective maternal pushing.

D2. True

D3. False *Reason:* Outlet forceps delivery has the same risk of perinatal morbidity as spontaneous vaginal delivery.

D4. True

D5. True

D6. A. The vacuum cup should be centered over the anterior fontanel.

D7. Every mid-forceps or mid-pelvis vacuum extractor delivery attempt should be considered a *trial*. If the procedure does not proceed *easily or smoothly,* you should be willing and prepared to perform a cesarean delivery promptly.

D8. 1. *The cervix is completely dilated* and
 2. *The fetal head is engaged.*

D9. _b_ Low forceps   a. Contraindicated before 35 weeks of gestation.
    _c_ Mid-forceps   b. Fetal head is below +2 station.
    _a_ Vacuum extraction   c. Use is seldom indicated.

Self-test E

E1. With rapid labor, abnormal fetal heart rate patterns may develop due to *frequent and strong compression of the placenta, which can interfere with normal oxygen exchange.*

E2. Yes | No
___ | _X_ Facial nerve palsy
___ | _X_ Maternal pulmonary edema
_X_ | ___ Fetal intracranial hemorrhage
_X_ | ___ Fetal distress
_X_ | ___ Broken clavicle
_X_ | ___ Uterine rupture
_X_ | ___ Perineal tears

E3. Yes | No
_X_ | ___ Postpartum hemorrhage
_X_ | ___ Postpartum endometritis
_X_ | ___ Birth canal lacerations
_X_ | ___ Neonatal infection
___ | _X_ Placental abruption
___ | _X_ Disseminated intravascular coagulation
___ | _X_ Maternal hypertension

UNIT 11: ABNORMAL LABOR PROGRESS AND DIFFICULT DELIVERIES

E4.
Yes	No	
X	___	Fetal intracranial hemorrhage
X	___	Cephalohematoma
X	___	Birth canal lacerations
___	X	Neonatal infection
X	___	Facial nerve palsy
X	___	Postpartum hemorrhage

E5.
Immediately	Within Several Minutes	Not Indicated	
___	X	___	Check the maternal blood pressure.
X	___	___	Stop oxytocin, if it is being infused.
___	X	___	Check the cervical dilation.
___	X	___	Check the fetal station.
___	___	X	Perform emergency cesarean delivery.
X	___	___	Check the fetal heart rate pattern.

Self-test F

F1.
Yes	No	
___	X	Maternal obesity
X	___	Premature rupture of membranes
X	___	Non-vertex presentation
X	___	Multifetal gestation
X	___	Preterm labor
X	___	Hydramnios
___	X	Growth-restricted fetus

F2. Elevate the fetal presenting part off the prolapsed cord by

1. Inserting a gloved hand into the vagina and elevating the presenting part.

   or

2. Placing a Foley catheter into the bladder and infusing 400 to 500 mL of sterile saline, then positioning the patient in the knee-chest position.

F3. False *Reason:* Meconium in the amniotic fluid *may* indicate fetal distress and should be considered a warning sign for possible distress. In utero passage of meconium may also occur in uncomplicated pregnancies and labors and is more common with post-term gestation and breech presentation.

F4. False *Reason:* If a baby has respiratory or neurological depression at birth, resuscitative measures should be done *first*. After the baby is stabilized, it may be appropriate to administer naloxone hydrochloride if excessive maternal opioid analgesia is the likely reason for the baby's status.

F5. False *Reason:* Shoulder dystocia is unpredictable and can occur with delivery of all but the smallest babies.

F6. True

F7. True

F8. True

F9. True

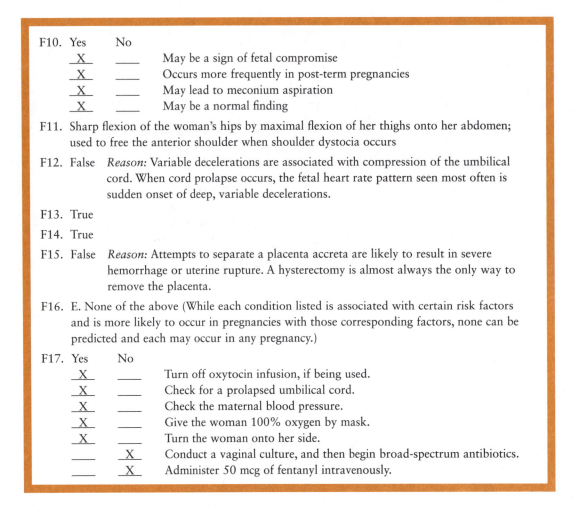

Unit 11 Posttest

After completion of each unit there is a free online posttest available at www.cmevillage.com to test your understanding. Navigate to the PCEP pages on www.cmevillage.com and register to take the free posttests.

Once registered on the website and after completing all the unit posttests, pay the book exam fee ($15) and pass the test at 80% or greater to earn continuing education credits. Only start the PCEP book exam if you have time to complete it. If you take the book exam and are not connected to a printer, either print your certificate to a .pdf file and save it to print later or come back to www.cmevillage.com at any time and print a copy of your educational transcript.

Credits are only available by book, not by individual unit within the books. Available credits for completion of each book exam are as follows: Book 1: 14.5 credits; Book 2: 16 credits; Book 3: 17 credits; Book 4: 9 credits.

For more details, navigate to the PCEP webpages at www.cmevillage.com.

Unit 12: Imminent Delivery and Preparation for Maternal/Fetal Transport

Objectives 404

Imminent Delivery

1. What is an imminent delivery? 407
2. How do you know delivery is imminent? 407
3. What should you do when you recognize delivery is imminent? 407
4. What should you do when the head crowns? 408
5. What should you do after the head delivers? 408
6. What should you do if the baby is breech? 409
7. What should you do after the baby is delivered? 411
8. What should you do if spontaneous delivery of the placenta does not occur within 30 minutes? 414

Table and Figure

    Table 12.1. Normal Values of Umbilical Cord Blood Gases 413

    Figure 12.1. The Bracht Maneuver 410

Preparation for Maternal/Fetal Transport

1. What is maternal/fetal transport? 416
2. Why is maternal/fetal transport important? 416
3. What are the goals of preparing a pregnant woman or fetus for transport? 416
4. Which women should be transported for delivery at a regional perinatal center? 417
5. Which pregnant women should *not* be transported? 418
6. What should you do to prepare a pregnant woman for transport? 418
7. How do you make an obstetric referral? 419

Recommended Routines 420

Objectives

In this unit you will learn

Imminent Delivery

A. How to safely support the mother and baby when delivery is about to occur unexpectedly

B. How to assist the woman in achieving a safe delivery with
- Vertex presentation
- Breech presentation

C. What to do after the baby is born

D. How to manage delivery of the placenta

E. How to recognize and respond to an abnormal third stage of labor

Preparation for Maternal/Fetal Transport

A. Which pregnant women may benefit from transport

B. Primary goals for preparing a pregnant woman for transport

C. Which pregnant women should not be transported

D. How to prepare a pregnant woman for transport

UNIT 12: IMMINENT DELIVERY AND PREPARATION FOR MATERNAL/FETAL TRANSPORT

Unit 12 Pretest

Before **reading the unit, please answer the following questions. Select the *one best* answer to each question (unless otherwise instructed). Record your answers on the test and check them with the answers at the end of the book.**

1. If the head of a baby delivers and the woman gives several strong pushes but the shoulders do not deliver, you should

Yes	No	
___	___	Move the woman immediately to the operating room.
___	___	Ask the woman to grasp her legs behind the knees and pull them to her chest.
___	___	Tell the woman to rest and try pushing again in several minutes.
___	___	Put the head of the bed flat.
___	___	Press down on the woman's abdomen, just above the pubic symphysis, while a second person places gentle downward traction on the baby's head.

2. All of the following signs indicate delivery of a baby is imminent, except:
   - **A.** A sudden gush of blood
   - **B.** The anus dilates, and the anterior wall of the rectum becomes visible.
   - **C.** The perineum bulges.
   - **D.** The woman states the baby is coming.

3. Which of the following actions is appropriate when imminent delivery is recognized?

Yes	No	
___	___	Tell the woman that she will need to push, or stop pushing, as you direct.
___	___	Ask the woman to assume the knee-chest position until her physician arrives.
___	___	Call for help, but do not leave the woman.
___	___	Assist the woman to deliver where she is.
___	___	Move the woman immediately to a delivery room.

4. **True** **False** When a woman with a known placenta previa, at 30 weeks of gestation, and on bed rest in your hospital begins to have bright red spotting, she should be transferred immediately to the regional perinatal center for delivery.

5. **True** **False** A gush of blood from the vagina normally follows placental separation.

6. **True** **False** If a baby is in breech presentation, you should wrap a dry towel around the baby's legs and hips and begin to pull gently but steadily.

(continued)

405

Unit 12 Pretest (*continued*)

7. The first thing to do after the baby's head delivers is to
   A. Begin delivery of the shoulders.
   B. Suction the baby's nose.
   C. Tell the mother to stop pushing.
   D. Check for a nuchal cord.

8. If the placenta does not separate within 30 minutes after the birth of a baby and there is no bleeding, which of the following actions should you take first?
   A. Pull gently but steadily on the umbilical cord.
   B. Do nothing while you wait for spontaneous separation.
   C. Call for anesthesia staff and start an intravenous line.
   D. Insert a gloved hand into the vagina, through the cervix, and into the uterus to remove the placenta.

9. **True   False**   Immediately after a baby is born, you should tug firmly on the placental end of the umbilical cord to begin delivery of the placenta.

10. **True   False**   It is best to transport a woman with severe preeclampsia for delivery at a regional perinatal center as soon as her blood pressure increase to 190/110 mm Hg is noted.

11. **True   False**   It would generally be considered safe to transport a woman in early labor at 32 weeks of gestation, 4 cm dilated, and 80% effaced to a regional perinatal center 1 hour away for delivery at the center.

UNIT 12: IMMINENT DELIVERY AND PREPARATION FOR MATERNAL/FETAL TRANSPORT

Imminent Delivery

1. What is an imminent delivery?

An imminent delivery is one that is about to occur, owing to labor progressing very rapidly. An imminent delivery may be accompanied by other, more emergent conditions, such as maternal hemorrhage or fetal bradycardia, but not necessarily so.

Help should be sought as soon as the situation of imminent delivery is recognized. If maternal complications occur, if the baby requires resuscitation, or if the baby is preterm, prompt and aggressive intervention may be needed immediately and would require additional personnel. Management of those situations is not covered in this unit but is covered in other maternal and fetal care or neonatal care units in the Perinatal Continuing Education Program series.

The material in this unit covers care of the woman and the baby during a very short period. If delivery and the third stage of labor are uncomplicated and the newborn is a healthy, term newborn, little additional care will be needed.

2. How do you know delivery is imminent?

Delivery will generally occur within moments when the
- Fetal presenting part is visible in the vagina (almost always the baby's scalp and hair)
- Perineum bulges
- Anus dilates and the anterior wall of the rectum is visible
- Woman reports the sensation that the baby is coming

3. What should you do when you recognize delivery is imminent?

A. Allow the woman to deliver where she is
   You can be most helpful to the woman and best assist her with the delivery by responding calmly to the situation when it occurs and getting the assistance of other team members. An imminent delivery does not require efforts to urgently move the woman to a delivery room or an operating room. You cannot help with the birth or care of the baby if you are pushing the bed to a delivery room. If the woman is already in a labor-delivery-recovery room and delivery is imminent, it is not always necessary to convert the bed to the "delivery" configuration (stirrups extended and bottom of the bed removed).

 Call for help, but stay with the patient.

   Talk with the woman about what you and she need to do together to ensure a safe delivery. Calmly explain the situation to the woman with clear, direct instructions. Be supportive and encouraging and acknowledge her pain and her emotions, which may include fear.

B. Allow the woman to deliver the baby without interference
   If your call for help was answered, ask for an emergency delivery kit to be brought to the room and opened.

An emergency delivery kit is a packaged bundle of sterile supplies that is kept readily available in the labor area and the emergency department at all times and contains
- Sterile gloves (several pairs)
- Bulb syringe
- Two Kelly clamps or cord clamps (for clamping the cord)
- Scissors (to cut the cord)
- Sterile gauze
- Towels (to dry the baby)
- Baby blankets
- Stocking cap
- Resuscitation equipment and supplies for the baby (may be packaged separately in some institutions)

Each responding team member assists the delivering woman according to their role and experience level. Inform the woman of what to expect and what she needs to do. Tell her she may need to push or to stop pushing, as directed. Reassure her that she will be able to do everything she needs to do to deliver the baby. Do *not* try to delay delivery by crossing the woman's legs or pushing in against the baby's head. Work with the woman to accomplish a safe delivery.

4. What should you do when the head crowns?

Allow the natural process of birth to proceed without interference. In nearly all cases, the head will deliver spontaneously, with minimal risk to the woman or baby. If it is clear the next push will be very forceful, ask the woman to push less vigorously and with more control. Ask her to breathe or "pant" and to stop pushing. She can push again with the next contraction. This will help keep the delivery from resulting in laceration. Use gentle counter-pressure to control fetal head extension, one of the final cardinal movements of labor, to help to prevent perineal lacerations. An episiotomy is rarely necessary.

5. What should you do after the head delivers?

A. Check for a nuchal cord
  - If the umbilical cord is wrapped around the baby's neck, see if you can loosen the loop. If you can, pull that over the baby's head and go on with the delivery.
  - If the cord is tight and will not loosen easily, ask the mother not to push until the cord is free.
  - Be very hesitant to clamp and cut the umbilical cord before delivery of the shoulders. If shoulder dystocia occurs, several minutes may elapse before the baby is delivered, and clamping the cord will have completely interrupted fetoplacental blood flow and gas exchange.

B. Monitor delivery of the shoulders
  - Encourage the woman to push, in control. Anytime it seems the baby is coming too fast, ask her to stop pushing.
  - In the situation of spontaneous, unexpected delivery, the shoulders will almost always deliver unaided and without difficulty.
  - If the shoulders do not deliver after 3 to 5 pushes, there may be shoulder dystocia. (See Unit 11, Abnormal Labor Progress and Difficult Deliveries, in this book.)

Quickly take the following actions if shoulder dystocia is present or suspected:
- Put the head of the bed flat (if not already flat).
- Have the woman grasp behind her knees and pull them to her chest (McRoberts maneuver).

These actions, by themselves, will usually bring about delivery of the shoulders.

If not, the perineum must be elevated far enough off the bed to allow gentle downward traction on the head by one person, while another person exerts pressure on the anterior shoulder by pressing on the woman's abdomen, just above the pubic symphysis. This is referred to as *suprapubic pressure,* and it should be applied correctly and from the correct side of the patient to avoid complications (see Unit 11, Abnormal Labor Progress and Difficult Deliveries, in this book). The McRoberts maneuver, suprapubic pressure, and gentle downward traction must be done in one orchestrated effort in conjunction with effective maternal effort. Elevation of the hips will not be needed if the woman is in a bed that can be instantly split to "delivery" configuration. That configuration allows room for gentle downward traction on the baby's head.

6. What should you do if the baby is breech?

With rapid labor in breech presentation, delivery usually occurs spontaneously, even if the baby is preterm. Let the woman push the body of the baby out as far as she can. Attempts to manipulate the baby or to prevent delivery from occurring are more likely to result in a problem than allowing delivery to occur spontaneously.

 Do not, at any time, pull on the baby.

A. Delivery up to the umbilicus

Do not pull on the baby's body. Pulling on the baby may cause the baby's arms and neck to extend ("deflex" the head), thereby impeding delivery. Pulling on the baby may also cause trauma to the spine and spinal cord. Until the baby's body is delivered past the umbilicus, the baby is getting enough blood flow through the cord to provide adequate oxygenation.

B. Delivery beyond the umbilicus

1. Let the woman deliver the baby

   If the woman can deliver the shoulders and head spontaneously, allow that to occur with minimal intervention. Avoid intervening until it is clear the woman cannot accomplish the delivery by herself.

2. Provide support to the baby's trunk
   - Wrap a dry towel around the baby. Hold the baby's legs and body together with both hands (Figure 12.1; towel not shown).

   Do not pull on the baby's legs, hips, or lower trunk.
   - Support the baby's body off the bed as rotation naturally occurs. Do not, however, attempt to rotate the baby. Just provide support as the natural process occurs.

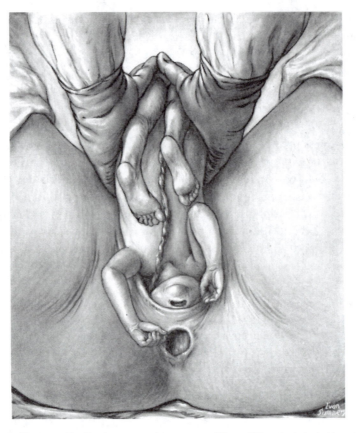

Figure 12.1. The Bracht Maneuver. The Bracht maneuver may seem as if it would hurt the baby but is actually the safest technique to use for a breech delivery in bed.
Based on Plentl AA, Stone RE. The Bracht maneuver. *Obstet Gynecol Surv.* 1953;8(3):313–325.

- *Elevate* the baby's hips and trunk upward as the arms and shoulders are being delivered. Do not apply traction.
- Continue to support the baby's body in a vertical position, with the baby's back held (not pressed) against the woman's symphysis (see Figure 12.1). Continue to lift, but *do not pull,* the baby while the woman pushes. The baby's head will deliver promptly.

7. What should you do after the baby is delivered?

A. One person takes care of the baby
   1. Assess the baby's condition
      Remember the ABCs of resuscitation. (See Book 1: Maternal and Fetal Evaluation and Immediate Newborn Care, Unit 5, Resuscitating the Newborn.) Follow standard neonatal resuscitation procedures to assess and ensure
      - Airway
      - Breathing
      - Circulation

      Suction first the baby's mouth and then the nose with the bulb syringe. If meconium is present, follow the standard procedure for neonatal resuscitation.

      Then
   2. Plan to prevent neonatal heat loss
      Do not overlook general support measures that are needed for every baby. In particular, it is important to keep the baby warm. Cold stress can severely compromise a preterm or sick baby. Even healthy term newborns can lose a tremendous amount of body heat and may have difficulty maintaining normal body temperature as they move from the warm, intrauterine environment to the cooler extrauterine environment.

      Heat loss and the danger of hypothermia should be minimized for *all* babies (preterm, term, post-term, healthy, at risk, or sick) by using the following procedures:
      - Maintain a relatively warm, draft-free delivery environment.
      - Before each delivery, turn on the radiant warmer and preheat the bed.
      - Use warm, dry towels to dry the baby immediately after delivery. (If possible, keep extra blankets and towels in a warmer immediately available to each room where deliveries occur.)
      - After delivery, place a term vigorous baby skin-to-skin with the mother and cover with warm, dry linens. Promptly remove any wet linens.
      - Dry the baby's head and put a cap on the baby.

      If the baby needs resuscitation measures, the initial steps of stimulation and drying can be performed on the mother's abdomen until the umbilical cord is clamped and cut. The infant may be transferred to the preheated radiant warmer for positive-pressure ventilation (PPV) and further intervention.

After delivery, all babies should be dried quickly, but thoroughly. Those requiring resuscitation should be placed on a preheated bed under a radiant warmer.

Take care not to *over*heat a baby, particularly if the baby requires resuscitation. *Hyper*thermia should be avoided because it may provoke apnea and worsen the extent of hypoxic brain injury in babies who experienced asphyxia before or during delivery. The general goal is to maintain a normal body temperature (36.5°C–37.5°C [97.7°F–99.5°F]).

Note: Therapeutic hypothermia instituted after resuscitation of a severely compromised newborn may reduce the extent of brain injury following hypoxia in term babies. This treatment is discussed in Book 1: Maternal and Fetal Evaluation and Immediate Newborn Care, Unit 5, Resuscitating the Newborn.

Then

3. Plan when to clamp and cut the umbilical cord

   Management of the umbilical cord after birth also requires coordination between obstetric and neonatal professionals. Leaving the umbilical cord intact while the newborn establishes spontaneous breathing facilitates the transition, as the lungs take over the function of oxygenation from the placenta and the heart changes from fetal to neonatal patterns of circulation. Providing an interval for physiological equilibration permits fetal blood that was circulating through the placenta to return to the newborn's circulation. This transfer of blood is especially valuable in preterm newborns to prevent low blood pressure immediately after birth and to help prevent anemia, the need for transfusion, and even intraventricular hemorrhage.

   - If the baby is vigorous, clamping and cutting the cord should be delayed. The ideal length of time to delay clamping has not been established, but it is clearly beneficial for the baby to cry and breathe before clamping the cord. The most rapid transfer of blood occurs in the first 1 to 3 minutes after birth. The baby may be dried on the mother's abdomen or on a surface at or below the level of the placenta. The initial steps of clearing the airway as needed and stimulating the baby to breathe can also be performed with the umbilical cord intact.
   - If a complication of pregnancy or delivery interferes with fetal-placental circulation, obstetric and neonatal professionals should agree on a plan before delivery and be prepared for rapid response to changes. For example, multiple gestation, placental bleeding, or a tight nuchal cord, in some cases, may be contraindications to delayed cord clamping.
   - If the baby needs PPV, the priority is to begin ventilation by 1 minute after delivery. Options for management include clamping the cord immediately or after the initial steps of drying and stimulating, then moving the baby to a radiant warmer for resuscitation. Other options, such as milking the umbilical cord prior to clamping or performing PPV with the umbilical cord intact, still have insufficient evidence to recommend them as routine procedures.

4. Obtain umbilical cord blood samples
   - After delivery of the baby, umbilical cord blood may be obtained for several purposes. Follow the protocol at your center for obtaining cord blood samples.
     a. Determine the baby's blood type and Rh(D) status.
        - If the mother is Rh(D) negative, umbilical cord blood should be collected to determine the newborn's Rh(D) status. If the baby is Rh(D) positive, administer Rh immunoglobulin to the mother prior to discharge to prevent Rh(D) alloimmunization. More information about this condition can be found in Unit 5, Obstetric Risk Factors: Prior or Current Pregnancy, in this book.
        - If the mother is blood type O, umbilical cord blood should be collected to determine the newborn's ABO status. A newborn whose blood group is A, B, or AB is at increased risk for hyperbilirubinemia and jaundice.

b. Determine the baby's umbilical cord blood pH level and acid-base status. Assessment of the pH level of arterial blood taken from the umbilical cord at the time of birth allows the obstetric care provider to identify the presence of severe acidemia (pH level < 7.00) at the time of birth, and assessment of a complete cord blood gas (including partial pressure of carbon dioxide and base deficit) allows the provider to determine if an acidotic fetus has a metabolic or respiratory acidosis. The presence of severe acidosis at the time of birth is essential to the diagnosis of intrapartum asphyxia. The absence of metabolic acidemia indicates that the cause of an adverse neonatal outcome is likely something other than an event that occurred during labor.

- There is no consensus on when an umbilical cord blood gas analysis should be performed. Clinical situations in which cord blood gases may be useful include persistently low Apgar scores (score < 4 at 5 minutes after birth), category III fetal heart rate tracings, urgent or emergency deliveries performed for indeterminate (category II) or abnormal (category III) fetal heart rate tracings, or sudden obstetric events, such as placental abruption, uterine rupture, or amniotic fluid embolism.
- Many providers clamp a 10- to 20-cm length of umbilical cord at each end and set it aside at the time of delivery. Blood may be drawn from the umbilical artery (and vein, if desired) for up to 60 minutes and still accurately reflect the baby's acid-base status at birth.
- Normal umbilical cord blood gas values are shown in Table 12.1.

c. Other blood tests may be performed from cord blood. Some centers have adopted the practice of obtaining neonatal intensive care unit admission laboratory tests, including complete blood count and blood cultures, by drawing blood from the vessels on the surface of the placenta. If a newborn requires blood samples for genetic testing, these may also be obtained from umbilical cord blood. In both cases, it is important to ensure that no maternal blood from the delivery is included in the sample.

Table 12.1. Normal Values of Umbilical Cord Blood Gases			
Component Name	**Unit of Measure**	**Reference Range for Arterial Cord Blood**	**Reference Range for Venous Cord Blood**
pH level	pH units	7.12 to 7.35	7.23 to 7.44
pO_2	mm Hg	6.2 to 27.6	16.4 to 40.0
pCO_2	mm Hg	41.9 to 73.5	28.8 to 53.3
Base excess	mmol/L	−9.3 to 1.5	−8.3 to 2.6
HCO_3	mmol/L	18.8 to 28.2	17.2 to 25.6

HCO_3, bicarbonate; pO_2, partial pressure of oxygen; pCO_2, partial pressure of carbon dioxide.

B. One person takes care of the mother
   1. Wait for the placenta to separate
      Hold the placental end of the clamped cord and maintain slight tension on the cord. There should be no attempt to pull the placenta out but just enough tension on the cord so you can feel when the placenta separates and the cord advances.
   2. Determine whether the placenta has separated
      Wait until there are indications that the placenta has separated. This usually occurs within 5 to 10 minutes after the cord is clamped. Indications of placental separation from the uterus include
      - A gush of blood from the vagina.
      - The cord advances from the vagina.
      - The placenta becomes visible at the introitus.
   3. Deliver the placenta
      Delivery of the placenta may occur after a few spontaneous pushes from the woman. If it does not, place a gloved finger in the vagina. If the placenta can be clearly felt or seen, pull gently on the cord and remove the placenta.

 Do not pull on the cord until you can see or feel the placenta in the vagina.

8. What should you do if spontaneous delivery of the placenta does not occur within 30 minutes?

A. If there is little or no bleeding
   Do nothing. If there is no bleeding, there is no reason for concern until more than 30 minutes after delivery of the baby has elapsed. During this time, do not pull on the cord. Do not push on the fundus. Be aware that retained placenta for more than 30 minutes after delivery may be a sign of placenta accreta, a condition in which the placenta is abnormally adherent to the uterine muscle. Attempts to manually remove a placenta accreta can result in significant, life-threatening blood loss. If there is minimal bleeding and the placenta has not yet delivered, await the arrival of an obstetric physician before attempting removal.

   Manual removal usually requires anesthesia.

   Preparations for manual removal include the following actions:
   - Start an intravenous (IV) line if one is not already in place; consider placing a second IV line.
   - Call for an anesthesiologist.
   - Manual removal may be attempted with regional anesthesia in the birthing suite, or you may consider moving the patient to a room where general anesthesia can be administered. The benefit of performing manual removal in the operating room under general anesthesia is that a laparotomy can be performed if necessary—for example, if placenta accreta is present.
   - Consider obtaining blood for possible transfusion.

UNIT 12: IMMINENT DELIVERY AND PREPARATION FOR MATERNAL/FETAL TRANSPORT

B. Whenever profuse bleeding is present or develops

Call for help. Anesthesia, volume expansion, and surgical and medical support are needed urgently.

If the patient is bleeding heavily or if profuse bleeding starts, the placenta must be removed. Do not attempt manual removal without anesthesia and surgical support unless the hemorrhage is so great that you fear the woman will soon bleed to death.

If you believe the woman's life is in danger, proceed immediately with manual removal. Simultaneously begin volume expansion and other measures to respond to maternal blood loss. The placenta must be removed from the uterus because the bleeding cannot be controlled until the placenta has been delivered.

See Unit 2, Obstetric Hemorrhage, and Unit 11, Abnormal Labor Progress and Difficult Deliveries, in this book, for additional information about management of obstetric hemorrhage and abnormal third stage of labor.

Self-test A

Now answer these questions to test yourself on the information in the last section.

A1. Give at least 2 signs the baby is coming.
_____
_____

A2. What is the first thing you should do after the head of a baby in vertex presentation is delivered?
_____

A3. What should you do immediately if the fetal shoulders of a vertex presentation do not deliver after 3 to 5 pushes?
_____
_____

A4. Give at least 2 indications the placenta has separated.
_____
_____

A5. A woman begins bleeding profusely after delivering a term newborn but before the placenta is delivered. The only way to control the bleeding is to
_____

Check your answers with the list that follows the Recommended Routines. Correct any incorrect answers and review the appropriate section in the unit.

Preparation for Maternal/Fetal Transport

1. What is maternal/fetal transport?

Maternal/fetal transport, sometimes called *intrauterine transport,* occurs when a pregnant woman is transferred to receive a higher level of care at a regional perinatal center. Depending on the woman's condition and available resources, she may be transported by private automobile, local rescue squad, community hospital ambulance and personnel, or specialized maternal transport vehicle and personnel based at the regional center.

2. Why is maternal/fetal transport important?

If the need for maternal/fetal or neonatal intensive care is anticipated, referral to a regional perinatal center is preferred for several reasons.
- Women or fetuses with certain conditions may require intensive care with highly specialized equipment and personnel for extended periods.
- Neonatal outcomes are significantly improved if delivery occurs at a regional perinatal center, instead of initiating neonatal transport to a regional perinatal center after delivery.
- Maternal/fetal transport allows a mother and baby to remain together after delivery.
- Maternal, fetal, and neonatal transport to a higher level of care provides cost-effective use of highly sophisticated, expensive medical equipment and resources for patients who also require high staff-to-patient ratios.

3. What are the goals of preparing a pregnant woman or fetus for transport?

The primary goal in preparing a pregnant woman and her fetus for transport to a regional perinatal center is to stabilize both of them. It is also important to decide which mode of transportation is most appropriate and make provisions for needed therapy en route.

A woman in active labor and a woman or fetus in unstable condition should not be transported, regardless of how close the regional perinatal center is to the referring hospital.

Likewise, the primary goal in preparing a baby for transport is to stabilize the newborn's condition. It is more important to stabilize a baby and wait for a regional center neonatal transport team to arrive at the birth hospital than to rush an unstable newborn to a regional center.

Stability of a baby's condition is far more important than speed of transport.

Transport of a newborn is covered in detail in Book 3: Neonatal Care, Unit 10, Preparation for Neonatal Transport.

4. Which women should be transported for delivery at a regional perinatal center?

Although each patient needs to be evaluated on an individual basis, general guidelines can be given for patients who are likely to require maternal/fetal or neonatal intensive care. Conditions for which maternal transfer might be advisable include, but are not limited to

- Maternal medical problems, such as cardiovascular, thyroid, or neurological conditions
- Preterm labor, unless in active labor
- Hypertensive disorder of pregnancy, including complications associated with chronic hypertension
- Rh or other red cell alloimmunization
- Maternal diabetes mellitus
- Third-trimester bleeding
- Preterm prelabor rupture of membranes
- Twin gestation at preterm gestational age or 3 or more fetuses at any gestational age
- Fetal growth restriction
- Severe maternal infection, such as hepatitis, pyelonephritis, influenza, HIV, or pneumonia
- Maternal kidney disease with deteriorating renal function
- Maternal substance use disorder
- Fetal malformation
- Hydramnios
- Oligohydramnios
- Abnormal results from tests of fetal well-being, provided immediate delivery is not indicated

 Whether maternal/fetal transport is advisable should be decided jointly by the patient's referring physician and the receiving regional perinatal center specialist. Never transport a patient unless she has been accepted at the regional center.

Points to discuss prior to transport include the following:

- Is transfer of this woman appropriate at this time, considering the specific circumstances and maternal/fetal condition? Can the resources available at the referring hospital meet the needs of the woman and the baby?
- When is the best time for transport to begin? (Now? After additional therapy is provided to the woman? Other time frame?)
- What mode of transport is most appropriate for this woman? Depending on the circumstances, options include a basic life support ambulance, an advanced life support ambulance, or air transfer.
- Are any specific preparations needed before transfer of this woman? Items to consider include
    - IV fluids and IV medications (as appropriate)
    - Medication administration (as appropriate)
    - Administration of the first dose of antenatal steroids
    - Blood transfusion
    - Recommended position for the woman during the transport
    - Fetal assessment

5. Which pregnant women should *not* be transported?

Generally, women in actively progressing labor should not be transported. Delivery under controlled circumstances at a referring hospital, with subsequent neonatal transfer, is almost always preferable to delivery en route during an attempted maternal transfer.

Exceptions may be made on an individual basis to allow transfer during actively progressing labor, with mutual agreement of the referring hospital and regional perinatal center staff. Such exceptions may be appropriate if there is a significant risk to the baby if delivered outside the regional center and usually only when there is a short transit time between the referring hospital and the regional center.

Transport should not be undertaken if a woman's condition cannot be stabilized. Examples of unstable maternal condition include uncontrolled hypertension or persistent vaginal bleeding. Transport also should not be undertaken if needed therapy cannot be provided during transfer. The level of care required in the hospital needs to be provided during transport.

Maternal transport should not be undertaken if there is a significant risk of delivery occurring during transfer or if essential care cannot be provided throughout the transfer process.

6. What should you do to prepare a pregnant woman for transport?

Maternal stability needs to be achieved before transport begins. This includes
- Stable vital signs
- Hemodynamic stability
- Cessation or stabilization of bleeding
- Suppression of seizure activity
- Control of metabolic status
- Control of hypertension

If maternal/fetal transport is undertaken for a woman whose condition might deteriorate during the journey, she should be accompanied by trained personnel with appropriate equipment. Minimal support for maternal transport in these circumstances includes
- Blood pressure monitoring equipment
- IV infusion apparatus, with an IV line in place before transport starts
- Appropriate medications
- Oxygen supply

Although maternal/fetal transport should not be undertaken if delivery during transit is likely to occur, complete neonatal resuscitation equipment should also be available. This should be specific neonatal equipment and separate from any equipment or supplies that might be needed for maternal care during transport.

UNIT 12: IMMINENT DELIVERY AND PREPARATION FOR MATERNAL/FETAL TRANSPORT

7. How do you make an obstetric referral?

Know how to contact your regional perinatal center for initiation of a maternal transfer. Communication between sending and receiving practitioners is essential prior to transfer. Both parties should agree on transfer, method of transport, and patient needs during transport. A paper or computer referral form, including one for a nurse-to-nurse report, to ensure standardization of communication about and process for a maternal/fetal or neonatal transport is recommended.

Self-test B

Now answer these questions to test yourself on the information in the last section.

B1. Give at least 3 reasons why maternal/fetal transport is important.
_____
_____
_____

B2. Name at least 6 conditions for which a maternal/fetal transport might be advisable.
_____
_____
_____
_____
_____
_____
_____

B3. A woman in _____ condition should not be transported.

B4. In addition to trained personnel, what equipment should be available during transport for the care of a pregnant woman who requires medical care during the transfer?
_____
_____
_____
_____
_____

Check your answers with the list that follows the Recommended Routines. Correct any incorrect answers and review the appropriate section in the unit.

IMMINENT DELIVERY AND PREPARATION FOR MATERNAL/FETAL TRANSPORT

Recommended Routines

All the routines listed below are based on the principles of perinatal care presented in the unit you have just finished. They are recommended as part of routine perinatal care.

Read each routine carefully and decide whether it is standard operating procedure in your hospital. Check the appropriate blank next to each routine.

Procedure Standard in My Hospital	Needs Discussion by Our Staff	Recommended Routine
_____	_____	1. Establish guidelines for an emergency • Standard contents • Designated storage locations (immediately accessible to, or in, each labor room and emergency department) • Maintenance of sterility of contents and replacement of kits
_____	_____	2. Establish a protocol for response to imminent deliveries, including a system for notifying obstetrics, pediatrics, anesthesia, and other personnel, as needed.
_____	_____	3. Ensure that information about how to make an obstetric referral is available at all times.
_____	_____	4. Establish guidelines for • Maternal condition prior to transport • Equipment and supplies to be available during transport

UNIT 12: IMMINENT DELIVERY AND PREPARATION FOR MATERNAL/FETAL TRANSPORT

Self-test Answers

These are the answers to the self-test questions. Please check them with the answers you gave and review the information in the unit wherever necessary.

Self-test A

A1. Any 2 of the following signs:
- The fetal presenting part is visible in the vagina (almost always the baby's scalp and hair).
- The perineum bulges.
- The anus dilates, and the anterior wall of the rectum is visible.
- The woman cries out that the baby is coming.

A2. Check for a nuchal cord.

A3. *Quickly* take the following actions:
- Put the head of the bed flat (if not already flat).
- Have the woman grasp behind her knees and pull them to her chest (McRoberts maneuver).

A4. Any 2 of the following indications:
- A gush of blood from the vagina
- The cord advances from the vagina.
- The placenta becomes visible at the introitus.

A5. A woman begins bleeding profusely after delivering a term newborn but before the placenta is delivered. The only way to control the bleeding is to *remove the placenta*.

Self-test B

B1. Any 3 of the following reasons:
- Allows highly specialized monitoring and evaluation for women or fetuses with uncommon conditions.
- Cost-effective use of medical equipment, personnel, and specialty services.
- Often less stressful for the baby than neonatal transport.
- Allows the mother to be near her baby soon after delivery.
- Recent data have shown improved maternal and neonatal outcomes when high-risk pregnant women give birth in regional perinatal centers.

B2. Any 6 of the following conditions:
- Maternal medical problems, such as cardiovascular, thyroid, or neurological conditions
- Preterm labor, unless in active labor
- Hypertensive disorder of pregnancy, including complications associated with chronic hypertension
- Rh or other red cell alloimmunization
- Maternal diabetes mellitus
- Third-trimester bleeding
- Preterm prelabor rupture of membranes
- Twin gestation at preterm gestational age or 3 or more fetuses at any gestational age
- Fetal growth restriction

- Severe maternal infection, such as hepatitis, pyelonephritis, influenza, HIV, or pneumonia
- Maternal kidney disease with deteriorating renal function
- Maternal drug dependency
- Fetal malformation
- Hydramnios
- Oligohydramnios
- Abnormal results from tests of fetal well-being, provided immediate delivery is not indicated

B3. A woman in *unstable* condition should not be transported.

B4. Blood pressure monitoring equipment
Intravenous (IV) infusion apparatus, with an IV line in place before transport starts
Appropriate medications
Oxygen supply
Neonatal resuscitation equipment

Unit 12 Posttest

After completion of each unit there is a free online posttest available at www.cmevillage.com to test your understanding. Navigate to the PCEP pages on www.cmevillage.com and register to take the free posttests.

Once registered on the website and after completing all the unit posttests, pay the book exam fee ($15) and pass the test at 80% or greater to earn continuing education credits. Only start the PCEP book exam if you have time to complete it. If you take the book exam and are not connected to a printer, either print your certificate to a .pdf file and save it to print later or come back to www.cmevillage.com at any time and print a copy of your educational transcript.

Credits are only available by book, not by individual unit within the books. Available credits for completion of each book exam are as follows: Book 1: 14.5 credits; Book 2: 16 credits; Book 3: 17 credits; Book 4: 9 credits.

For more details, navigate to the PCEP webpages at www.cmevillage.com.

Glossary

ABO incompatibility: A condition that may lead to neonatal hemolytic disease. The pregnant woman has group O red blood cells and antibodies to group A and B red blood cells. These antibodies are transferred to the fetus and cause destruction of fetal red blood cells. While this process is similar to Rh incompatibility, the hemolytic disease resulting from ABO incompatibility is less severe than the disease caused by Rh incompatibility. Unlike Rh incompatibility, ABO incompatibility cannot be prevented by giving the mother Rh immune globulin.

Acidosis: Abnormally *low* pH of the blood. The range of blood pH in a healthy neonate is between 7.25 and 7.35. A blood pH of 7.20 or lower is considered severe acidosis. Acidosis may result from metabolic disturbances in which the serum bicarbonate is low or inadequate respiratory efforts in which serum carbon dioxide is high. Often metabolic and respiratory factors simultaneously influence the blood pH. Acidotic babies are usually lethargic and may have mottled or grayish colored skin. If extremely acidotic, babies typically take deep, regular gasping breaths. If a baby is gasping, the pH is probably 7.00 or less. Acidosis should be corrected promptly, most commonly with assisted ventilation when due to inadequate respiratory effort or occasionally by administration of sodium bicarbonate if due to metabolic factors.

Acoustic stimulation: A test in which fetal response to a sound when produced by a device placed against the maternal abdomen and triggered to give a loud, 1-second buzz is used as an estimate of fetal well-being. This test may be used during a nonstress test or labor.

Adrenaline: Official British Pharmacopoeia name for epinephrine. The trademark name for epinephrine preparations is *Adrenalin*.

AGA: *See* Appropriate for gestational age.

Age, adjusted: *See* Age, corrected.

Age, chronological: Number of days, weeks, months, or years that have elapsed since birth.

Age, conceptional: Time elapsed between the day of conception and day of delivery. *Note:* The term *conceptual age* is incorrect and should not be used. *Conceptional age* may be used when conception occurred as a result of assisted reproductive technology, but should *not* be used to indicate the age of a fetus or newborn. *See also* Age, gestational.

Age, corrected: Chronologic age in weeks or months reduced by the number of weeks born before 40 weeks of gestation. It is used only for children up to 3 years of age who were born preterm. It is the preferred term to use after neonatal hospitalization, and should be used instead of *adjusted age*. *Example:* A 24-month-old child born at 28 weeks' gestation has a corrected age of 21 months.

Age, gestational: Number of completed weeks between the first day of the woman's last menstrual period and the day of delivery (or the date an assessment is performed if the woman has not yet delivered). If pregnancy was achieved using assisted reproductive technology and, therefore, the date of fertilization or implantation is defined, gestational age may be calculated by adding 2 weeks to the conceptional age.

Age, postmenstrual: Weeks of gestational age plus chronologic age. It is the preferred term to describe the age of preterm infants during neonatal hospitalization. *Note: Postconceptional age* should *not* be used. *Example:* A baby born at $33^{1}/_{7}$ weeks with a chronologic age of $5^{4}/_{7}$ weeks has a postmenstrual age of $38^{5}/_{7}$ weeks.

AIDS: Symptomatic stage of the illness caused by HIV.

Albumin: The major protein in blood.

Alkalosis: Abnormally *high* pH of the blood. Range of blood pH in a healthy neonate is between 7.25 and 7.35. Alkalosis may result from a high serum bicarbonate or, more commonly, when the carbon dioxide concentration in a baby's blood is lowered by hyperventilation (assisting the baby's breathing at an excessively fast rate). Babies who are alkalotic may not respond to stimulation intended to increase their breathing efforts until their blood carbon dioxide level rises toward the reference range.

Alpha fetoprotein: A normal fetal serum protein. When a fetus has an open neural tube defect, such as anencephaly or meningomyelocele, increased amounts of this protein pass into the amniotic fluid and the pregnant woman's blood, thus providing the basis for an antenatal screening test. Low or high maternal serum alpha fetoprotein levels may also indicate certain other fetal chromosomal defects or congenital malformations.

ALT: Alanine transaminase. The serum level of this enzyme is used as a measure of liver function. When liver cells are destroyed by disease or trauma, transaminases are released into the bloodstream. The higher the ALT, the greater the number of destroyed or damaged liver cells.

Alveoli: The numerous, small, saclike structures in the lungs where the exchange of oxygen and carbon dioxide between the lungs and blood takes place.

Amniocentesis: A procedure used to obtain amniotic fluid for tests to determine genetic makeup, health, or maturity of the fetus. Using ultrasound guidance, a needle is inserted through a pregnant woman's abdominal wall and into the uterus where a sample of amniotic fluid is withdrawn, usually at 16 to 20 weeks' gestation. If done earlier (11–13 weeks), there is often insufficient amniotic fluid and the complication rate is higher.

Amnioinfusion: Infusion of fluid into the amniotic cavity. Amnioinfusion may be done by either of the following procedures: after membranes have ruptured, by passing a catheter through the cervix and into the uterus and infusing physiologic (normal) saline solution or otherwise by infusing saline through an amniocentesis needle placed through the maternal abdominal wall and into the uterus. Amnioinfusion may be used to reduce cord compression (as indicated by variable fetal heart rate decelerations) during labor when oligohydramnios is present.

Amnion: The inner membrane surrounding the fetus. The amnion lines the chorion but is separate from it. Together these membranes contain the fetus and amniotic fluid.

Amniotic fluid: Fluid that surrounds the fetus and makes up the "water" in the "bag of waters." It provides a liquid environment in which the fetus can grow freely and serves as insulation, protecting the fetus from temperature changes. It also protects the fetus from a blow to the uterus by distributing equally in all directions any force applied to the uterus. Amniotic fluid is composed mainly of fetal urine, but also contains cells from the fetus's skin and chemical compounds from the fetus's respiratory passages.

Amniotic fluid analysis: Evaluation of various compounds in the amniotic fluid that relate to fetal lung maturity and fetal health. Fetal skin cells that normally float in the amniotic fluid may also be obtained with amniocentesis and grown in a culture to allow determination of fetal chromosomal status.

Amniotic fluid embolism: Amniotic fluid that escapes into the maternal circulation, usually late in labor or immediately postpartum. Rather than causing a mechanical blockage in the circulation as emboli of other origin might do, amniotic fluid embolism is thought to cause an anaphylactic-type response in susceptible women. This response is dramatic and severe, with sudden onset of hypoxia and hypotension. Seizures or cardiac arrest may occur. If a woman survives the initial phase, disseminated intravascular coagulation often follows. Although rare, it is associated with a high maternal mortality rate.

Analgesia: Relative relief of pain without loss of consciousness. Administration of specific medications is the most common way to provide analgesia.

Anemia: Abnormally low number of red blood cells. The red blood cells may be lost because of bleeding, destroyed because of disease process, or produced in insufficient numbers. Anemia is determined by measuring the hemoglobin or hematocrit.

Anencephaly: A lethal congenital defect of neural tube development in which there is partial or complete absence of the skull and brain.

Anesthesia: Total relief of pain, with or without loss of consciousness. Usually requires more invasive techniques than that required for analgesia. General inhalation anesthesia produces loss of consciousness, while major conduction anesthesia, such as spinal or epidural injection of long-lasting local anesthetics, produces total loss of pain in a specific area of the body without loss of consciousness.

Anomaly, congenital: Malformation resulting from abnormal development during embryonic or fetal growth. For example, a cleft lip is a congenital anomaly, as is gastroschisis, anencephaly, and countless others. Used synonymously with *congenital malformation*.

Antenatal: Period during pregnancy before birth. Synonymous with *prenatal*.

Antenatal testing: Techniques used to evaluate fetal growth and well-being prior to the onset of labor. Examples include nonstress test, biophysical profile, and ultrasonography.

Antepartum: Period of pregnancy before delivery. Most often used for period of pregnancy preceding the onset of labor. (*Intrapartum* is used to refer to the time during labor.) Used in reference to the woman.

Antibody: A type of blood protein produced by the body's lymph tissue in response to an antigen (a protein that is foreign to the bloodstream). Each specific antibody is formed as a defense mechanism against a specific antigen.

Antibody screening test: A test of maternal serum against a large variety of blood group antigens as a screening test for possible blood group incompatibility between a pregnant woman and her fetus. If the antibody screening test result is positive, the individual blood group incompatibility should be identified. *See also* Coombs test.

Antibody titers: A test used to indicate the relative concentration of a particular antibody present in a person's blood. *Example:* A high rubella titer indicates a person has been exposed to rubella (German measles) and formed a significant amount of antibody against the rubella virus and, therefore, will most likely be able to ward off another attack of the virus without becoming ill.

Anticonvulsants: Drugs given to prevent the occurrence of seizures (convulsions). The most common anticonvulsants used in infants are phenobarbital and phenytoin (Dilantin). Anticonvulsant therapy, with certain medications, for a pregnant woman with a seizure disorder may affect health of the fetus.

Antiphospholipid antibody syndrome (APS): Development of antibodies to naturally occurring phospholipids in the blood, causing abnormal phospholipid function. Antiphospholipid antibodies may be present in healthy women but are more commonly associated with a generalized disease (eg, lupus erythematosus). They have a strong association with recurrent miscarriage, fetal growth restriction, preeclampsia, and other factors adversely affecting fetal or maternal health.

Aorta: Main artery leaving the heart and feeding the systemic circulation. It passes through the chest and abdomen, where it branches into smaller arteries. In a newborn, an umbilical arterial catheter passes through one of the arteries in the umbilical cord and into the abdominal section of the aorta.

Apgar score: A score given to newborns and based on heart rate, respiratory effort, muscle tone, reflex irritability, and color. The score is given 1 minute after the baby's head and feet are delivered (not from the time the cord is cut) and again when the baby is 5 minutes of age. If the 5-minute score is less than 7, additional scores are given every 5 minutes for a total of 20 minutes. The 1-minute Apgar score indicates a baby's immediate condition; the 5-minute score reflects the baby's condition and effectiveness of resuscitative efforts. A low 5-minute score is a worrisome sign. It is not, however, a certain indicator of damage. Likewise, a high score is not a guarantee of a healthy baby. The score is named for Dr Virginia Apgar, who developed it. The 5 letters of her name may also be used to signify the 5 components of the score: A = appearance (color), P = pulse (heart rate), G = grimace (reflex irritability), A = activity (muscle tone), and R = respirations.

Apnea: Stoppage of breathing for 15 seconds or longer, or stoppage of breathing for less than 15 seconds if also accompanied by bradycardia or cyanosis.

Appropriate for gestational age (AGA): Refers to a baby whose weight is above the 10th percentile and below the 90th percentile for babies of that gestational age.

APS: *See* Antiphospholipid antibody syndrome.

Arrhythmia: Abnormal rhythm of the heartbeat. *Fetal* arrhythmias are rare. One of the more common ones is congenital heart block, which occurs almost exclusively with maternal systemic lupus erythematosus, although it is uncommon even in that situation. With a *maternal* arrhythmia, the more persistent the arrhythmia and farther the rate is from normal (either faster or slower), the more likely it is there will be a deleterious effect on maternal cardiac output and, thus, on blood flow to the uterus.

Artery: Any blood vessel that carries blood away from the heart.

Asphyxia: A condition resulting from inadequate oxygenation or blood flow and characterized by low blood oxygen concentration, high blood carbon dioxide concentration, metabolic acidosis, and organ injury.

Aspiration: (1) Breathing in or inhaling of a fluid (eg, formula, meconium, or amniotic fluid) into the lungs. Aspiration usually interferes with lung function and oxygenation. If inhaled, meconium is irritating as well as obstructing, resulting in meconium aspiration syndrome, which often causes serious and sometimes fatal lung disease. (2) Removal of fluids or gases from a cavity, such as the stomach, by suction. *Example:* A nasogastric tube is inserted and an empty syringe is attached to the tube and used to suck out or aspirate air and gastric juices from the stomach.

Assisted ventilation: Use of mechanical devices to help a person breathe. Bag and mask with bag breathing, endotracheal tube with bag breathing, or a respirator machine may each be used to assist ventilation.

AST: Aspartate transaminase. The serum level of this enzyme is used as a measure of liver function. As with alanine aminotransaminase, liver damage causes transaminases to be released into the bloodstream.

Atelectasis: Condition in which lung alveoli have collapsed and remain shut.

Atony: Loss of muscle tone or strength. Uterine atony is a leading cause of postpartum hemorrhage.

Axillary: Refers to the axilla, or armpit.

Bacteriuria: Presence of bacteria in the urine.

Bag breathing: Artificially breathing for a person by inflating the lungs with a resuscitation bag and mask or resuscitation bag and endotracheal tube.

Ballooning of lower uterine segment: A sign of impending labor, either term or preterm. The process leading to labor produces thinning of the lower uterine segment of myometrium, so that the lower segment "balloons out" into the anterior fornix of the vagina. The ballooned segment may be seen during speculum examination or palpated during digital examination.

BCG: Bacille Calmette-Guérin. Vaccine made from the Calmette-Guérin strain of *Mycobacterium bovis* for immunization against tuberculosis.

Beneficence: Acting for the benefit of a patient.

β-human chorionic gonadotropin (β-hCG): A hormone produced by trophoblastic cells of the chorionic villi. It is the first biochemical marker of pregnancy and produced in increasing amounts until maximal levels are reached at 8 to 10 weeks. When β-hCG is present in the blood or urine of a woman, she is pregnant. High titers are found with multifetal gestation and erythroblastosis fetalis; extremely high titers may be seen with hydatidiform mole and choriocarcinoma, while declining or low levels are found with spontaneous abortion and ectopic pregnancy.

Betamimetic: A drug that stimulates β-adrenergic receptors of smooth muscle, such as the myometrium (uterine muscle), causing decreased contractions. Used to suppress the onset of premature labor. A betamimetic drug is also called a *β-adrenergic receptor agonist*. An example is terbutaline.

Bilirubin: A substance produced from the breakdown of red blood cells. High blood bilirubin level causes the yellow coloring of the skin (and sclera) that is termed *jaundice*.

Biophysical profile (BPP): A combination of measures used to evaluate fetal well-being. Each of the 5 components (nonstress test, ultrasound evaluation of amniotic fluid volume, fetal body movements, muscle tone, and respirations) is scored. Each measure is given 2 points if present, zero if absent (there is no score of 1). The scores are added together for the final BPP score.

GLOSSARY

Biparietal diameter (BPD): Diameter of the skull, measured as the distance between the parietal bones, which lie just above each ear. Ultrasonography is used to determine BPD of the fetal skull. Serial BPD measurements are used to assess fetal growth and estimate fetal gestational age.

Bishop score: A system that scores cervical dilation, effacement, consistency, and position, as well as station of the presenting part to assess the "readiness" of a cervix for labor. Scores correlate with the likelihood that an attempt at induction of labor will be successful.

Blood gas measurement: Determination of the pH and concentration of oxygen, carbon dioxide, and bicarbonate in the blood.

Blood glucose screening test: Any of several commercially available, small, thin, plastic reagent strips designed to estimate blood glucose level with a single drop of blood. A color change caused by a drop of blood placed on the reagent pad provides an estimate of the blood glucose level. In addition, several handheld devices are designed to draw in a tiny amount of blood and give a digital readout of the glucose level.

Blood group: Numerous blood groups are in humans, each defined by their antigenic responses. The major blood groups are A, B, AB, and O, which are then further defined by their Rh type, positive or negative, as well as various other minor antigens. *Note:* Every person is exposed to the major blood group antigens (A and B) soon after birth, because the antigens are found in air, food, and water. Each person who lacks one or both of the major blood group genes (A or B) will make antibodies against the antigens they lack. Thus, persons with blood group O develop anti-A and anti-B antibodies and keep them throughout life. If given a blood transfusion with group A or B blood, a person with group O blood will have a transfusion reaction, which may in some cases be fatal. Similar reactions occur when a person with group B blood is given group A blood, or vice versa. Group "AB" persons do not make antibodies against either A or B because they have both antigens on their red blood cells. Persons with group AB blood can receive blood from people with any major blood group, but AB blood should be transfused only into persons with AB blood. Persons with group O blood should receive only blood transfusions with O blood, but O blood may be used to transfuse a person with any major blood group. This is why a person with AB blood is called a *universal recipient* and a person with O blood is called a *universal donor*.

Blood pressure, diastolic: Lowest point of the blood pressure between heartbeats, when the heart is relaxed.

Blood pressure, mean: The diastolic blood pressure plus one-third of the difference between the systolic and diastolic blood pressure.

Blood pressure, systolic: Highest point of the blood pressure. The blood pressure during the heartbeat, when the heart is contracted.

Blood smear: A thin layer of blood spread across a glass slide and studied under a microscope to determine the types of blood cells present.

Blood type: *See* Blood group.

Bloody show: Bloody mucus passed from the vagina in late pregnancy, usually associated with cervical effacement. It often heralds the onset of labor and is a normal finding. Any bleeding in pregnancy, however, should be investigated.

BPD: *See* Biparietal diameter.

BPP: *See* Biophysical profile.

Brachial plexus nerve injury: Paralysis of the arm that results from injury to the upper brachial plexus. Is associated with shoulder dystocia or a difficult breech delivery when traction is applied to the shoulder, stretching the nerve trunks exiting from the cervical spinal cord (brachial plexus). However, about one-half of these injuries occur in children in whom there was no evidence of either shoulder dystocia or breech delivery. The injury, therefore, may be initiated before birth by deformation of the neck and shoulder by abnormal positioning of the fetus. Many such palsies will recover within the first few years after birth.

Bracht maneuver: A method of delivering breech presentations in cases in which delivery is imminent and neither a practitioner skilled in vaginal breech delivery nor cesarean delivery is immediately available.

Bradycardia: Slow heart rate. (1) *Fetal:* Considered to be a baseline heart rate of less than 110 beats/min for 2 minutes or longer. Bradycardia alone may or may not indicate fetal distress. (2) *Neonatal:* Considered to be a sustained heart rate less than 100 beats/min.

Breech presentation: The feet- or buttocks-first presentation of a fetus. (1) *Frank:* Buttocks presenting, with the fetus's legs extended upward alongside the body. (2) *Footling:* One foot can be felt below the buttocks. (3) *Double footling:* Both feet can be felt below the buttocks. (4) *Complete:* Buttocks presenting, with the knees flexed.

Bronchopulmonary dysplasia (BPD): Also called *chronic lung disease.* A form of chronic lung disease sometimes seen in infants who have required ventilator therapy for any of a variety of lung problems, including respiratory distress syndrome and meconium aspiration syndrome. Bronchopulmonary dysplasia is thought to result from the combined effects of oxygen free-radical injury of premature lungs and trauma to the lungs produced by high airway pressures generated by ventilators.

Brow presentation: The brow (forehead) of the fetus is the presenting part. On vaginal examination, the anterior fontanel can be felt, but the posterior fontanel cannot. Management depends on whether the presentation stays brow or changes to face or the baby's neck flexes and the presentation becomes vertex.

Caput succedaneum: Edema of the fetal scalp that develops during labor. This swelling crosses suture lines of the skull. Caput succedaneum may occur with a normal, spontaneous vaginal delivery, but a lengthy labor or delivery by vacuum extraction increases the risk of occurrence.

Cardiac massage: *See* Chest compressions.

Cardiac output: Output of the left ventricle in milliliters per minute.

Central nervous system depression: Condition in which the body is less reactive than normal to stimuli, such as a pinprick. Central nervous system depression may be characterized by delayed reflexes, lethargy, or coma. It may result from a variety of causes, including certain drugs, certain metabolic disorders, or asphyxia.

Cephalhematoma: Also called *cephalohematoma.* Hematoma under the periosteum of the skull and limited to one cranial bone (does not cross suture lines) of the newborn. It is usually seen following prolonged labor and difficult delivery, but may also occur with uncomplicated birth. Delivery with forceps or vacuum extraction increases the risk of occurrence.

Cephalopelvic disproportion (CPD): *See* Fetopelvic disproportion.

Cerclage of the cervix: The procedure of placing a suture around the cervix to prevent it from dilating prematurely. There are several different techniques for placing the suture. Cervical cerclage is used as a treatment for incompetent cervix.

Cervix: The lower, narrow end of the uterus, which opens into the vagina.

Cesarean delivery: Surgical delivery of the fetus through an abdominal incision. The uterine incision may be classical (vertical, cutting through both the contractile and non-contractile segments) or confined to the non-contractile lower uterine segment (either vertical or transverse incision).

Chest compressions: Artificial pumping of blood through the heart by a bellows effect created from intermittent compression of the sternum, over the heart, during resuscitation.

Chickenpox: *See* Varicella-zoster virus.

Chlamydia: A type of microorganism with several species. Capable of producing a variety of illnesses, including eye infection, pneumonia, and infection of the genitourinary tract.

Choanal atresia: Congenital blockage of the nasal airway. Because babies breathe mainly through their noses, a baby with choanal atresia will have severe respiratory distress at birth. The immediate treatment is insertion of an oral airway. Surgical repair when the baby is stable is required for permanent correction.

GLOSSARY

Chorioamnionitis: Inflammation of the fetal membranes, also known as *intra-amniotic infection,* or IAI. The fetus may also become infected.

Chorion: Fetal membrane that surrounds the amnion, but is separate from it, and lies against the decidual lining of the uterine cavity (endometrium). During embryonic development, the chorion gives rise to the placenta.

Chorionic villus sampling (CVS): A highly specialized technique in which a tiny portion of the chorionic villi, which contain the same genetic material as the fetus, is obtained in a manner similar to a needle biopsy. The cells obtained may be analyzed for chromosomal defects. Chorionic villus sampling may be done as early as 10 weeks' gestation, with preliminary results available within as little as 2 days, allowing earlier and more rapid detection of chromosomal disorders than is possible with amniocentesis. The incidence of complications is similar to the risks associated with amniocentesis.

Chromosome: The material (DNA protein) in each body cell that contains the genes, or information regarding hereditary factors. Each normal cell contains 46 chromosomes. Each chromosome contains numerous genes. A baby acquires one-half of chromosomes from the mother and one-half from the father. A chromosomal defect results from an abnormal number of chromosomes or structural damage to the chromosomes. *Example:* Each cell in the body of a baby with Down syndrome (trisomy 21) contains 47 instead of 46 chromosomes.

Chronic lung disease (CLD): *See* Bronchopulmonary dysplasia.

Circulatory system: The system that carries blood through the body and consists of the heart and blood vessels. The systemic circulatory system carries blood to and from the head, arms, legs, trunk, and all body organs except the lungs. The pulmonary circulatory system carries blood to the lungs, where carbon dioxide is released and oxygen is collected, and returns the oxygenated blood to the systemic circulatory system.

Cirrhosis: Chronic degeneration of the hepatic cells, replacing them with fibrosis and nodular tissue and resulting in liver failure. Chronic hepatitis and alcoholism are common causes.

CLD: Chronic lung disease. *See* Bronchopulmonary dysplasia.

CMV: *See* Cytomegalovirus.

Coagulation: The process of blood clot formation.

Colon: The large intestine, which is between the small intestine and rectum.

Colonization: Persistent, asymptomatic presence of bacteria in a particular area of the body. If symptoms develop, it becomes an infection. *Example:* Many women have vaginal or rectal colonization with group B β-hemolytic streptococci but are entirely without symptoms, although maternal group B β-hemolytic streptococci colonization poses a risk for life-threatening neonatal infection.

Compliance (of lung): Refers to elastic properties of the lungs. Babies with certain lung diseases have decreased compliance (stiff lungs) and thus cannot expand their lungs well during inhalation.

Comprehensive ultrasound: Detailed ultrasound examination designed to review all parts of fetal anatomy. Done when congenital malformations are suspected.

Condyloma: Warty growth of skin in the genital area caused by human papillomavirus.

Congenital: Refers to conditions that are present at birth, regardless of cause. Congenital defects may result from a variety of causes, including genetic factors, chromosomal factors, diseases affecting the pregnant woman, and drugs taken by the woman. The cause, however, of most congenital defects is unknown. *Note: Congenital* and *hereditary* are not synonymous. *Congenital* means present at birth. *Hereditary* means the genetic transmission from parent to child of a particular trait, which may be the trait for a specific inheritable disease and associated malformations. Some defects are congenital and hereditary, but many are simply congenital with no genetic link.

Congenital rubella syndrome: A group of congenital anomalies resulting from an intrauterine rubella infection. Anomalies commonly include cataracts, heart defects, deafness, microcephaly (abnormally small head), and intellectual disability.

Congestive heart failure: A condition that develops when the heart cannot pump as much blood as it receives. As a result, fluid backs up into the lungs and other tissues, causing edema and respiratory distress. Congestive heart failure may result from a diseased or malformed heart, severe lung disease, or too much fluid given to the patient.

Conjugation of bilirubin: Process that occurs in the liver and combines bilirubin with another chemical so it may be removed from the blood and pass out of the body in the feces. Failure of bilirubin conjugation is one cause of jaundice.

Conjunctivitis: Inflammation of the membrane that covers the eye and lines the eyelids. Certain genital tract infections, particularly *Chlamydia* and gonorrhea, in a pregnant woman can cause severe conjunctivitis and eye damage in a newborn, unless proper neonatal treatment is given.

Continuous positive airway pressure (CPAP): A steady pressure delivered to the lungs by means of a special apparatus or mechanical ventilator. Continuous positive airway pressure may be used for babies with respiratory distress syndrome to prevent alveoli from collapsing during expiration.

Contraction stress test (CST): Termed *oxytocin challenge test* when oxytocin is used to induce contractions. A brief period of uterine contractions (either spontaneous or induced with nipple stimulation or intravenous oxytocin administration) during which the fetal heart rate and uterine contractions are monitored with an external monitor. It is a test used in certain high-risk pregnancies to assess fetal well-being.

Coombs test: Test to determine the presence of antibodies in blood or on red blood cells. There are 2 forms of the test. The direct Coombs test detects antibodies attached to the red blood cells; the indirect Coombs test detects antibodies within the serum. *Example:* The direct test is used to detect antibodies present on the red blood cells of Rh-positive babies born to Rh-negative sensitized women. The indirect test is used on a woman's blood to detect antibodies to fetal Rh-positive cells. *See also* Antibody screening test.

Cord presentation: Also referred to as *funic presentation*. A situation in which the umbilical cord lies against the membranes over the cervix, beneath the fetal presenting part. This poses a risk for cord injury or prolapse when the membranes rupture.

Cordocentesis: *See* Percutaneous umbilical blood sampling.

Corticosteroids: Refers to any of the steroids of the adrenal cortex. Betamethasone and dexamethasone are artificially prepared steroids that may be given to a woman to speed up the process of lung maturation in her fetus when preterm delivery is unavoidable.

COVID-19: Coronavirus disease 2019, the clinical illness caused by infection with SARS-CoV-2 (severe acute respiratory syndrome coronavirus 2), a novel coronavirus that caused a global pandemic beginning in late 2019.

CPAP: *See* Continuous positive airway pressure.

CPD: Cephalopelvic disproportion. *See* Fetopelvic disproportion.

Creatinine: A chemical in the blood excreted in urine and used as an indication of renal function.

Cryoprecipitate: A concentrated form of plasma. In a much smaller volume, it contains fibrinogen, coagulation factor VIII, and some, but not all, of the other coagulation factors found in fresh frozen plasma. Used in the treatment of severe disseminated intravascular coagulation.

CST: *See* Contraction stress test.

CVS: *See* Chorionic villus sampling.

Cyanosis: Bluish coloration of the skin. (1) *Central cyanosis:* Bluish coloration of the skin and mucous membranes due to inadequate arterial blood oxygen concentration. Sometimes babies with central cyanosis are described as appearing dusky. (2) *Acrocyanosis:* Cyanosis of the hands and feet only, which is generally not associated with low blood oxygen concentration.

Cytomegalic inclusion disease: An infection with cytomegalovirus. Maternal infection may go unnoticed, but fetal infection, especially early in gestation, can damage every organ system. The disease commonly causes an enlarged liver and spleen, encephalitis, microcephaly, intracranial calcification, and visual or hearing defects.

Cytomegalovirus (CMV): The virus that causes cytomegalic inclusion disease.

Debridement: Removal of dead tissue and foreign matter from a wound.

Deceleration: *See* Fetal heart rate deceleration.

Decidua: Endometrium that has been modified by the hormonal effects of pregnancy; the endometrium during pregnancy.

Deflexed head: The fetal head is not round. It is longer from front to back (occipitomental diameter is approximately 13.5 cm at term) than it is from side to side (biparietal diameter is approximately 9.5 cm at term). When the fetal head is well flexed with the chin on the chest, the top of the head, with a maximum diameter of 9.5 to 10 cm, is presented to the pelvis. In most cases, the pelvis is larger than this, allowing the head (largest part of the fetus) to pass through it. When the head is deflexed, as it is in brow and face presentations, the farther the chin is from the chest, the larger the diameter is presented to the pelvis. These presentations make vaginal delivery difficult or impossible without risk of serious damage to the fetus or woman.

Deformation: Structural defect of a fetus caused by mechanical force, rather than abnormal embryonic development or an inherited disease. External factors, such as uterine fibroids or amniotic bands, may produce a deformity by compressing parts of the fetus. Prolonged oligohydramnios can also cause deformities, due to lack of the amniotic fluid cushion normally provided to a growing fetus. Sometimes these deformities, such as an angulated spine or flattened head, resolve spontaneously over time. In other cases, cosmetic surgery will be needed for correction. Malformation and deformation are not synonymous. *Malformation* is the term used when a congenital anomaly is due to *abnormal development* of the fetus. *Deformation* is the term used when a congenital anomaly is due to *external mechanical force* applied to a growing fetus.

Dehiscence: Separation of an incision that had been surgically united. The separation may be partial, involving only the outer layer, or complete through all tissue layers. In perinatal care, this term is most commonly applied to the postoperative separation of an abdominal incision or development of an opening in a uterine scar from a previous cesarean delivery.

Diabetes, gestational: Also called *glucose intolerance of pregnancy* or *gestational diabetes mellitus*. Disturbance of glucose metabolism that mimics diabetes mellitus and first appears during pregnancy and, in many cases, disappears after delivery. Women with this condition are more likely than the general population, however, to develop insulin-dependent diabetes later in life. Because normal control of blood glucose during pregnancy is important for fetal well-being, and because this metabolic problem is fairly common, screening tests for abnormal glucose tolerance are recommended for every prenatal patient.

Diabetes mellitus: A metabolic disorder in which the body's ability to use glucose is impaired because of a disturbance in normal production of or response to insulin. This leads to high blood glucose levels and other metabolic imbalances. Diabetes mellitus during pregnancy places the woman and fetus at risk for certain serious problems and may affect health of the newborn.

Diaphragm: The primary muscle of breathing that separates the chest cavity from the abdominal cavity.

Diaphragmatic hernia: A defect in the diaphragm through which abdominal organs slip and enter the chest, where they compress the lungs. If abdominal organs enter the chest cavity early in gestation, development of one or both of the lungs can be severely inhibited.

DIC: *See* Disseminated intravascular coagulation.

Digital examination: Examination of the cervix and, during labor, the presenting part of the fetus, with a gloved hand inserted in the vagina (examination is done using your fingers, or digits), as opposed to a speculum examination to view the cervix.

Digitalis: A drug that increases the contraction force of the heart while at the same time decreasing the rate at which the heart beats. Sometimes used to treat congestive heart failure.

Dilation: The condition of being stretched beyond normal dimensions. In perinatal care this most commonly refers to the degree of opening in the cervical os.

Dipstick: Thin, narrow paper or plastic strip (or "stick") with chemical reagents that change color in the presence of certain conditions in the liquid being tested. Different types of dipstick test for different substances, and some dipsticks have several reagent patches to test for several substances on the same stick. Dipsticks are used to test body fluids, such as vaginal secretions, gastric aspirate, and urine. Examples of their use in perinatal care include testing vaginal secretions for pH to help identify rupture of the membranes and urine for protein in women with hypertension.

Disseminated intravascular coagulation (DIC): An acquired disturbance of the body's blood coagulation processes in which coagulation factors are consumed, leaving the blood incapable of coagulating. Certain serious illnesses may trigger the onset of DIC in neonates or adults. Most commonly in neonates, DIC may accompany severe sepsis, hypoxia, acidosis, or hypotension. In pregnant women, DIC may accompany placental abruption, retained dead fetus syndrome, or sepsis. Blood platelets and coagulation factors are activated abnormally by the release of thromboplastic substances into the circulation. As a result, numerous fibrin clots are formed in the capillaries. Red blood cells may be broken down as blood flow pushes the cells through the clogged capillaries, which may lead to hemolytic anemia. In addition, oozing from puncture sites, surgical incisions or other wounds, and easy bruising may occur as the platelets and coagulation factors are consumed by the fibrin clots and are no longer available to maintain normal blood coagulation. Neonates with DIC, especially preterm babies, are also at risk for pulmonary or intracranial hemorrhage. Treatment, which is complex, is directed at correcting the underlying disease process and providing emergency management to correct the coagulation deficit.

Diuretics: Drugs (eg, furosemide, thiazides, spironolactone) given to prevent or decrease fluid buildup in the lungs and body by increasing urine output.

DNA testing: Also called *genetic testing*. Samples of tissues (eg, blood, urine, skin) are treated, using a highly technical process, to extract the DNA of chromosomes (and mitochondria). Tests can then reveal defective genes that cause specific diseases. Most disease-causing genes, however, have not yet been identified.

Dolichocephalic: Long headed; typically refers to the elongated head of a fetus in breech position when ultrasonography is used to measure the fetal skull biparietal diameter. This head shape reduces the accuracy of biparietal diameter measurements.

Doppler instrument: A device used to detect changes of blood flow through a blood vessel. A Doppler instrument may be used to detect fetal heartbeats.

Double setup: A vaginal examination performed in an operating room, with everything in readiness for either a vaginal or cesarean delivery. Used in cases of suspected placenta previa during labor, in which the examination itself may trigger such profuse hemorrhage that immediate surgery is required.

Down syndrome: Also called *trisomy 21*. A chromosomal abnormality resulting in a typical facial appearance, intellectual disability, and sometimes other congenital defects, particularly cardiac defects. Individuals with Down syndrome have 47 instead of the normal 46 chromosomes, with one additional copy of chromosome 21 in each cell.

Ductus arteriosus: A blood vessel in the fetus that connects the pulmonary artery and aorta. This allows less blood to go to the fetal lungs and more blood to go to the systemic and placental circulation. Normally this vessel closes shortly after birth, thus redirecting blood flow to the lungs. A *patent ductus arteriosus* means the ductus arteriosus persistently remains open after birth. As a result, and with changes in pressure that occur within the circulatory system once placental circulation is eliminated, blood may flow from the aorta into the pulmonary artery, resulting in too much blood directed to the lungs. This may cause congestive heart failure in the baby.

Dusky: *See* Cyanosis.

Dye test: In perinatal care, this usually refers to a test done to determine if the amniotic membranes are ruptured. There is no indication for a dye test unless there is reason to suspect that rupture of membranes has occurred, other tests are negative, *and* the diagnosis of ruptured membranes will affect clinical management. Amniocentesis is done under ultrasound guidance. If indicated, a sample of amniotic fluid is withdrawn for testing. A dye, usually indigo carmine, is then introduced through the amniocentesis needle. A sterile gauze pad (4 × 4 in) is placed high in the woman's vagina. If no dye appears on the pad after 20 to 30 minutes of sitting or walking, it is most likely that the membranes are intact and have not ruptured.

Dyspnea: Difficult breathing, labored. This may accompany any variety of disease states or be a result of physical exertion in a healthy person.

Dystocia: Difficult labor. (1) *Uterine:* Abnormal labor, particularly prolonged. Used to refer to weak or ineffective uterine contractions. Usually used to describe a labor that has ceased progressing such that a cesarean delivery is necessary. (2) *Shoulder:* Situation in which the shoulders of a baby in vertex presentation become trapped after delivery of the head. This is an emergency, requiring immediate intervention to avoid severe fetal hypoxia.

ECG: *See* electrocardiograph.

Eclampsia: Term used to describe the condition in which convulsions or coma develop in a pregnant or postpartum woman with pregnancy-related hypertension. The condition of preeclampsia becomes eclampsia whenever seizures or coma develop.

EDD: Estimated date of delivery. *See* Pregnancy due date.

Edema: Swelling due to an excessive amount of fluid in the tissues.

Effacement: The process of thinning of the cervix prior to and after the onset of labor.

Electrocardiograph: Also called *electrocardiogram, electronic cardiac monitor*. A device used for recording the heart's electrical activity.

Electrolyte: A substance that dissociates into ions when in solution (and thereby makes the solution capable of conducting electricity). Commonly refers to sodium, potassium, chloride, and bicarbonate in blood.

Embolus: A blood clot or other plug (eg, an air bubble) carried by the blood from a larger to smaller blood vessel, where it lodges and obstructs the blood flow. Plural: emboli.

Embryo: Term used for the product of conception, from the time a fertilized egg is implanted until all major structures and organs are defined. In humans, this is the first 8 weeks of development after conception (10 weeks after the last menstrual period). After 8 weeks and until birth, the term *fetus* is used.

Endocrine system: Refers to organs that release hormones into the blood.

Endometritis: Infection of inner lining of the uterine cavity, the endometrium.

Engagement, engaged: Term applied during late pregnancy or in labor that indicates that the largest diameter of the presenting part is at or below the smallest diameter of the pelvis. Usually the presenting part is the fetal head, which is said to be engaged when a vaginal examination reveals the head to be at or below the ischial spines.

Environmental oxygen: *See* Inspired oxygen.

Epidural: A technique for providing anesthesia during labor. A hollow needle is inserted between 2 vertebrae in the woman's spine, and a catheter is threaded through the needle and into the epidural space of the spinal column. A local anesthetic is then injected through the catheter into the epidural space. This eliminates all sensation for the nerve roots that the drug contacts. The greater the volume of anesthetic medication injected, the greater the number of nerve roots affected and, therefore, the larger the area of body that is anesthetized. By anesthetizing only some of the spinal nerve roots, epidural anesthesia provides pain relief during labor but, at the same time, may also permit walking. As with spinal anesthesia, the anesthetic medication also blocks the sympathetic nerves leaving the spinal cord. Because of this, blood pressure of the woman may decline and requires careful monitoring. (For this reason, a loading dose of 500–1,000 mL of physiologic [normal] saline solution may be given intravenously prior to introduction of the anesthetic.)

Epigastric: Area immediately below the tip of the sternum in the center of the upper abdomen. Pain felt here is usually related to liver or gallbladder disease. Of most importance in pregnant women with pre-eclampsia, the onset of epigastric pain indicates swelling of the liver capsule. This often precedes the onset of the first convulsion of eclampsia.

Epiglottis: The flap of cartilage that overlies the larynx. The epiglottis is open during breathing and closes over the larynx during swallowing to prevent food from entering the trachea.

Epinephrine: A natural body hormone that is released by adrenal glands into the blood during stress. It may also be used as a drug during resuscitation to constrict blood vessels and increase blood pressure, and to increase heart rate and volume of blood pumped.

Erb palsy: The most common form of brachial plexus nerve injury in newborns.

Erythema: Redness of the skin produced by dilation of the smallest blood vessels. *Example:* The redness that occurs around an infected wound.

Erythroblastosis fetalis: Hemolytic anemia resulting from the passage of antibodies between the pregnant woman and the fetus across the placenta during pregnancy. Red blood cell alloantibodies may develop in a woman when fetal red blood cells enter the maternal circulation during a prior pregnancy (most commonly at the time of delivery), or as a result of a blood transfusion (less common). The placenta transfers immunoglobulin G antibodies from mother to fetus during pregnancy. If the fetal red blood cells exhibit the specific antigen to which the mother has an alloantibody, the interaction between the antibody and antigen leads to breakdown (hemolysis) of the fetal red blood cells. As the fetal blood-forming organs produce red blood cells more rapidly than normal to replace those undergoing hemolysis, immature fetal red blood cells (erythroblasts) are released into the fetal circulation. The consequences of untreated fetal hemolytic anemia can include fetal hydrops and stillbirth.

Esophagus: The muscular tube that connects the throat and stomach.

Etiology: The cause of anything. *Example:* Sepsis may be the etiology of hyperbilirubinemia in a newborn.

Exchange transfusion: Process during which a baby's blood is removed and replaced with donor blood so that when the exchange transfusion is completed, most of the baby's blood has been replaced by donor blood. Most often, exchange transfusions are used as a treatment for severe hyperbilirubinemia.

Expiration: (1) Period during the breathing cycle when the person is breathing out or exhaling. (2) The end of a period of usefulness, validity, or effectiveness, such as the expiration date for a product or medication, after which time the item should not be used. (3) Death.

Face presentation: The face is the presenting part. The chin (mentum) is the reference point, and it may rotate either anteriorly (mentum anterior), in which case vaginal delivery is likely if the pelvis is normal in size, or posteriorly. When the chin rotates posteriorly into the hollow of the sacrum (mentum posterior), vaginal delivery is impossible unless the forces of labor or use of obstetric forceps are successful in rotating the chin to the anterior position. Cesarean delivery is usually performed for mentum posterior position.

FAD: *See* Fetal activity determination.

FAE: *See* Fetal alcohol effects.

Familial: Used to describe a disease or defect that affects more members of a family than would be expected by chance.

FAS: *See* Fetal alcohol syndrome.

Fat, brown: Fat tissue that has a rich blood and nerve supply. Babies have proportionally more brown fat than do adults and metabolize or "burn" it as their main source of heat production, while adults produce heat mainly by shivering. Extra oxygen and calories are used when brown fat is metabolized.

Fat, white: Type of fat that has few blood vessels and appears whitish. It is used mainly for insulation and as a reserve supply of energy and is not nearly as metabolically active as brown fat.

Fatty acids: Substances resulting from the breakdown of fat. Fatty acids decrease binding of bilirubin to albumin, thus increasing the chance of brain damage from hyperbilirubinemia.

Femoral pulse: Pulse felt in the groin, over the femoral artery.

Fern test: A test for amniotic fluid in the vagina, used when rupture of membranes is suspected. When there is a pool of fluid in the vagina, a drop of it is smeared on a glass slide and allowed to dry in the air. Salt content of the amniotic fluid will dry in a typical pattern, resembling a fern, while other fluids (eg, urine) will not. If a fern pattern is seen, the membranes are ruptured.

Fetal activity determination (FAD): A noninvasive means to monitor fetal well-being that may be used by either low- or high-risk pregnant women. Approximately 80% of gross fetal movements observed on ultrasound are felt by the pregnant woman. Beginning at approximately 28 weeks' gestation, a pregnant woman records fetal activity daily according to one of several accepted protocols. Any significant decrease in activity warrants prompt (the same day) investigation of fetal condition.

Fetal alcohol effects (FAE): The effects of maternal alcohol ingestion during pregnancy may be seen in a baby without the baby having all the findings typical of fetal alcohol syndrome.

Fetal alcohol syndrome (FAS): Constellation of findings, including intellectual disability, that may occur in fetuses of women who ingest alcohol during pregnancy, especially early in gestation.

Fetal echocardiogram: An ultrasonographic technique that shows movements of the walls and valves of the beating heart of a fetus. Certain valvular and other abnormalities of the fetal heart may be seen. Used only when there is some reason to suspect that the fetus may have an abnormal heart.

Fetal heart rate, baseline: Approximate average fetal heart rate during any 10-minute period that is free of accelerations, decelerations, and marked variability (>25 beats/min). The reference baseline range is between 110 and 160 beats/min.

Fetal heart rate acceleration: Abrupt increase (at least 15 beats/min) in fetal heart rate (onset to peak rate occurs in <30 seconds) that lasts at least 15 seconds but less than 2 minutes.

Fetal heart rate deceleration: A decrease in the fetal heart rate that then returns to baseline. There are 3 types of decelerations (early, late, and variable), which are defined by their shape and relationship to uterine contractions.

Fetal heart rate variability: Fluctuations in baseline fetal heart rate that are irregular in amplitude and frequency. Visual inspection is used to classify the peak-to-trough beats per minute difference as absent (no detectable change from baseline), minimal (fluctuation of ≤5 beats/min), moderate (fluctuation of 6–25 beats/min), or marked (fluctuation of ≥25 beats/min).

Fetal lung maturity: Analysis of a sample of amniotic fluid for the presence of surfactant components. The lecithin to sphingomyelin ratio is one such test. *See also* Pulmonary maturity.

Fetal membranes: The amnion and chorion.

Fetal monitoring, external: Refers to continuous electronic monitoring using a device strapped to the woman's abdomen to detect the fetal heart rate, periodic rate changes, and timing of the uterine contractions.

Fetal monitoring, internal: Refers to continuous electronic monitoring using a wire attached to the fetal presenting part to detect fetal heart rate and a pressure transducer placed inside the uterus to detect onset and intensity of uterine contractions.

Fetal pole: A term used to describe the appearance of either end of the fetal body when the fetus is so small the head cannot be distinguished from the breech.

Fetopelvic disproportion (FPD): Condition in which the internal size of the maternal pelvis is too small or the fetal head is too large to allow vaginal delivery. Because exact measurements of the fetal head and maternal pelvis cannot be made, this is a relative term.

Fetoscope: A specially constructed stethoscope used to listen to fetal heart rate.

Fetus: After development of organ systems (after the first 8 weeks from conception/10 weeks from the last menstrual period), an embryo is called a *fetus* until delivery.

FIO_2: Fractional inspired oxygen. The percentage of oxygen being inhaled. An environmental oxygen concentration of 55% may also be written FIO_2 = 55%. The FIO_2 of room air is 21%.

Flaccid: Limp.

Flexion: Bending of a body part. *Example:* Flexion of the arm occurs when the elbow is bent. By contrast, *extension* means the straightening of a body part.

Flip-flop phenomenon: Flip flop is caused by lowering the environmental oxygen concentration too rapidly, or allowing a baby requiring oxygen therapy to breathe room air for even a short period. In response, the arteries to the lungs constrict, thus limiting the amount of blood that can be oxygenated in the lungs. The baby then requires an environmental oxygen concentration even higher than that breathed previously to achieve the same arterial blood oxygen concentration.

Foramen ovale: The opening between the 2 upper chambers (atria) of the heart in the fetus. It consists of redundant tissue in the interatrial wall that results in a functional closure of the opening when left atrial pressure exceeds right atrial pressure shortly after birth.

Forceps: Obstetric forceps are 2 metal instruments, made in mirror image of each other, curved laterally to follow the shape of the fetal head and vertically to fit the curve of the maternal pelvis. Used to assist vaginal delivery of the fetal head and shorten the second stage of labor, for either maternal or fetal reasons. They are made in a variety of sizes and shapes, including forceps designed to help deliver the aftercoming head in breech presentations. When forceps are used, the delivery is classified as *midforceps, low forceps,* or *outlet forceps,* depending on fetal station and position when the forceps are applied.

FPD: *See* Fetopelvic disproportion.

Fundal height: During pregnancy, the fundus of the uterus can be felt higher and higher in the maternal abdomen. The distance between the fundus and symphysis pubis (front pelvic bone) is the fundal height. It is used as an estimate of gestational age of the fetus. Consistency in the technique used (preferably by the same examiner) throughout pregnancy is important for accurate results.

Fundus: The broad top two-thirds of the uterus.

Gastroschisis: A defect of the abdominal wall during embryonic development, allowing abdominal organs to protrude into amniotic fluid. As opposed to omphalocele, no peritoneal sac covers the organs with gastroschisis.

GBS: *See* Group B β-hemolytic streptococcus.

GDM: Gestational diabetes mellitus. *See* Diabetes, gestational.

General inhalation anesthesia: An anesthetic technique that produces loss of consciousness. The patient is usually given barbiturates or narcotics to induce anesthesia, followed by paralyzing drugs, endotracheal intubation, and artificial ventilation. Anesthetic gases are used to continue the anesthetic state until the surgical procedure is completed. Because the gases are quickly cleared from the blood by the lungs, the patient "wakes up" within a few minutes after the anesthetic gases are stopped. With this type of anesthesia, the drugs and gases used can cross the placenta and may depress a fetus. Anesthesia provided to an obstetric patient must consider the unique physiological state of a pregnant woman as well as the potential effect drugs given to her may have on the fetus.

Geneticist: A physician who specializes in knowing how genes are inherited by children from their parents and the association between certain genetic abnormalities and specific physical characteristics.

Genitourinary tract: Pertaining to the reproductive organs and urinary organs.

Gestational diabetes mellitus (GDM): *See* Diabetes, gestational.

Glottis: The vocal cords and opening between them that leads to the trachea.

Glucose tolerance test (GTT): A test for abnormal glucose metabolism. A fasting patient is given a standard dose of glucose orally, with the blood level of glucose determined at standard intervals.

Glycogen: Main storage form of glucose in the body. It is changed to glucose and released to the bloodstream as needed.

Glycosylated hemoglobin (hemoglobin A_{1C}): Reflects circulating blood glucose for the previous 3 months. It is used as an indicator of long-term glucose control.

Gonorrheal ophthalmia, neonatal: Eye infection in newborns that results from gonorrhea bacteria acquired by a baby during the birth process, if the woman has gonorrhea. Silver nitrate drops or erythromycin ointment placed in the baby's eyes shortly after delivery prevents the development of this potentially damaging infection.

Gram stain: A specific stain for bacteria that separates gram-positive bacteria (which stain blue) from gram-negative bacteria (which stain red). These 2 categories of bacteria vary in the types of disease they cause and their antibiotic sensitivity. Gram stain of an infected body fluid (eg, urine, pus, amniotic fluid) may identify the type of organism causing the infection and allow appropriate antibiotic therapy to begin before culture and sensitivity studies can be completed.

Gravidity: Number of pregnancies a woman has had, regardless of pregnancy outcome. With her first pregnancy, a woman is a *primigravida*. With her second pregnancy, a woman is, technically, a *secundigravida,* and with her third or subsequent pregnancies, a *multigravida*. In practice, however, *secundigravida* is rarely used and *multigravida* is used to refer to any woman with her second, or subsequent, pregnancy. *See also* Parity.

Group B β-hemolytic streptococcus (GBS): A type of streptococcal bacteria that can cause serious or fatal neonatal illness. Some women, without evidence of infection, have chronic GBS vaginal or rectal colonization, which may infect the fetus before delivery or the baby at the time of delivery.

Growth restriction: Describes fetuses that, on serial examination, are significantly smaller than would be expected, with their growth falling below the 10th percentile for their gestational age.

Grunting: A sign of respiratory distress in a neonate. The grunt or whine occurs during expiration as a result of the baby exhaling against a partially closed glottis. The baby grunts in an attempt to trap air in the lungs and hold open the alveoli. Grunting sometimes may be normal immediately following birth; after 1 to 2 hours it is always abnormal.

GTT: *See* Glucose tolerance test.

HBIG: Hepatitis B immune globulin. Administration of HBIG soon after delivery is part of the treatment for newborns whose mothers are hepatitis B surface antigen–positive (test for hepatitis B).

HBsAg: *See* Hepatitis B surface antigen.

HCT: *See* Hematocrit.

Heart murmur, functional: A heart murmur that does not result from disease or an abnormality of the heart. A functional heart murmur is *not* associated with abnormal functioning of the heart.

HELLP syndrome: Hemolysis, elevated liver enzymes, low platelet count occurring in association with preeclampsia. An uncommon and severe form of pregnancy-related hypertension.

Hematocrit (Hct): A blood test showing the percentage of red blood cells in whole blood. *Example:* An Hct of 40 means that 40% of the blood is red blood cells and 60% is plasma and other cells.

Hemoglobin (Hgb): (1) Blood test showing the concentration of Hgb in blood. (2) Oxygen-carrying part of red blood cells.

Hemoglobinopathy: A genetic disorder that causes a change in the molecular structure of hemoglobin in the red blood cells and results in certain typical laboratory and clinical changes, frequently including anemia. Sickle cell disease is one type of hemoglobinopathy.

Hemolysis: Breakdown of red blood cells. Hemolytic anemia, therefore, is anemia that results from the destruction of red blood cells, rather than loss of blood or inadequate production of red blood cells.

Hemorrhage: Bleeding; most often used to indicate severe bleeding.

Heparin lock: A technique used to prevent blood clot formation in an arterial or venous catheter, when a continuous infusion of fluids is not being used. A solution of intravenous fluids with a specific concentration of heparin is flushed through the catheter and then the stopcock is closed to the catheter.

Hepatitis: Serious inflammation of the liver usually caused by a viral infection. There are several forms of hepatitis, depending on the specific causative agent and mode of transmission. Infection may be acute or chronic.

Hepatitis B surface antigen (HBsAg): Term for protein on the surface of the hepatitis B virus. Screening all prenatal patients for this antigen identifies women who are carriers for hepatitis B, and therefore at risk for passing the virus to their fetuses before birth. Such newborns should be given hepatitis B immune globulin and hepatitis B vaccine soon after birth.

Hepatosplenomegaly: Enlargement of the liver and spleen.

Hereditary: Used to describe a condition that is transmitted by the genes, from parents to their children. *Example:* Cystic fibrosis is a hereditary disease, and eye color is a hereditary trait.

Heredity: Genetic transmission from parent to child of traits and characteristics. *Example:* A baby with brown eyes can be said to have that color of eyes as part of his or her heredity.

Herpes: Refers to diseases caused by herpesvirus. Maternal herpes may have serious consequences for the newborn.

Hgb: *See* Hemoglobin.

HIE: *See* Hypoxic-ischemic encephalopathy.

HIV: The virus that causes AIDS, which attacks and eventually overcomes the body's immune system.

HPV: Human papillomavirus.

Hyaline membrane disease: Older name for *neonatal respiratory distress syndrome.*

Hydatidiform mole: A pregnancy characterized by grossly abnormal development of the chorionic villi, which eventually form a mass of cysts. Usually, but not always, no fetus is present. Excessive secretion from the trophoblast cells leads to very high levels of β-human chorionic gonadotropin. Vaginal bleeding during the first trimester is common and may be the presenting sign. Uterine size does not usually correspond to expected size for the dates of a pregnancy: larger than expected in about 50% of cases and smaller than expected in about 30% of cases.

Hydramnios: Also called *polyhydramnios*. Abnormally large amount of amniotic fluid. It may be associated with fetal abnormalities (particularly gastrointestinal tract abnormalities that prevent amniotic fluid from being swallowed into the gastrointestinal tract of the fetus) or certain maternal medical illnesses; however, in most cases, the cause of hydramnios is unknown.

Hydrocephalus: Enlargement of the head due to abnormally large collection of cerebrospinal fluid in the brain. It may be congenital or acquired after birth. Accumulation of cerebrospinal fluid may be caused by a blockage in the normal flow of fluid around the brain and spinal cord or by a decrease in the normal absorption of the fluid.

Hydrops fetalis: Edema in the entire body of a fetus, accompanied by at least one effusion in a body cavity (pleural, pericardial, or peritoneal). Usually a result of severe hemolytic anemia caused by Rh disease or other alloimmunizations, but may (rarely) be caused by certain other serious in utero conditions or viral infections. In many cases the cause for hydrops is not clear.

Hyperbilirubinemia: Excess amount of bilirubin in the blood.

GLOSSARY

Hyperbilirubinemia, physiological: Hyperbilirubinemia due to a baby's immature liver, which has a limited ability to excrete bilirubin from the body, rather than hyperbilirubinemia due to a disease process such as ABO incompatibility.

Hyperkalemia: High blood potassium level.

Hypernatremia: High blood sodium level.

Hyperosmolar: Used to describe a liquid with a higher concentration of particles than found in a physiological fluid. For example, an intravenous solution may be hyperosmolar compared to blood, or formula may be hyperosmolar compared to human (breast) milk.

Hypertension: High blood pressure. In adults, generally defined as higher than 130/80 mm Hg.

Hyperthermia: High body temperature; fever. In adults, generally defined as greater than or equal to 38.0°C (100.4°F).

Hypertonic: Used to describe a solution that is more concentrated than body fluid and therefore will draw water out of the body's cells, causing the cells to shrink.

Hypocalcemia: Low blood calcium level.

Hypoglycemia: Low blood glucose level.

Hypotension: Low blood pressure.

Hypothermia: Low body temperature.

Hypovolemia: Low blood volume.

Hypoxemia: Low concentration of oxygen in the arterial blood.

Hypoxia: A deficiency of oxygen and perfusion in the body tissues resulting in compromised metabolism and injured tissue.

Hypoxic-ischemic encephalopathy (HIE): Neonatal brain injury that presents at birth and is caused by a newborn experiencing a hypoxic and/or ischemic event around the time of delivery.

IAI: *See* Intra-amniotic infection.

Icterus: *See* Jaundice.

Ileitis: Inflammation of the ileum, the distal portion of the small bowel (between the jejunum and cecum). Usually represents Crohn disease, a chronic inflammation of the intestinal tract, most often affecting the terminal ileum (may also involve the colon). Cause is unknown, complications are frequent (eg, abscess, obstruction, fistula formation), and recurrence after treatment is common.

Ileus: Obstruction of the intestines. Commonly used to refer to a dynamic or functional ileus in which there is an absence of peristalsis resulting from postsurgical inhibition of bowel motility but frequently not associated with a mechanical blockage of the intestines.

Immune thrombocytopenic purpura (ITP): A disease of unknown cause in which the body destroys its own platelets, causing thrombocytopenia and resulting in coagulation disorders and easy bruising. The fetus of a woman with ITP may also have thrombocytopenia. Formerly called *idiopathic thrombocytopenic purpura*.

In utero: Latin for "inside the uterus."

In utero resuscitation: Term applied to measures taken to improve fetal oxygenation when there is a non-reassuring fetal heart rate pattern during labor. These measures include provision of 100% oxygen by mask to the woman, correction of maternal hypotension (turn woman on her side or from one side to the other, give fluids, or elevate legs), and reduction of uterine activity (stop oxytocin; consider use of tocolytics).

Incompetent cervix: A condition in which the cervix (lower part of the uterus and entrance to the birth canal) dilates prematurely, causing a spontaneous abortion or preterm delivery. A woman with an incompetent cervix is at risk for a preterm delivery with each pregnancy. *See also* Cerclage of the cervix.

Infant death rate: Number of babies that die within the first year after birth (365 days) per 1,000 live births.

Infective endocarditis: An infectious inflammatory process in which the infecting bacteria form growths on the heart valves or endocardium. The process may have an acute or subacute course. Diagnosis is usually made during the subacute, longer-lasting stage. Heart tissue is permanently damaged, and the infection can be difficult or impossible to treat effectively. Patients with heart valve malformations are particularly prone to developing these infective growths on the abnormal valves and surrounding endocardium.

Inferior vena cava: The major vein returning blood from the lower body to the right side of the heart.

Infiltration of intravenous fluids: Occurs when an intravenous catheter or needle in a peripheral vein perforates the wall of the vein and the intravenous fluids infuse into the surrounding tissue instead of bloodstream. Swelling and tenderness develop near the tip of the catheter. An infiltrated intravenous catheter should be removed immediately because some intravenous fluids can cause severe tissue damage.

Infusion pump: A machine used to push fluid at a controlled, preset rate into an artery or vein. All neonatal infusions should use a pump so the volume infused can be controlled precisely. Some pumps infuse fluids by means of small, regular pulses, while other pumps, particularly syringe pumps, infuse continuously.

INH: Isoniazid hydrazide. Generic name for an antituberculosis medication.

Insensible water loss: Body fluid lost through the skin and respiratory passages.

Inspired oxygen: The oxygen concentration that is being inhaled (*not* the concentration in the blood). Also called *environmental oxygen*.

Intra-amniotic infection (IAI): Formerly known as *chorioamnionitis,* or infection of the fetal membranes, which puts the fetus at risk for also becoming infected with the same organism.

Intra-arterial infusion: An infusion of fluid into an artery (eg, via a peripheral or an umbilical arterial catheter).

Intracardiac: Inside the heart.

Intrapartum: Period of pregnancy during labor.

Intrauterine: Inside the uterus.

Intubation, endotracheal: Insertion of a hollow tube (endotracheal tube) into the trachea to suction foreign matter, such as meconium, from the trachea or deliver air or oxygen under pressure directly into the lungs by assisted ventilation.

Iron: A mineral important for the formation of red blood cells. Iron deficiency is a common cause of anemia.

Isosmolar: Of the same particle concentration as body fluid.

ITP: *See* Immune thrombocytopenic purpura.

IUGR: In utero growth restriction. *See* Growth restriction.

Jaundice: Also called *icterus*. Yellow coloration of the skin and mucous membranes resulting from hyperbilirubinemia.

Karyotype: The complete set of chromosomes of the nucleus of a cell. Also used to refer to the photomicrograph of the chromosomes arranged in a standard order. The process of identifying a karyotype uses a technique that stops cells in their reproductive cycle and causes the individual chromosomes to swell, thus allowing each chromosome to be identified and counted. This technique is used to identify conditions, such as Down syndrome (trisomy 21) or Turner syndrome (monosomy X), that are caused by an excess or deficiency of one or more chromosomes. The technique cannot identify individual genes that comprise each chromosome.

Lactic acid: A by-product from one of the body's metabolic pathways. During periods of poor oxygenation, metabolism may be incomplete and lactic acid may build up, thus resulting in low blood pH or acidosis.

Large for gestational age (LGA): Refers to an infant whose weight is above the 90th percentile for infants of that gestational age.

Laryngoscope: An instrument used to visualize the glottis during endotracheal intubation.

Larynx: The area containing the vocal cords and located between the base of the tongue and the trachea.

Leopold maneuvers: A method of systematically palpating the abdomen of a pregnant woman to determine fetal presentation and position.

Lethargy: Condition of diminished activity due to drowsiness, medication, or illness.

LGA: *See* Large for gestational age.

Lie: Relationship of the long axis of the fetus's body with that of the maternal spine (transverse, oblique, or longitudinal).

Lightening: The feeling of decreased abdominal distension a pregnant woman has as the fetus and uterus descend into the pelvic cavity during the last 4 weeks of a term pregnancy.

Macrosomia: Large body size. A newborn weighing more than 4,000 g (8 lb 13 oz) at birth is considered macrosomic.

Maladaptation: Failure to adapt to stresses of the environment.

Malformation, congenital: A defect that occurs during embryonic or fetal development. Used synonymously with *congenital anomaly* but not *deformation*. *See also* Deformation.

Maternal serum alpha fetoprotein (MSAFP): *See* Alpha fetoprotein.

Maternal-fetal medicine (MFM): The subspecialty of obstetrics and gynecology that deals specifically with the care of high-risk pregnancies.

Maximum vertical pocket (MVP): A way of estimating the relative volume of amniotic fluid using ultrasound identification and measurement of the single deepest pocket of amniotic fluid of at least 1 cm in width.

McRoberts maneuver: Used to relieve shoulder dystocia by elevating and flexing the woman's legs so her knees and thighs are held as closely as possible against her abdomen and chest. This extreme flexion of the maternal hips rotates the pelvis in such a way that there is more room for the anterior shoulder to slip under the symphysis pubis, allowing delivery.

Meconium: The dark green-brown sticky material that makes up a baby's first stools. It is formed by the fetus in utero from intestinal secretions and swallowed amniotic fluid. The rectum may relax and release meconium into the amniotic fluid in post-term gestations and during periods of fetal stress. Meconium-stained amniotic fluid may therefore be a worrisome sign but does not always indicate fetal jeopardy.

Meningitis: Inflammation of the membranes that surround the brain and spinal cord.

Meningomyelocele: Congenital defect of the spinal column. Part of the spinal cord and surrounding membranes protrude through an opening in the spine and form a sac on the baby's back. The sac may be large or small, and located anywhere along the baby's spine. There may be various degrees of neurologic impairment occurring below the level of the meningomyelocele. It may be detected in the fetus by assessment of maternal serum alpha fetoprotein.

Metabolism: All the physical and chemical processes that produce and maintain body tissue.

Methimazole: A mercaptol-imidazole compound used to treat hyperthyroidism.

MFM: *See* Maternal-fetal medicine.

Morbidity: Any complication or damage that results from an illness.

Mortality: Death.

Motility: Movement.

MSAFP: Maternal serum alpha fetoprotein. *See* Alpha fetoprotein.

Multifetal gestation: More than one fetus. Multifetal gestation may be used to describe a pregnancy involving twins, triplets, quadruplets, quintuplets, or more.

Multigravida: Precise term for a pregnant woman who has had 2 or more previous pregnancies. Commonly used, however, to refer to a pregnant woman who has had one or more previous pregnancies. (*Secundigravida* is the precise term for a woman in her second pregnancy.)

MVP: *See* Maximum vertical pocket.

Myometrium: The muscular wall of the uterus.

Naloxone hydrochloride (Narcan): A drug that counteracts the depressant effects of narcotics. Naloxone may be given to a depressed baby whose mother received narcotic pain medication shortly before delivery. Adequate oxygenation with assisted ventilation, as necessary, should be provided *before* time is taken to give this drug. Naloxone should be used with caution if maternal drug addiction is suspected.

Narcan: *See* Naloxone hydrochloride.

NAS: *See* Neonatal abstinence syndrome.

Nasal flaring: A sign of neonatal respiratory distress. Edges of the nostrils fan outward as the baby inhales.

Nasogastric tube: A pliable tube that is inserted through the baby's nose, down the esophagus, and into the stomach. It is used for feeding or to decompress the stomach by intermittent or constant suctioning of air or gastric juices out of the stomach.

NEC: *See* Necrotizing enterocolitis.

Necrotizing enterocolitis (NEC): A serious disease in which sections of the intestines are injured and may die. Medical treatment may result in complete resolution, but in some cases portions of the intestines must be surgically removed. It occurs more often in preterm infants, but the cause is unclear.

Neonatal: Refers to the time period from delivery through the first 28 days.

Neonatal abstinence syndrome (NAS): Constellation of findings, including jitteriness, irritability, hypertonia, seizures, sneezing, tachycardia, difficulty with feedings, or diarrhea, often occurring in babies born to women who used heroin or methadone during pregnancy. These findings result from the baby's sudden withdrawal from maternal drugs following delivery.

Neonate: Baby from birth through the first 28 days of age.

Neonatal opioid withdrawal syndrome (NOWS): A condition that results from newborns being exposed to opioids in the womb. NOWS symptoms can include tremors, excessive crying and irritability, and problems with sleeping, feeding, and breathing.

Neonatologist: A pediatrician who specializes in caring for newborns, particularly at-risk and sick babies.

Nephrosis: General term used for any noninfectious disease of the kidney.

Neural tube defect: Used to describe any congenital defect in the brain or spinal cord (structures that developed from the neural tube of the embryo), including anencephaly, encephalocele, and meningomyelocele.

Neutral thermal environment: The very narrow environmental temperature range that keeps a baby's body temperature normal, with the baby having to use the least amount of calories and oxygen to produce heat.

Nitrazine: Trade name for phenaphthazine.

GLOSSARY

Nonhemolytic jaundice: Hyperbilirubinemia not resulting from an excessive breakdown of red blood cells.

Nonmaleficence: Avoiding harm to a patient.

Nonstress test (NST): One of several measures used to assess fetal well-being in high-risk pregnancies, during which spontaneous fetal heart rate accelerations in relation to fetal activity are monitored with an external electronic monitor. The pregnant woman is resting during the procedure and receives no medication.

NOWS: *See* Neonatal opioid withdrawal syndrome.

NST: *See* Nonstress test.

OCT: Oxytocin challenge test. *See* Contraction stress test.

Oligohydramnios: An abnormally low amount of amniotic fluid. It may be associated with abnormalities of the fetal kidney, ureter, or urethra (fetal urine is the primary component of amniotic fluid); certain fetal chromosomal defects; fetal growth restriction; uteroplacental insufficiency; positional deformities (due to prolonged uterine pressure in the absence of a fluid cushion); and umbilical cord compression (particularly during labor). Oligohydramnios may also result from early, prolonged rupture of membranes.

Omphalocele: A congenital opening in the abdominal wall allowing the abdominal organs, covered with a peritoneal membrane, to protrude and form a sac outside the abdominal cavity. *See also* Gastroschisis.

Ophthalmia: General term for any disease of the eye.

Oral airway: A device that allows babies with blocked nasal passages to breathe through their mouths. It is inserted into the mouth and keeps the tongue forward, preventing it from obstructing the airway.

Orogastric tube: A pliable tube that is inserted through the baby's mouth, down the esophagus, and into the stomach. It is used for the same purposes as a nasogastric tube.

Orthopnea: Shortness of breath while lying down. It is usually caused by heart or lung failure and is characterized by the patient sitting up to sleep.

Osmolarity: Concentration of particles in a solution. Synonymous with *osmolality*.

Ovulation: Release of an egg, ready for fertilization, from an ovary.

Ovum: Female reproductive cell that, after fertilization and implantation, becomes an embryo.

Oximeter: A device that reads the color of blood and reports the percentage saturation of hemoglobin with oxygen (Spo_2). The probe of an oximeter emits a light that is sensed by a detector. *See also* Pulse oximetry.

Oxygen hood: Also called *oxyhood*. A small plastic box with a neck space designed to fit over a baby's head and allow precise control of a baby's inspired (environmental) oxygen concentration.

Oxyhemoglobin saturation: Hemoglobin is the oxygen-carrying component of red blood cells. The amount of oxygen attached to hemoglobin is measured as percent saturation and called *oxyhemoglobin saturation* (commonly shortened to "% sat" or "O_2 sat"). The degree of saturation can range from 0% to 100%.

Oxytocin: A hormone occurring naturally in the body and also used to induce labor, enhance weak labor contractions, and cause contraction of the uterus after delivery of the placenta.

Oxytocin challenge test (OCT): *See* Contraction stress test.

$Paco_2$ or Pco_2: Concentration of carbon dioxide in the blood (*a* specifies arterial blood).

Palate: Roof of the mouth. The structure that separates the oral and nasal passages. A cleft palate is one that is split from front to back, sometimes with an opening so deep that the mouth and nasal passages are connected.

Pao_2 or Po_2: Concentration of oxygen in the blood (*a* specifies arterial blood).

Parens patriae: The duty of the state to protect the vulnerable or incompetent.

Parenteral: Taking something into the body in a manner other than through the digestive canal (which is enteral).

Parity: The condition of a woman with respect to having had one or more pregnancies reach a gestational age of viability. Parity is determined by the number of pregnancies that reached viability, whether the fetuses were live-born or stillborn, and not the number of fetuses. Twins, triplets, or more do not increase a woman's parity. *Nulliparity* is the condition of having carried no pregnancies to an age of viability; *primiparity,* of having carried one pregnancy to an age of viability; *secundiparity,* of having 2 pregnancies reach viability; and *multiparity,* of having had 3 or more pregnancies reach viability. In practice, however, *secundiparity* is rarely used and *multiparity* is used for any woman who has had 2 or more pregnancies reach an age of viability. *Example:* A woman whose first pregnancy ended in stillborn twins at 30 weeks' gestation, second pregnancy ended in a single, healthy fetus born at 39 weeks, and third pregnancy ended in spontaneous abortion at 10 weeks has a parity of 2. She is now pregnant for the fourth time, at 32 weeks' gestation, and therefore has a gravidity of 4. She may be described as a gravida 4, para 2. When she delivers the current pregnancy, she will become a G4 P3.

Pelvis, contracted: Smaller than normal-sized pelvis. The pelvis may be too small to allow the vaginal birth of a baby.

Percutaneous umbilical blood sampling (PUBS): Also called *cordocentesis*. A highly specialized technique during which a needle is inserted through a pregnant woman's abdominal wall into the uterus and then directly into an artery or vein of the umbilical cord, usually near the base of the cord at the placenta. Ultrasound visualization of the fetus, placenta, and umbilical cord is used throughout the procedure. A sample of fetal blood is obtained. Percutaneous umbilical blood sampling may be used to detect congenital infections, isoimmune diseases, and chromosomal defects (for chromosomal defects, fetal blood can yield results in a few days, while amniotic fluid cell culture may take several weeks). Percutaneous umbilical blood sampling may also be used to give a direct blood transfusion to a fetus in cases of severe anemia.

Perfusion: The flow of blood through an organ or tissue.

Pericarditis: Inflammation of the pericardium, the sac of fibrous tissue surrounding the heart. Pericarditis is sometimes caused by infection and other times by an inflammatory, noninfectious disease such as systemic lupus erythematosus.

Perinatal: The time surrounding a baby's birth. The perinatal period begins at 22 completed weeks and ends 7 completed days after birth.

Perinatologist: Technically, a subspecialist physician who cares for the fetus and neonate. Often used, incorrectly, to refer to an obstetrician with subspecialty training in maternal-fetal medicine.

Perinatology: Now more commonly referred to as *maternal-fetal medicine,* perinatology is a subspecialty of obstetrics and gynecology that focuses on the care of patients with complicated pregnancies and the diagnosis and care of conditions that affect the fetus before birth.

Periodic heart rate changes: Fetal heart rate accelerations and decelerations. Their occurrence and relationship to fetal activity or uterine contractions is used as an estimate of fetal well-being, for antenatal testing, and during labor.

Peripheral: The outward and surface parts of the body. *Example:* Peripheral circulation is the blood flow in the skin, arms, and legs.

pH level: Refers to the acidity or alkalinity of a liquid. A blood pH level outside the reference range indicates metabolic or respiratory disturbance.

Pharynx: Throat above the esophagus and below the nasal passages.

Phenaphthazine (Nitrazine): A pH-sensitive dye embedded in paper that, when dipped into fluids, estimates pH of the fluid. Used primarily to distinguish amniotic fluid (which has an alkaline pH) from urine or vaginal secretions (which are acidic) in pregnant patients with symptoms of premature rupture of the membranes.

Phototherapy: Use of fluorescent, tungsten-halogen, or fiberoptic lights to treat hyperbilirubinemia in neonates by breaking down bilirubin accumulated in the skin. The color of phototherapy lights ranges from nearly white to deep blue, depending on the type and brand of lights.

Pierre Robin syndrome: A group of congenital anomalies that include a small jaw, a cleft palate, and backward displacement of the tongue. Babies with Pierre Robin syndrome may have great difficulty breathing or eating.

Placenta: Organ that joins the woman and fetus during pregnancy. The umbilical cord is implanted on one side, while the other side is attached to the uterus. Maternal and fetal blood does not mix directly, but nutrients and waste products are exchanged across a thin membrane that separates maternal and fetal blood.

Placenta accreta: Term used to describe a rare condition of implantation in which the implanting trophoblasts not only penetrate the endometrium but continue into the myometrium as well. This eliminates the normal cleavage plane in the decidua (endometrium during pregnancy) that allows normal spontaneous separation of the placenta following delivery. Attempts to remove a placenta accreta by manual separation usually result in excessive hemorrhage. Hysterectomy may be the only way to remove the placenta, as separation from the myometrium may be impossible, and emergency surgery may be required if heavy bleeding begins.

Placenta previa: Abnormally low implantation of the placenta in the lower segment of the uterus. As the placenta grows with pregnancy, it spreads so that it partially or completely covers the internal cervical os at term. The resultant position of the placenta is in front of the fetus. Thus, a vaginal delivery would require delivery of the placenta before the fetus. Painless vaginal bleeding during the third trimester is the most common sign of placenta previa. If not identified earlier, severe hemorrhage with maternal and fetal compromise may occur as the cervix dilates during labor. Whether placenta previa is identified prenatally or not until after labor has begun, cesarean delivery is required for the health of the woman and fetus. *Note:* Early in gestation a placenta may appear to be low lying, but not be later in pregnancy. A diagnosis of placenta previa cannot be made until after 20 weeks' gestation and should be reconfirmed at 26 to 28 weeks.

Placental abruption: Premature separation of a normally placed placenta. Placental separation can occur at any time during pregnancy, but is most likely to occur during late pregnancy and before the onset of labor. Several risk factors are associated with placental abruption, but usually the cause is unknown. Depending on the degree of separation, bleeding may be slight or severe. If severe, both the woman and fetus may go into shock. Bleeding, even severe bleeding, can be completely hidden behind the placenta. In the most severe cases, the uterus is tense, boardlike, and tender. The woman's blood pressure may fall, and symptoms of shock or disseminated intravascular coagulation may develop. Fetal distress is common, and fetal death may occur. Placental abruption requires an emergency response.

Placental perfusion: Blood from the uterine artery flows into the intervillous space, bathing the placental villi that protrude into this space with nutrients and oxygen. Flow of blood through the intervillous space allows perfusion of nutrients and oxygen into the fetus from the maternal blood and waste products of fetal metabolism to pass from the fetus to the maternal circulation. Fetal and maternal blood does not mix. Nutrients and waste are exchanged across the thin membrane of the placental villi.

Pneumonia: Inflammation of the lungs. Neonatal pneumonia has many possible causes, such as bacterial infection, aspiration of formula, or aspiration of meconium.

Pneumothorax: Rupture in the lung that allows air to leak outside the lung, form a collection of air between the lung and chest wall, and thereby compress the lung so it cannot expand fully. Often when a pneumothorax develops, a baby suddenly becomes cyanotic and shows signs of increased respiratory distress. There are decreased breath sounds over the affected lung. Insertion of a tube or needle into the chest is required to remove the air pocket and allow the lung to re-expand. Plural: pneumothoraces (rupture in both lungs).

Polycythemia: Abnormally high number of red blood cells. It is more common in infants of diabetic mothers and in newborns small for gestational age.

Polyhydramnios: Synonymous with *hydramnios*, although *hydramnios* is now the preferred term for this condition.

Position, fetal: Relationship of the fetal-presenting part to the maternal pelvis. In vertex presentations, the posterior fontanel is the reference point. With breech presentations, it is the tip of the fetal sacrum; with face presentations, the chin; and with brow presentations, the anterior fontanel. Position is not the same as presentation. A fetus in vertex presentation may be in any of several positions. *Example:* Left occiput anterior position indicates that the fetal occiput, as determined by position of the posterior fontanel, is located on the left side of the anterior part of the woman's pelvis.

Positive-pressure ventilation: Artificial breathing for a person by forcing air or oxygen into the lungs under pressure by bag and mask, bag and endotracheal tube, T-piece resuscitator, or mechanical ventilator.

Post-term: Refers to a fetus or baby whose gestation has been longer than 42 completed weeks.

Postnatal: The time after delivery, used in reference to the baby.

Postpartum: The time after delivery, used in reference to the mother.

Potter syndrome: A rare, fatal congenital malformation with characteristic facial appearance and absent or hypoplastic kidneys. Oligohydramnios may be noted in the mother. These babies are often born at term, are frequently small for gestational age, and may have hypoplastic lungs.

Preconceptional: Before conception. Refers to counseling women or families *before* conception regarding the risks of various problems during pregnancy. This is particularly important when a woman has a disease known to affect pregnancy or fetal development or a family history of such problems or pregnancy carries increased risks for a woman because of an illness or condition she has.

Preeclampsia: New-onset hypertension in pregnancy with excretion of protein into the urine, with or without other laboratory abnormalities or symptoms.

Pregnancy due date: Expected date for the onset of labor. On average, the date of delivery will occur 280 days, or 40 weeks, after the first day of the last menstrual period. The reference range of variation is 2 weeks before or after the calculated due date. Babies delivered between 37 and 42 weeks' gestation are considered *term*. Babies delivered prior to the onset of the 37th week are designated *preterm,* and those delivered after $41^{6/7}$ weeks are considered *postterm*. Inaccuracies can occur with calculating the due date because the date of the menstrual period may not be recalled correctly or there are variations in the length of the preovulatory phase of a menstrual cycle. In some women with irregular periods, the preovulatory phase may be prolonged several weeks or even months.

Premature rupture of membranes (PROM): Rupture of the membranes ("bag of waters") before the onset of labor.

Prenatal: The time during pregnancy and before birth of the baby. Synonymous with *antenatal*.

Presentation: Refers to that part of the fetus that is in the birth canal and will deliver first. The normal presentation, near term and during labor and delivery, is vertex (headfirst). Any other presentation at that time is considered abnormal.

Preterm: Refers to that part of pregnancy between $20^{0/7}$ weeks and $36^{6/7}$ weeks (eg, preterm labor, preterm rupture of the membranes, or an infant born before 37 weeks' gestation).

Primary infection: First episode of a given infection. Some infections, such as cytomegalovirus or herpes, remain latent, without symptoms, in a person but may recur from time to time. The primary infection, however, is the most severe and likely to be the most damaging to a fetus or newborn. Other infections, such as syphilis or gonorrhea, may be cured, but if reinfection occurs, it will be as severe as the first infection.

Primigravida: A woman pregnant for the first time. *See also* Gravidity.

Primipara: A woman who has had one pregnancy carried to viability. *See also* Parity.

Prodromal labor: Refers to a patient having contractions but without sufficient cervical changes to make the diagnosis of true labor.

Prodrome: The time before a disease or process reaches its full strength. *Example:* The prodrome of a herpes infection may be mild itching in the area where the vesicles will later appear. This could be described as prodromal itching.

Prognosis: A forecast of the most likely outcome of an illness.

Prolapse: Falling out of a viscus. For example, an umbilical cord that slips through the cervix ahead of the fetus is a prolapsed cord, or a uterus that falls partially or completely into the vagina has prolapsed.

Prolapsed cord: Premature expulsion of the umbilical cord during labor and before the fetus is delivered. This is an emergency situation because a prolapsed cord is likely to be compressed, which may cause severe fetal compromise.

PROM: *See* Premature rupture of membranes.

Propylthiouracil (PTU): An antithyroid agent used to treat hyperthyroidism during the first trimester of pregnancy.

Proteinuria: Condition in which proteins from the blood are present in the urine. Also called *albuminuria*.

Psychosis: Any major mental disorder in which a person loses contact with reality and is unable to process information rationally.

PTU: *See* Propylthiouracil.

PUBS: *See* Percutaneous umbilical blood sampling.

Pudendal block: Nerve block by injection of local anesthetic into the area of the pudendal nerve. Used primarily for anesthesia of the perineum for delivery.

Pulmonary: Refers to the lungs.

Pulmonary hypoplasia: Underdevelopment of the fetal lungs, usually related to in utero compression of the fetal chest or lungs that prevents appropriate growth. This is seen with diaphragmatic hernia and with severe oligohydramnios, such as may occur with Potter syndrome.

Pulmonary maturity: Refers to relative ability of the fetal lungs to function normally if the fetus were to be delivered at the time a test for pulmonary maturity is performed. As the lungs mature, various chemicals produced by the fetal lungs appear in the amniotic fluid. Lecithin to sphingomyelin ratio, phosphatidyl glycerol detection, or lamellar body count may be performed on a sample of amniotic fluid to assess fetal lung maturity.

Pulse oximetry: Uses a noninvasive device that allows continuous measurement of the saturation of hemoglobin with oxygen. Hemoglobin changes color from blue to red as it becomes increasingly saturated with oxygen. A pulse oximeter uses a tiny light to shine through the skin and a light detector to measure the color of light coming through the skin. The color of light coming through the skin is determined by the amount of oxygen carried by hemoglobin in the red blood cells. From this the percentage of saturation is calculated (Spo_2). The percentage of saturation is not the same as a Pao_2 value, which measures the amount of oxygen dissolved in plasma.

Quickening: The first time fetal movements can be felt by the pregnant woman. This usually occurs between 16 and 20 weeks of gestation. Quickening generally occurs later in pregnancy for a primigravida than a woman who has had a previous pregnancy.

Radiant warmer: A servo-controlled heating device that is placed over a baby and provides radiant heat to keep body temperature normal.

RDS: *See* Respiratory distress syndrome.

Respiratory distress syndrome (RDS): Formerly called *hyaline membrane disease*. A disease mainly affecting preterm infants, due to immaturity of the lungs and lack of surfactant. Without surfactant, the alveoli collapse during exhalation and are difficult to open with the next breath.

Resuscitation: The process of restoring or supporting cardiac function, blood pressure, and respiration so as to provide adequate oxygenation and perfusion to a baby, child, or adult who is apparently dead or near death. For newborns, resuscitation is needed most often in the delivery room; for adults, resuscitation may be needed after any of a number of life-threatening events.

Resuscitation team: This concept refers to the fact that more than one person is needed to provide resuscitation. At least 2, preferably 3, health care professionals, skilled in the techniques of resuscitation, are needed for each resuscitation.

Reticulocyte count: Estimation of the number of newly formed red blood cells (reticulocytes) in a blood sample.

Retinopathy of prematurity (ROP): Abnormal blood vessel growth in the eye that may lead to detachment of the retina and partial or complete blindness. Blood vessel changes may result from many factors, including excessively high arterial blood oxygen concentrations for a period that can be as short as a few hours. The more preterm a baby, the more likely the baby is to develop ROP. Often ROP resolves spontaneously, but if permitted to proceed unchecked, scarring may occur and the retina may detach. It is critical that babies with ROP be followed by an ophthalmologist trained in examining babies so that laser therapy may be used to check the progression.

Retractions: A sign of respiratory distress. These occur with each breath as the skin is pulled inward between the ribs as a baby tries to expand stiff lungs.

Retrolental fibroplasia (RLF): Scarring phase of retinopathy of prematurity.

Rh alloimmunization: Formerly referred to as Rh sensitization. (1) Development of antibodies by an Rh-negative woman pregnant with an Rh-positive fetus. The antibodies cross the placenta into the fetus's blood, thus causing hemolysis of the fetus's red blood cells. (2) Development of antibodies against the Rh-positive red blood cells following a transfusion of Rh-positive blood unintentionally given to an Rh-negative person.

Rh blood type: Besides the major blood groups of A, B, O, and AB, there are a number of minor groups, of which the Rh system is the most important for perinatal care. Prevalence of the Rh factor varies by ethnic and racial groups. In the white population, 85% have the Rh antigen and are said to be Rh positive, while 15% lack the Rh antigen and, therefore, are Rh negative. Regardless of ethnic or racial heritage, persons who lack a blood antigen can make antibodies against that blood group. This means that Rh-negative persons can make antibodies against Rh-positive blood, if their immune system has been exposed to that blood (from external transfusion or transplacental transfer). Persons who have developed such antibodies are said to be alloimmunized, or sensitized to that blood group. *See also* Rh alloimmunization and Erythroblastosis fetalis.

Rh disease: *See* Erythroblastosis fetalis.

RhIg: Rh immune globulin (RhoGAM is one commercial name for Rh immune globulin products). The antibodies from sensitized Rh-negative persons can be harvested, purified, and prepared for safe injection into another Rh-negative, but unsensitized, woman. The product is called Rh immune globulin, or RhIg. The injected antibodies contained in RhIg prevent alloimmunization by reacting with the antigens on the few Rh-positive blood cells that may have escaped from the fetus into the maternal circulation. Rh-negative, unsensitized women should receive RhIg at 28 weeks' gestation and again following delivery. Rh-negative, unsensitized women should also receive RhIg within 72 hours of an abortion or an episode of vaginal bleeding during pregnancy. Protection lasts for 12 weeks. Therefore, depending on the course of the pregnancy, subsequent doses may also be needed. Use of RhIg protects fetuses in future pregnancies from Rh disease.

Rhinitis: Inflammation of mucous membranes of the nasal passages, causing a characteristic runny or stuffy nose. Although generally uncommon in newborns, rhinitis is frequently found in babies with congenital syphilis.

RLF: *See* Retrolental fibroplasia and Retinopathy of prematurity.

ROP: *In neonatal care*, retinopathy of prematurity. *In obstetric care*, an abbreviation for a specific position (right occiput posterior) of a vertex presentation during labor. *See also* Retinopathy of prematurity.

Rotation (of the fetal head): Gradual turning of the fetus during labor for the fetal head to accommodate size and shape of the maternal pelvis as the fetus descends through it.

Rubella: A mild viral infection, also called *German measles*. A rubella infection in a pregnant woman during early pregnancy may result in infection of the fetus and cause rubella syndrome.

SARS-CoV-2: Severe acute respiratory syndrome coronavirus 2, a novel coronavirus that caused a global pandemic of COVID-19 (coronavirus disease 2019), beginning in late 2019.

Scalp stimulation test: Test in which fetal heart rate response to mechanical stimulation of the fetal scalp (by examiner's gloved finger or sterile instrument) is assessed. Used as an estimate of fetal well-being during labor.

Scaphoid abdomen: Sunken or hollow-looking abdomen, occurring when there is a diaphragmatic hernia, which allows the intestines to slip from the abdomen through a hole in the diaphragm and into the chest cavity.

Secondary infection: Recurrent infection. *See also* Primary infection.

Sepsis: Infection of the blood. Also referred to as *septicemia*.

Serum bicarbonate: Also called *blood* or *plasma bicarbonate*. Concentration of bicarbonate in the blood. Bicarbonate is the main body chemical responsible for the acid-base balance of the blood.

Serum urea nitrogen: A blood chemistry test of renal function. The higher the serum urea nitrogen, the more urinary excretion has been impaired.

Servo control: A mechanism that automatically maintains skin temperature at a preset temperature. A thermistor probe is taped to the baby, registers the skin temperature, and in turn activates a radiant warmer or incubator to continue to produce heat, or to stop heating.

Sexually transmitted infection (STI): An infection that is transmitted from one partner to another during sexual activity. Many infections can be transmitted in this way, but certain STIs can have significant effect on the fetus or newborn, including syphilis, gonorrhea, *Chlamydia*, and HIV.

SGA: *See* Small for gestational age.

Shock: Collapse of the circulatory system due to inadequate blood volume, cardiac function, or vasomotor tone. *In babies*, the causes are most often hypovolemia, sepsis, or severe acidosis. Symptoms are hypotension, rapid respirations, pallor, weak pulses, and slow refilling of blanched skin. *In pregnant women*, the cause is most often hemorrhage. Because of the expanded blood volume of pregnancy and vasoconstrictive capabilities of most (young, healthy) pregnant women, blood loss may be severe before symptoms of shock (hypotension, weak and rapid pulse, rapid respirations, anxiousness or confusion, and cold, clammy, pale skin) become evident.

Short bowel syndrome: A syndrome of weight loss and dehydration related to having less than the normal length of intestine. The less intestine a baby has, the less well nutrients can be absorbed. Short bowel syndrome may result from a baby being born with an abnormally short bowel or may be the result of a portion of the intestines having been removed for treatment of certain types of bowel disease.

Shoulder dystocia: Situation in which the baby's shoulders become wedged between the maternal symphysis and sacrum after delivery of the fetal head. The head may be pulled back against the perineum as the woman relaxes her push that delivered the head (the "turtle sign"). Various procedures may be tried to free the shoulders. Severe asphyxia or fetal death can occur if there is significant delay in delivery of the shoulders and trunk.

Shunt: A diversion of fluid from its normal pathway. (1) *Blood:* In some sick babies, blood will be shunted from the right side of the heart to the left (baby will be blue); in other babies, the shunt will be from the left side of the heart to the right (baby will be in congestive heart failure). Commonly seen in babies with congenital heart disease or severe lung disease in which the blood cannot be normally oxygenated. (2) *Cerebrospinal fluid:* An artificial pathway for the flow of cerebrospinal fluid when blockage is in the normal pathway, resulting in hydrocephalus. Typically, cerebrospinal fluid is shunted through a one-way valve from the ventricles into a small tube tunneled under the skin and empties into the abdominal cavity. This is called a *ventriculoperitoneal*, or V-P, shunt.

Sickle cell anemia: A genetic hemoglobinopathy causing chronic anemia. Crises, resulting from infarction of various body areas clogged by the sickled cells obstructing small blood vessels, may occur periodically. Management during pregnancy is particularly complicated.

Sickle cell–hemoglobin C disease: A hemoglobinopathy similar to sickle cell anemia.

Sickle cell–thalassemia disease: Sickle cell disease and thalassemia are genetically transmitted anemic diseases caused by abnormal hemoglobin. *See* Hemoglobinopathy.

Sims position: The patient rests on one side, with the upper leg drawn up so that the knee is close to the chest. Often used with an emergency delivery in bed or outside the hospital. This position does not allow for much assistance by an attendant but has the advantage of placing less tension on the perineum during delivery and, therefore, may result in fewer lacerations.

SLE: Systemic lupus erythematosus.

Small for gestational age (SGA): A baby whose weight is lower than the 10th percentile for infants of that gestational age.

"Sniffing" position: Proper position of a baby's head during bag-and-mask ventilation or endotracheal intubation. The head and back are in straight alignment, with the chin pulled forward as if sniffing. This position is different from the one used for endotracheal intubation of an adult because the relative size and relationship of anatomic structures is different between babies and adults. The neck is *not* hyperextended (bent backward to an extreme degree) during endotracheal intubation in babies.

Sodium bicarbonate: Drug used to counteract metabolic acidosis. After being given to a baby, it rapidly changes to carbon dioxide and water. Therefore, it should be given only to babies who are breathing adequately on their own or receiving adequate assisted ventilation. These babies can "blow off" the excess carbon dioxide formed. If sodium bicarbonate is given to a baby with a high $Paco_2$, it will make the $Paco_2$ go even higher and thereby worsen the acidosis.

Spinal (block): An anesthetic technique in which a local anesthetic is introduced into the subarachnoid space of the spinal canal through a hollow needle placed (temporarily) in the spine. It is technically easier to perform placement of an epidural catheter because spinal fluid in the subarachnoid space will flow out through the hollow needle and, thereby, identify proper placement of the needle before injection of the anesthetic. Because the anesthetic also blocks sympathetic nerves leaving the spinal cord, the blood pressure of the woman may decline. (For this reason, a loading dose of 500–1,000 mL of physiologic [normal] saline solution may be given intravenously prior to introduction of the anesthetic.) Spinal anesthetics are not ordinarily given until the second stage of labor has begun because the anesthetics used do not remain effective for longer than 2 hours.

Spo_2: The percentage of saturation of hemoglobin by oxygen as detected by a pulse oximeter, which reads and reports how red the blood is. Fully saturated hemoglobin appears bright red, while desaturated hemoglobin appears blue.

Sterile vaginal examination: Vaginal examination with a speculum, using sterile technique. In this situation, sterility obviously cannot be ensured. When a woman is pregnant and rupture of membranes is known or suspected, the goal is to minimize the risk of introducing bacteria during examination.

Sternum: The breastbone. The chest bone that joins the left and right ribs.

STI: *See* Sexually transmitted infection.

Stopcock: Small device with 3 openings and a lever to close any 1 of the 3 openings. One opening is designed to fit the hub of an intravenous catheter, umbilical catheter, or similar catheter. The other 2 are designed to connect with a syringe or intravenous fluid tubing.

Stylet: Slender metal probe with a blunt tip that may be inserted inside an endotracheal tube to make the tube stiffer during intubation. Also, the solid, removable center within certain needles.

Succenturiate lobe of placenta: A malformation of the placenta in which the placenta has a second lobe, with the umbilical blood vessels traversing membranes between the main placenta and accessory or succenturiate lobe. Umbilical vessels between the 2 lobes may lie over the cervical os (creating the condition known as vasa previa) and can be torn, particularly if the membranes are ruptured artificially. Also, the succenturiate lobe may produce a placenta previa if it lies over the os, even though a previous ultrasound may have reported a normally placed placenta, which may be accurate for the main portion of the placenta.

Superimposed preeclampsia: Development of preeclampsia in a woman who already has chronic hypertension. Sometimes it is difficult to tell if the increase in blood pressure is due to poor control of existing hypertension or development of preeclampsia. If the blood pressure increases and there is increasing proteinuria, superimposed preeclampsia is most likely. This complication increases the risk of development of eclampsia.

Supine: Position of a person when he or she is flat on his or her back.

Supine hypotension: In late pregnancy, the enlarged uterus may compress the vena cava when a woman lies on her back. This reduces return of blood to the heart and, thus, reduces cardiac output. This then causes a reduction in blood pressure and in the perfusion of body tissues. The woman may feel faint. Most pregnant women lie on their sides to sleep. During labor it may be helpful to have a woman lie on her side as much as possible. If supine hypotension develops with a woman resting on her back, uterine blood flow may be affected, which might result in a non-reassuring fetal heart rate pattern. One measure to take if a non-reassuring fetal heart pattern occurs during labor is to turn a woman onto her side (if on her back) or from one side to the other to relieve pressure on the vena cava.

Suprapubic puncture: A technique used to tap the bladder of a newborn. A needle is inserted into the center of the lower abdomen, above the pubic bone, and into the bladder to obtain a sterile urine specimen for culture.

Surfactant: A group of substances, including lecithin, that contributes to compliance (elasticity) of the lungs by coating the alveoli and allowing them to stay open during exhalation. Without surfactant, the alveoli collapse during expiration and are difficult to open with the next breath.

Symphysis pubis: Connection between the right and left hip bones in front of the body, in the pubic area.

Systemic: Refers to the whole body.

Tachycardia: Rapid heart rate. (1) *Fetal* tachycardia is considered to be a sustained heart rate faster than 160 beats/min. (2) *Neonatal* tachycardia is considered to be a sustained heart rate faster than 180 beats/min while a baby is quiet and at rest.

Tachypnea: Rapid respiratory rate. In a neonate, tachypnea is considered to be a sustained breathing rate faster than 60 breaths/min.

Tent: Small cone-shaped device made of material that can expand. Used to dilate an orifice or keep a wound open. In obstetrics, tents may be used for cervical ripening and may also be called osmotic dilators.

Teratogen: A substance that causes malformations in the developing embryo. Certain medications are known teratogens and should not be taken during pregnancy. Most congenital malformations, however, cannot be traced to a teratogen but are instead due to unknown factors (most common) or hereditary factors.

Thalassemia: Any one of several hereditary hemolytic anemias caused by abnormal hemoglobin.

Thermistor probe: A small sensing device that measures temperature continuously and is able to detect very small changes. Servo-control devices operate by a thermistor probe attached to the baby and then the radiant warmer or incubator.

Thrombocytopenia: Abnormally low number of blood platelets.

Thrombophlebitis: Inflammation of a vein associated with the formation of a thrombus. In a superficial blood vessel, a thin red streak will form in the skin directly over the path of the blood vessel and the area will feel warm to the touch. Thrombophlebitis may develop at the site of a peripheral intravenous catheter, in which case the catheter should be removed and the intravenous catheter restarted into another vein. Further treatment is rarely needed. If thrombophlebitis develops in deep veins, however, it is a serious condition, generally requiring treatment with intravenous heparin.

Thrombosis: The process involved in formation of a thrombus (blood clot in a vessel).

Thrombus: A blood clot that gradually forms inside a blood vessel and may become large enough to obstruct blood flow. If a thrombus separates from the blood vessel and is carried in the blood, it becomes an embolus. Plural: thrombi.

Thyroid storm: A sudden worsening of adult hyperthyroidism, usually triggered by trauma or surgery and characterized by marked tachycardia and fever.

Thyroid-stimulating hormone (TSH): A protein secreted by the anterior pituitary gland that stimulates thyroid function.

Thyroid-stimulating immunoglobulin (TSI): An antibody produced by lymphocytes that, for unknown reasons, stimulates the thyroid to release thyroxin. These antibodies may cross the placenta and cause hyperthyroidism in the fetus.

Tocolysis: Administration of a drug to stop uterine contractions.

Tonus: The amount of continuous contraction of muscle. *Uterine tonus* refers to how tightly the muscle of the uterus is contracted between labor contractions. With an internal monitor, it is measured as the resting pressure in the uterus between contractions. *Hypertonus* refers to a uterus that remains excessively tense and does not relax normally between labor contractions.

TORCH: Toxoplasmosis, other agents, rubella, cytomegalovirus, and herpes simplex. A specific group of infections that can cause in utero fetal infection (usually resulting in severe damage) or, in the case of herpes, life-threatening neonatal infection. The "other" category includes less common, serious infections such as varicella, coxsackievirus B, and syphilis.

Toxemia: Term formerly used to refer, collectively, to all forms of hypertensive disorders of pregnancy.

Toxoplasmosis: Disease caused by a type of protozoa (a type of microscopic organism). Toxoplasmosis in a woman may go unnoticed but may infect the fetus, thus causing congenital toxoplasmosis. Congenital toxoplasmosis damages the central nervous system of the fetus and may lead to blindness, brain defects, or death.

Trachea: The windpipe or tube of stacked cartilaginous rings that descends into the chest cavity from the larynx and branches into the right and left bronchi, which branch further into smaller bronchioles inside the lungs.

Transfusion, fetal-fetal: Situation that may occur, in utero, between fetuses of a multifetal gestation, when there is a connection between an artery of one fetus and a vein of the other in a monochorionic placenta. The fetus on the arterial side becomes a chronic blood donor to the fetus on the venous or recipient side. When born, the donor twin may be pale, severely anemic, and small for gestational age. The recipient twin may be red, polycythemic, and, occasionally, large for gestational age.

Transfusion, fetal-maternal: Situation that may occur in utero if an abnormal connection develops between the fetal and maternal circulation in the placenta. The reverse direction of maternal-fetal transfusion apparently does not occur. The newborn may present with findings similar to the "donor" fetus described in fetal-fetal transfusion. To diagnose this condition, the woman's blood can be tested for the presence of fetal cells with the Kleihauer-Betke test.

Transverse lie: The body of the fetus lies horizontally across the maternal pelvis and hence across the birth canal entrance. A cesarean delivery is required for safe delivery of a fetus in transverse lie.

Trendelenburg position: A position of the body that may be used for surgery or examination. The patient lies supine on an inclined surface, with the head lowered below the level of the feet.

Trimester: A period of 3 months. The time during pregnancy is often divided into the first trimester (first through third month), second trimester (fourth through sixth month), and third trimester (seventh through ninth month).

Trisomy: Chromosomal abnormality in which there is an extra (third) chromosome of one of a normal pair of chromosomes. The most common is trisomy 21 (three 21 chromosomes), which is also called Down syndrome. Other trisomies also occur, such as trisomy 13 (three 13 chromosomes) and trisomy 18 (three 18 chromosomes), both of which have a characteristic set of multiple congenital anomalies.

TSH: *See* Thyroid-stimulating hormone.

TSI: *See* Thyroid-stimulating immunoglobulin.

Turner syndrome: A chromosomal abnormality in which there are 45 chromosomes, with the absent chromosome being one sex chromosome (45,X) instead of the typical 46,XX (female) or 46,XY (male). These individuals are phenotypically female and may have physical abnormalities including webbed neck, low hairline, and certain skeletal, urinary tract, lymph system, and cardiac abnormalities. The baby will have female external genitalia, but the ovaries may be completely absent and sexual development will be severely impaired.

Twin-twin transfusion: *See* Transfusion, fetal-fetal.

Twins, conjoined: Twin fetuses joined together, usually at the chest or abdomen but may be at almost any site, and sharing one or more organs. This results from incomplete separation during the process of twinning of single ovum (which, if completely split, would have become identical twins). The greater the degree of organ sharing, the less likely one or both twins can survive surgical separation.

Twins, fraternal: Two fetuses created from the fertilization and implantation of 2 separate ova.

Twins, identical: Two fetuses created from the division of one fertilized ovum.

Ultrasonography (US): A technique used to visualize the fetus and placenta by means of sound waves, which bounce off of these structures and are turned into a picture outline. Used to assess fetal growth, fetal well-being, congenital abnormalities, multifetal gestation, placental location, location of structures during percutaneous umbilical blood sampling and amniocentesis, and volume of amniotic fluid.

Urine drug screening: Commonly available test in which the metabolic breakdown products of recently taken drugs can be identified in the urine.

US: *See* Ultrasonography.

Uterine atony: Failure of the uterine muscle (myometrium) to contract in the immediate postpartum period. A leading cause of postpartum hemorrhage.

Uterine dysfunction: Abnormal progress of labor due to uterine contractions that are inadequate in strength or occur in an uneven, uncoordinated pattern.

Uterine fibroids: Tumors of the uterus made up of fibrous connective tissue and smooth muscle. Also called *leiomyomas*. These myomas may become very large, occasionally interfering with implantation. Other risks, although uncommon, include placenta previa, obstructed labor, preterm labor, postpartum hemorrhage, and endometritis.

Uterine inertia: Inadequate labor caused by uterine contractions that are too short, too weak, and too infrequent to produce adequate progress.

Uteroplacental: Refers to the uterus and placenta together as a functioning unit.

Uteroplacental insufficiency: An inexact term suggesting a placenta that is functioning poorly, with inadequate transfer of nutrients and oxygen to the fetus, and used to explain some cases of in utero growth restriction or fetal distress during labor.

Uterus: A hollow, muscular organ in which the fetus develops, often called the *womb*.

Vacuum extractor (VE): An instrument used to assist delivery, in which a plastic cup is placed over the fetal occiput, suction is applied so the cup is sealed to the scalp, and then traction is applied to the cup. There are risks, benefits, and specific indications for use of vacuum extraction.

Vagus nerve: A major nerve with branches to the heart and gastrointestinal tract. Something that stimulates one branch of the vagus nerve may also affect another branch. *Example:* Suctioning deep in the back of a baby's throat directly stimulates part of the vagus nerve to the gastrointestinal tract and indirectly may affect the branch to the heart and cause bradycardia (termed *reflex bradycardia*).

Varicella-zoster virus: The virus that causes chickenpox in children. Adults who were not infected as children and, therefore, did not acquire immunity may also develop chickenpox, which, in adults, can cause life-threatening pneumonia. Infection in a pregnant woman early in pregnancy can cause severe fetal malformations and serious neonatal illness at term. *Note:* Reactivated infection in adults is herpes zoster. This occurs in a small percentage of individuals who had chickenpox as children and causes pain and the formation of vesicles along specific nerve tracks. These symptoms are known as *shingles*.

VariZIG: Varicella-zoster immune globulin. Specific antibodies to the varicella-zoster virus obtained from persons who have had the disease. Principally used to attenuate infection in the newborn of a mother who has the infection.

Vasa previa: An abnormality of placental development. Instead of joining together at a point over the placenta, the vessels that form the umbilical cord join some distance from the edge of the placenta. The vessels lie on the membranes and, if the vessels lie across the cervical os, are exposed when the cervix dilates. This is a dangerous situation because when the membranes rupture or are artificially ruptured, the vessels may tear open. The fetal hemorrhage that results is often fatal.

Vasoconstriction: Tightening of the blood vessels, allowing less blood flow through the vessels. *Example:* When a significant volume of blood is lost, the small blood vessels in the skin will constrict, thus allowing the remaining blood to be directed to the brain and other vital organs.

VBAC: Vaginal birth after cesarean.

VE: *See* Vacuum extractor.

Vein: Refers to blood vessels that return blood to the heart. In most veins, this blood is dark red because it has a low oxygen concentration because most of the oxygen from the arterial blood has been transferred to the body's cells for metabolism. The pulmonary veins, however, carry oxygenated blood as it flows from the lungs to the heart.

Vertex: Top of the head. A fetus in vertex presentation is headfirst in the maternal pelvis. This presentation is identified on vaginal examination by palpation of the posterior fontanel in the center of the birth canal.

Vital signs: Refers to the group of clinical measures that includes respiratory rate, heart rate, temperature, and blood pressure.

Vitamin E: A vitamin important for maintaining red blood cell stability. When a baby is deficient in vitamin E, the red blood cells may break down more rapidly than normal and the baby may become anemic.

Volume expander: Fluid used to replace blood volume, and thereby increase blood pressure, in cases of hypotension thought to be due to hypovolemia. Blood or physiologic (normal) saline solution are examples of volume expanders.

Woods maneuver: Maneuver for management of shoulder dystocia in which the fetus is rotated 180 degrees so the posterior shoulder becomes the anterior shoulder.

Zavanelli maneuver: Maneuver for management of shoulder dystocia in which the fetal head is replaced into the vagina and a cesarean delivery is done.

Index

Page numbers followed by *f* indicate a figure.
Page numbers followed by *t* indicate a table.
Page numbers followed by *b* indicate a box.

A

ABCs (airway, breathing, circulation), 411
Abnormal blood clotting, 66
Abnormal labor progress and difficult delivery, 345–402
   anesthesia and, 373
   causes, 359–360
   clinical clues, 357
   congenital malformation and, 372
   curve, 358*f*
   fetal heart rate abnormalities, 387–388
   fetal presentation or position and, 367–372
   fetopelvic disproportion and, 373
   handling emergent or potentially emergent conditions, 387–393
   ineffective pushing and, 373
   investigating, 360–364
   labor diagnosis, 351
   labor progress curve, 357–358
   maternal analgesia or anesthesia, 388–389
   maternal risks, 383
   meconium-stained amniotic fluid, 387
   normal progress of labor vs, 351–353
   obstetric hemorrhage (*See* Obstetric hemorrhage)
   operative vaginal deliveries, 377–382
   posttest, 402
   pretest, 348–350
   prolapsed umbilical cord and, 254, 389–390
   prolonged labor, 354, 383–384, 386
   rapid labor, 354, 384–385, 386
   recommended routines, 397
   responses to, 374–375
   risks of, 354–355
   self-test, 356, 365–366, 376, 395–396, 398–402
   shoulder dystocia, 390–393
   third stage of labor, 394–395
   treatment, 366–375
   uterine dysfunction and, 366–367
   what constitutes, 354
   when to suspect, 357–358
ABO status, 412
Action stage, 214
Acute pyelonephritis, 137–138
AIM Hypertension bundle, 19–22
AIM Obstetric hemorrhage bundle, 43*f*
Alcohol use, 222–223
Alloimmunization, 62, 186–187
Amantadine, 91
Aminoglycosides, 91
Amniocentesis, 192
   for prelabor rupture of membranes (PROM), 256
Amnioinfusion, 260, 261, 262, 264, 266
Amniotic fluid
   abnormal amount, 194–198
   embolism, 59
   meconium-stained, 387
Amniotic fluid index (AFI) method, 194
Amniotomy, 327–328
Amphetamines, 220–221
Analgesia, 388–389
Anemia, severe, 162
Anesthesia and abnormal labor progress, 373, 388–389, 395
Antenatal steroids, 260, 263, 265, 267
   preterm labor and delivery and, 302–306
Antibiotics for prelabor rupture of membranes (PROM), 259–260
Antihypertensive management, 12, 13*t*, 24*b*
Antimicrobial medications, 90–91
Antiphospholipid antibody syndrome (APS), 166–168
Antiretroviral therapy, HIV, 100–103
Anxiety, 217–218
Apgar scores, 413
APS. *See* Antiphospholipid antibody syndrome (APS)
Arrested labor, 354
Arterial vasospasm, 70
Asthma, 173
Augmentation. *See* Labor augmentation

B

Bacterial vaginosis, 137
Barnum maneuver, 392
Bishop score, 321–322
   amniotomy for high, 327–328
   calculation of, 322*t*
   cervical ripening for low, 322–326
   midrange, 327
Bleeding
   excessive, 394
   little or no, 394
   placenta delivery and, 414–415
Blood gas analysis, 413
Blood loss. *See* Obstetric hemorrhage
Blood samples, umbilical cord, 412–414
Bloody show, 46, 48
Boggy uterus, 68
Bracht maneuver, 410*f*
Breastfeeding Handbook for Physicians, 216
Breech presentation, 370, 409–410

C

Carboprost tromethamine (Hemabate), 70
Cardiovascular disease, 154–157
Cell-free DNA screening, 191
Cephalic replacement, 392–393
Cerclage, 295
Cervical bleeding, 51
Cervical dilation, 351
   ineffective pushing and, 373
Cervical insufficiency, 295
Cervical length screening, 293
Cervical ripening, 322–327
Cesarean delivery
   disseminated intravascular coagulation (DIC) and, 61
   fetal presentation and, 370–371
   gestational diabetes (GDM) and, 242
   HIV and, 100
   late term and post-term, 201
   prelabor rupture of membranes (PROM) and, 259, 260
   risks associated with previous, 184–185
   risks of, 383
Chickenpox, 113, 133–134

INDEX

Chlamydia, 92–95
Chorionic villus sampling, 192
Chronic hypertension, 6
    management during pregnancy, 11–14
Coagulation factor replacement, 60
Coagulopathy, 66
Cocaine, 221
Code sheets, 75
Combination antiretroviral therapy (cART), 100
Compound presentation, 369
Compression, umbilical cord, 254
Congenital malformations
    abnormal labor progress and, 372
    genetic screening for, 190–192
    history of previous, 183
Contemplation stage, 214
Coronavirus disease 2019 (COVID-19), 135
COVID-19. *See* Coronavirus disease 2019 (COVID-19)
Crowning, 408
Cryoprecipitate, 60
Cytomegalovirus (CMV), 110, 114–115

D

Deep tendon reflexes (DTRs), 22–23
Dehydration, 297
Delivery of twins, 193t
Depression, 217–218
Diabetes mellitus, 159–160, 235. *See also* Gestational diabetes (GDM)
DIC. *See* Disseminated intravascular coagulation (DIC)
Diethylstilbestrol, 295
Diet therapy, gestational diabetes (GDM), 238
Difficult delivery. *See* Abnormal labor progress and difficult delivery
Dinoprostone cervical gel (Prepidil), 325
Disseminated intravascular coagulation (DIC), 59–62
Documentation, obstetric hemorrhage management, 75
Drugs in Pregnancy and Lactation, 216

E

Early delivery and gestational diabetes (GDM), 241
Early pregnancy bleeding in Rh(D)-negative women, 62
Eclampsia, 7–8t, 9
    labor management for, 22–25
    management guidelines, 17–19
    stabilized, 27
Ectopic pregnancy, 47–48
Edinburgh Postnatal Depression Scale, 217
Electronic cigarettes, 224–225
Emergency care for obstetric hemorrhage, 42–45
Empty uterus, 47
Endocrine disorders, 157–160. *See also* Gestational diabetes (GDM)
    diabetes mellitus, 159–160
    hyperthyroidism, 157–158
    hypothyroidism, 158–159
Escherichia coli, 138
Excessive bleeding, 394
Exercise and gestational diabetes (GDM), 238

F

Face presentation of the fetus, 368f
Fallopian tubes, 72
False labor, 351
Fertility preservation, 71–72
Fetal death, 47
    disseminated intravascular coagulation (DIC) and, 59
    history of previous, 183
    infectious diseases in pregnancy and, 88
    late term and post-term, 201
    umbilical cord complications and, 254
Fetal fibronectin, 297–298
Fetal growth assessment, 12–13
Fetal growth restriction
    diagnosis and management, 199–200
    infectious diseases in pregnancy and, 88
Fetal heart rate
    abnormalities in, 387–388
    labor induction/augmentation and, 331, 335–336
Fetal hydrops, 186–187
Fetal hyperglycemia, 236
Fetal lie, 361
Fetal malformations, infectious diseases in pregnancy and, 88
Fetal monitoring, gestational diabetes (GDM) and, 241–242
Fetal positioning during labor, 362f
Fetal presentation, 307, 330, 361, 362, 367–372
    breech, 370, 409–410
Fetal size and gestational diabetes (GDM), 241, 242
Fetopelvic disproportion, 373
FFP. *See* Fresh frozen plasma (FFP)
First-trimester nuchal translucency screening, 191
5 A's Intervention for Tobacco Use in Pregnancy, 225t
5 P's questionnaire, 218
Fluoroquinolones, 91
Forceps, 377–378
    risks and safety of, 379–381
4 P's questionnaire, 218
Fresh frozen plasma (FFP), 60–61

G

GAS. *See* Group A streptococcus (GAS)
GBS. *See* Group B streptococcus (GBS)
GDM. *See* Gestational diabetes (GDM)
Genetic screening, 190–192
German measles, 112, 120–121
Gestational age
    late term and post-term, 200–202
    prelabor rupture of membranes (PROM) management and, 261–262
Gestational diabetes (GDM), 231–248
    caring for women with, 237–239
    causes, 235
    diagnosis, 237
    diet therapy, 238
    exercise and, 238
    fetal monitoring, 241–242
    home blood glucose monitoring and, 238
    importance of identifying women with, 236
    insulin for, 239
    long-term care and advice, 243
    postpartum follow-up, 242

INDEX

posttest, 248
versus pregestational diabetes, 159–160, 235
preparation for delivery, 242
pretest, 233–234
recommended routines, 245
screening, 236–237
self-test, 240, 244, 246–247
Gestational hypertension, 7–8t, 8. *See also* Hypertension in pregnancy
Gestational thrombocytopenia, 164
Gonorrhea, 93, 95–96, 284
Group A streptococcus (GAS), 140
Group B streptococcus (GBS), 112, 123–128
 algorithm for screening, 126f, 127f
 intrapartum prophylaxis, 128f
 prelabor rupture of membranes (PROM) and, 261–264
 preterm labor and delivery and, 306

H

Heat loss, neonatal, 411
HELLP syndrome, 7–8t, 9
 disseminated intravascular coagulation (DIC) and, 59
 management, 29
Hematologic disease, 162–166
 hemoglobinopathy, 162–164
 severe anemia, 162
 thrombocytopenia, 164–165
 thromboembolic disease, 165–166
Hemoglobinopathy, 162–164
Hemorrhage, obstetric. *See* Obstetric hemorrhage
Hepatitis A virus, 115
Hepatitis B virus, 111, 115–117
Hepatitis C virus, 117
Hereditary disease, 183
Herpes simplex virus (HSV), 92, 93, 96–98
High parity, 184
High-risk conditions, 151–176
 cardiovascular disease, 154–157
 endocrine disorders, 157–160
 hematologic disease, 162–166
 immunologic disease, 166–170
 neurological disease, 172–173
 posttest, 176
 preconception counseling, 154

pretest, 153
renal disease, 170–171
respiratory disease, 173
self-test, 161, 174–176
History, obstetric, 181–188
HIV, 92, 93, 100–104
Home blood glucose monitoring, 238
HPV. *See* Human papillomavirus (HPV)
HSV. *See* Herpes simplex virus (HSV)
Human chorionic gonadotropin (hCG) test, 46
Human papillomavirus (HPV), 92, 93, 104–105
Hyperglycemia, 236
Hypertension in pregnancy, 1–35
 classification of, 5–10
 eclampsia, 7–8t
 gestational, 7–8t
 HELLP syndrome, 7–8t, 9, 29
 hospital measures for, 19–22
 labor management for, 22–25
 management during stages of pregnancy, 11–14
 management guidelines, 16–17
 maternal condition stabilized, 27–28
 posttest, 35
 preeclampsia, 7–8t
 preeclampsia and eclampsia management guidelines, 17–19
 preeclampsia with severe features, 7–8t
 pretest, 3–4
 recommended routines, 31
 risks after delivery, 29
 risks of, 5
 seizures, 22–23, 26–27
 self-test, 10, 15, 19, 25, 30, 32–34
 stabilized eclampsia or preeclampsia, 27
 types and characteristic findings, 7–8t
 women at increased risk for development of, 15–16
Hypertensive disorders of pregnancy, 6
Hyperthermia, 411
Hyperthyroidism, 157–158
Hypertonic uterine dysfunction, 331, 366–367
Hyponatremia, 336

Hypothermia, 411–412
Hypothyroidism, 158–159
Hypotonic contractions, 361
Hypotonic uterine dysfunction, 330, 367
Hysterectomy, 56, 70–72

I

Imminent delivery, 403–422. *See also* Maternal/fetal transport
 breech presentation, 409–410
 defined, 407
 placenta delivery, 414–415
 pretest, 405–406
 recognizing, 407
 recommended routines, 420
 self-test, 415
 what to do after baby is delivered, 411–414
 what to do after head delivers, 408–409
 what to do on, 407–408
 what to do when head crowns, 408
Immune thrombocytopenic purpura (ITP), 164–165
Immunologic disease, 166–170
 antiphospholipid antibody syndrome (APS), 166–168
 systemic lupus erythematosus (SLE), 168–170
Induction. *See* Labor induction
Ineffective pushing, 373
Infectious diseases in pregnancy, 83–149
 bacterial vaginosis, 137
 chlamydia, 92–94
 coronavirus disease 2019 (COVID-19), 135
 cytomegalovirus (CMV), 110, 114–115
 disseminated intravascular coagulation (DIC) and, 59
 fetal effects, 88–91
 gonorrhea, 93, 95–96
 group A streptococcus (GAS), 140
 group B streptococcus, 112, 123–128
 hepatitis A virus, 115
 hepatitis B virus, 111. 115–117
 hepatitis C virus, 117
 herpes simplex virus (HSV), 93, 96-98

463

INDEX

Infectious diseases in pregnancy (*continued*)
    HIV, 93, 100–104
    human papillomavirus (HPV), 92, 93, 104–105
    intra-amniotic infection, 139
    listeriosis, 111, 118–119
    management, 92–141
    mastitis, 141
    parvovirus B19, 111, 119–120
    posttest, 149
    prelabor rupture of membranes (PROM) and, 253–254, 258, 262–263
    preterm labor and, 293
    pretest, 86–87
    puerperal endometritis, 139–140
    recommended routines, 143–144
    risks associated with, 88
    rubella, 112, 120–121
    self-test, 99, 109, 122, 136, 142, 145–148
    syphilis, 93, 105–108
    toxoplasmosis, 112, 129–130
    tuberculosis, 113, 130–132
    urinary tract infection (UTI) and acute pyelonephritis, 137–138
    varicella-zoster virus, 113, 133–134
Insulin, 239
Intervention for tobacco use in pregnancy, 225t
Intimate partner violence (IPV), 214–216
Intra-amniotic infection, 139
    prelabor rupture of membranes (PROM) and, 258, 259–260, 269
Intrauterine pregnancy, 47
IPV. *See* Intimate partner violence (IPV)
Isoniazid, 91
ITP. *See* Immune thrombocytopenic purpura (ITP)

L

Labor
    abnormal progress of (*See* Abnormal labor progress and difficult delivery)
    active, characteristics of, 351t, 355t
    contraction pattern, 351
    delay of progress, 360t, 374–375t
    diagnosis of, 351
    face presentation, 368f
    fetal positioning during, 362f
    latent, characteristics of, 351t, 355t
    normal progress, 351–353, 355t, 358f
    prolonged, 354, 383–384, 386
    rapid, 354, 384–385, 386
    responses to delay of, 374–375
    stages, 352–353, 355t
    third stage of, 355t, 394–395
    time of onset, 351
Labor augmentation
    complications of oxytocin, 335–336
    contraindications, 330–331
    defined, 319
    how long to use oxytocin for, 337
    oxytocin administration, 331–333
    posttest, 343
    pretest, 317–318
    reasons, 330
    recommended routines, 339
    self-test, 334, 338, 340–342
Labor induction, 13–14, 315–343
    amniotomy, 327–328
    Bishop score and, 321–328
    cervical ripening, 322–327
    contraindications, 320
    defined, 319
    how long to use oxytocin, 336–337
    posttest, 343
    for prelabor rupture of membranes (PROM), 266
    preparation for, 321
    pretest, 317–318
    reasons, 319–320
    recommended routines, 339
    self-test, 329, 338, 340–342
    successful, 321–322
Lacerations, genital tract, 66
Lactation and antimicrobial medications, 91t
Laparotomy, 71–72
Late-pregnancy bleeding
    causes of, 53–54
    in Rh(D)-negative women, 63
Late-term gestational age, 200–202
Limited or no prenatal care, 213–214
Listeriosis, 111, 118–119
Lithium, 216
Low placental implantation, 49f

M

Macrosomia
    gestational diabetes (GDM) and, 241
    labor augmentation contraindication, 330
    previous, 181–182
    prolonged labor and, 383
Magnesium
    levels, 22–23
    prelabor rupture of membranes (PROM) and, 263, 267
    preterm labor and delivery and, 302
Maintenance stage, 214
Manual compression of the uterus, 69f
Marijuana, 223–224
Mastitis, 141
Maternal age, 190
Maternal death, infectious diseases in pregnancy and, 88
Maternal/fetal transport, 416–422. *See also* Imminent delivery
    contraindications, 418
    defined, 416
    importance of, 416
    obstetric referral and, 419
    preparation for, 416, 418
    reasons for, 417
    recommended routines, 420
    self-test, 419, 421–422
Maternal illness, infectious diseases in pregnancy and, 88, 110–113t
Maternal serum α-fetoprotein, 191
Maximum vertical pocket method, 194–195
McRoberts maneuver, 390–391
Meconium-stained amniotic fluid, 387
Medications
    antenatal steroids, 260, 263, 265, 267, 302–306
    antimicrobial, 91t
    antihypertensive, 13t, 24b
    to be avoided during pregnancy and lactation, 91t
    carboprost tromethamine (Hemabate), 70
    cardiovascular disease, 156

INDEX

dinoprostone cervical gel (Prepidil), 325
group A streptococcus, 140
group B streptococcus, 112, 123–128, 261–264, 306
HIV, 103*t*
hyperthyroidism, 157
insulin, 239
intra-amniotic infection, 259–260
misoprostol (Cytotec), 70, 325–326
mood stabilizer, 216
oxytocin (*See* Oxytocin)
preterm labor and delivery, 302–306
prostaglandins, 322, 323, 324–325, 326
tocolytic, 263, 265, 266, 299–300, 306
uterotonic, 66–67, 70
Medications and Mothers' Milk, 216
Mental health disorders, 216–217
Methimazole, 157
Methylergonovine maleate (Methergine), 70
Metronidazole, 91
Misoprostol (Cytotec), 70, 325–326
Mood disorders, 217–218
Motivational interviewing, 214
Multifetal gestations, 192–194
Multiple markers, 192
Multiple previous births, 184
Myomectomy, 181

N

National Institute on Drug Abuse (NIDA) Quick Screen, 218
Neonatal death, history of previous, 183
Neonatal resuscitation, 308
Neurological disease, 172–173
Newborns
  congenital malformations in, 183
  head crowning, 408–409
  infectious diseases in pregnancy and, 88
  macrosomic (*See* Macrosomia)
  managing heat loss in, 411
  obstetric hemorrhage and, 62
  prelabor rupture of membranes (PROM) and, 269
  shoulder dystocia in, 390–393, 408–409
  what to do after delivery of, 411–414

New York Heart Association Functional Classification of heart disease, 155–157
Nitrofurantoin, 91
Non-vertex presentation, 307
Normal progress of labor, 351–353
Nuchal cord, 408, 412

O

Obstetric hemorrhage, 37–81
  AIM bundle, 43*f*
  causes, 46–51, 53–54
  defined, 41–42
  disseminated intravascular coagulation (DIC), 59–62
  documentation, 75
  emergency care, 42–45
  management, 42, 56–57
  newborn care, 62
  postpartum hemorrhage, 65–72
  posttest, 81
  pretest, 39–40
  recommended routines, 76
  Rh(D)-negative women and, 62–63
  self-test, 46, 52, 55, 64, 74, 77–80
  uterine inversion, 72–73
Obstetric history, 181–188
Obstetric referral, 419
Obstetric risk factors, 177–208
  abnormal amount of amniotic fluid, 194–198
  current pregnancy, 189–202
  fetal growth restriction, 199–200
  genetic screening, 190–192
  high parity, 184
  high-risk conditions (*See* High-risk conditions)
  history of previous congenital malformation(s) or hereditary disease, 183
  history of previous fetal or neonatal death, 183
  history of previous macrosomic newborn, 181–182
  increased maternal age, 190
  late term and post-term gestational age, 200–202
  multifetal gestations, 192–194
  obstetric history, 181–188
  posttest, 208
  pretest, 179–180
  previous cesarean delivery, 184–185
  previous uterine surgery, 181
  recommended routines, 204
  red blood cell alloimmunization, 62, 186–187
  self-test, 188, 198–199, 203, 205–207
  teen pregnancy, 189–190
  women of increased maternal age, 190
Occiput posterior, 371
OGTT. *See* Oral glucose tolerance test (OGTT)
Oligohydramnios, 197–198, 254
Operative vaginal deliveries
  forces and vacuum extractor used in, 377–378
  safety and risks of, 379–381
  self-test, 382
Opioids, 219–220, 307, 388
Oral glucose tolerance test (OGTT), 237
O Rh-negative red blood cells, 187
Osmotic dilator, 322, 324
Ovaries, 72
Oxytocin
  administration of, 331–333
  complications, 335–336
  how long to use, 336–337
  labor augmentation contraindication, 330–331
  in labor induction, 327
  in multifetal delivery, 194
  obstetric hemorrhage and, 66–67, 70
  preparing for use of, 331
  standard guideline for dosage and rate advancement, 332–333
  uterine dysfunction, 366
  water intoxication and, 336

P

Palpation, uterus, 68–69
Parvovirus B19, 111, 119–120
Patient Health Questionnaire-9, 217
Pelvic size, 363–364
Pelvimetry, clinical, 363*f*
Penicillin, treatment of syphilis, 107*t*
Perinatal mood and anxiety disorders, 217–218
pH level, 413
Placenta delivery, 414–415

465

INDEX

Placental abruption, 48t, 50–51
  disseminated intravascular coagulation (DIC) and, 59
  grades of placental separation, 50t
  management, 57
  prelabor rupture of membranes (PROM) and, 254
Placental bleeding, 48–51
Placental fragments, retained, 65
Placental implantation, low, 49f
Placenta previa, 48t, 49–50
  management, 56
Platelets in disseminated intravascular coagulation (DIC), 60–61
Polyhydramnios, 195–196
Positioning of the fetus during labor, 362f
Positive-pressure ventilation (PPV), 411, 412
Posterior arm, delivery of, 393f
Postpartum care, gestational diabetes (GDM), 242
Postpartum depression, 217–218
Postpartum hemorrhage
  causes of, 65–66
  defined, 65
  routine prevention or reduction, 66–67
  treatment, 67–72
Postpartum psychosis, 218
Post-term gestational age, 200–202
Posttests
  abnormal labor progress and difficult delivery, 402
  gestational diabetes (GDM), 248
  high-risk conditions, 176
  hypertension in pregnancy, 35
  imminent delivery and maternal/fetal transport, 422
  labor induction and augmentation, 343
  obstetric hemorrhage, 81
  obstetric risk factors, 208
  perinatal infections, 149
  prelabor rupture of membranes (PROM), 274
  preterm labor and delivery, 314
  psychosocial risk factors, 229
PPV. See Positive-pressure ventilation (PPV)
Preconception counseling, 154
Precontemplation stage, 214

Preeclampsia, 7–8t, 8
  labor management for, 22–25
  management guidelines, 17–19
  with severe features, 7–8t, 9, 11
  stabilized, 27
  superimposed, 9–10, 11
Pregestational diabetes mellitus, 159–160, 235
Pregnancy
  genetic screening in, 190–192
  high-risk conditions (See High-risk conditions)
  late term and post-term, 200–202
  maternal age in, 190
  multifetal gestations, 192–194
  psychosocial risk factors effects on, 214–225
  risk factors (See Obstetric risk factors)
  teen, 189–190
  weight gain, recommended, 182t
Prelabor rupture of membranes (PROM), 249–284
  amniocentesis, 256
  assays for amniotic proteins in vaginal secretions, 255
  examination, 255
  history, 254–255
  intra-amniotic infection and, 258, 259–260, 269
  management, 258
  maternal-fetal risks affected by, 253–254
  posttest, 274
  preterm, management of, 268t
  pretest, 251–252
  recommended routines, 271
  risk factors, 253
  self-test, 257, 270, 272–273
  sterile speculum examination, 275–280
  tests for suspected or proven, 281–284
  ultrasonography for, 255–256
  without intra-amniotic infection, 261–268
Premature labor, infectious diseases in pregnancy and, 88
  postdelivery care, 269
Preterm labor and delivery, 192–193, 285–314
  causes of, 289–290
  evaluation, 296–300
  interventions to reduce risk of, 291–293, 295–296

  management, 306–308
  medications, 304–305t
  posttest, 314
  prelabor rupture of membranes (PROM) and, 262–263, 264, 266, 268t
  preterm labor, 287–288
  pretest, 287–288
  recommended routines, 310
  risks of, 289
  self-test, 294, 301, 309, 311–313
  tocolytic medications, 304–305t
  treatment, 302–306
Pretests
  abnormal labor progress and difficult deliveries, 348–350
  gestational diabetes (GDM), 233–234
  high-risk conditions, 153
  hypertension in pregnancy, 3–4
  imminent delivery, 405–406
  infectious diseases in pregnancy, 86–87
  labor induction and augmentation, 317–318
  obstetric hemorrhage, 39–40
  obstetric risk factors, 179–180
  prelabor rupture of membranes (PROM), 251–252
  psychosocial risk factors, 211–212
Prolapsed umbilical cord, 254, 389–390
Prolonged labor, 354, 383, 386
  fetal and neonatal risks, 383–384
PROM. See Prelabor rupture of membranes (PROM)
Prostaglandins, 322, 323, 324–325, 326
Protracted labor, 354
Psychosis, postpartum, 218
Psychosocial risk factors, 209–229
  defined, 213–214
  effects on pregnancy, 214–225
  intimate partner violence (IPV), 214–216
  limited or no prenatal care, 213–214
  mental health disorders, 216–217
  perinatal mood and anxiety disorders, 217–218
  postpartum psychosis, 218
  posttest, 229
  pretest, 211–212
  recommended routines, 227

INDEX

screening, brief intervention, and referral for treatment (SBIRT) and motivational interviewing for, 214
self-test, 226, 228
substance use disorders, 218–225
Puerperal endometritis, 139–140
Pushing, ineffective, 373

Q

Questionnaires
Alcohol Quantity and Drinking Frequency, 223*t*
T-ACE, 223*t*

R

Rapid labor, 354, 384–385, 386
Red blood cell alloimmunization, 62, 186–187
Referral, obstetric, 419
Rehydration, 297
Relapse stage, 214
Renal disease, 170–171
Repeat cesarean delivery, 184–185
Respiratory disease, 173
Resuscitation, 308
Retained placental fragments, 65
Rh(D)-negative women, 62–63, 412
Rh(D)-positive women, 412
Ribavirin, 91
Rubella, 112, 120–121
Rubin maneuver, 392

S

SBIRT. *See* Screening, brief intervention, and referral for treatment (SBIRT)
Screening, brief intervention, and referral for treatment (SBIRT), 214
Secondary arrest of labor, 330, 367
Second maneuver, 68
Seizures, 22–23, 26–27, 172–173
Self-tests
abnormal labor progress, 356, 365–366, 376, 395–396, 398–402
gestational diabetes (GDM), 240, 244, 246–247
high-risk conditions, 161, 174–176
hypertension in pregnancy, 10, 15, 19, 25, 30, 32–34
imminent delivery, 415, 421–422

labor induction and augmentation, 329, 334, 338, 340–342
maternal/fetal transport, 419, 421–422
obstetric hemorrhage, 46, 52, 55, 58, 64, 74, 77–80
obstetric risk factors, 188, 198–199, 203, 205–207
operative vaginal deliveries, 382
perinatal infections, 99, 109, 122, 136, 142, 145–148
prelabor rupture of membranes (PROM), 257, 270, 272–273
preterm labor and delivery, 294, 301, 309, 311–313
psychosocial risk factors, 226, 228
rapid and prolonged labor, 386
Severe anemia, 162
Sexually transmitted infections (STIs), 92–98
Short cervix, 293
Shoulder dystocia, 390–393, 408–409
Shoulders, delivery of, 408–409
Sickle cell disease, 163
Skill units
sterile speculum examination, 275
tests for suspected or proven rupture of membranes, 281–284
SLE. *See* Systemic lupus erythematosus (SLE)
Smoking, 224–225
Spontaneous miscarriage, 47
Sterile speculum examination, 275–280, 297
STIs. *See* Sexually transmitted infections (STIs)
Stripping of membranes, 322, 323, 324
Substance use disorders, 218–225, 388
alcohol, 222–223
amphetamines, 220–221
cocaine, 221
marijuana, 223–224
opioids, 219–220
tobacco products and electronic cigarettes, 224–225
Sulfonamides, 91
Superimposed preeclampsia, 9–10, 11

Syphilis, 93, 105–108
Systemic lupus erythematosus (SLE), 168–170

T

T-ACE questionnaire, 223*t*
Tachysystole, 324, 335–336
Teen pregnancy, 189–190
Tetracyclines, 91
Third stage of labor, 394–395
Thrombocytopenia, 164–165
Thromboembolic disease, 165–166
Thromboplastins, disseminated intravascular coagulation (DIC) and, 59
Tobacco products, 224–225
Tocolysis, 263, 265, 266, 299–300, 304–305*t*, 306
TOLAC. *See* Trial of labor after cesarean delivery (TOLAC)
Toxoplasmosis, 112, 129–130
Transmission route and timing, prenatal infection, 88–89
Transport. *See* Maternal/fetal transport
Transverse lie, 369–370
Trial of labor after cesarean delivery (TOLAC), 184–186
Triplet pregnancy, 192
True labor, 351
Tuberculosis, 113, 130–132
Twin gestations, 192–194
Twins, delivery, 193*t*

U

Ultrasonography (US)
abnormal labor progress, 363
amniotic fluid index (AFI) method, 194
comprehensive, 192
maximum vertical pocket method, 194–195
prelabor rupture of membranes (PROM), 255–256
preterm labor and delivery, 298
Umbilical cord
blood gases, 413*t*
complications, 254, 389–390, 408
obtaining blood samples from, 412–414
when to clamp and cut, 412

INDEX

Unknown cause, obstetric bleeding of, 51
Urinary tract infection (UTI), 137–138
   preterm labor and delivery and, 295
US. *See* Ultrasonography (US)
Uterine atony, 65, 68
Uterine dysfunction, 361*t*
Uterine inversion, 66, 69*f*, 72–73
Uterine replacement, 72–73
Uterine rupture, 66
Uterine surgery, previous, 181
Uterotonic medication, 66–67, 70
Uterus
   manual compression of, 69*f*
   palpation of, 68–69
   quadrants for amniotic fluid measurements, 195*f*
UTI. *See* Urinary tract infection (UTI)

V

Vacuum extractor, 377–378
   risks and safety of, 379–381
Vaginal delivery
   disseminated intravascular coagulation (DIC) and, 61
   fetal presentation and, 370–371
   late term and post-term, 201
   multifetal gestations, 194
Valproate, 216
Varicella-zoster virus (VZV), 113, 133–134
Venous thromboembolism (VTE), 165–166
Venous vasospasm, 70
Vertex presentation, 307
VTE. *See* Venous thromboembolism (VTE)
VZV. *See* Varicella-zoster virus (VZV)

W

Water intoxication, 336
Weight gain in pregnancy, recommended, 182*t*
Woods screw maneuver, 391–392

Z

Zavanelli maneuver, 392–393